Health Care Education in Nigeria

This book provides a comprehensive and authoritative assessment of the training of health professionals in Nigeria, looking back to how health care education has evolved in the country over time, before investigating new and emerging trends.

The book begins with a discussion of the fundamentals of health care education, the art of teaching health care students, and modeling professionalism in health care. The book highlights the work of pioneer Nigerian health care academics, and explores the administration of health care education at the departmental level. Finally, it highlights the role of elite Nigerian health care academics in the diaspora, chronicles contemporary challenges in health care education, and makes recommendations for reform.

This book will be of interest to students, scholars, and practitioners working on health care education in Africa.

Joseph A. Balogun is a Distinguished University Professor at the College of Health Sciences, Chicago State University, USA, and Emeritus Professor of Physiotherapy and Associate Director of Research Development and Innovation at the University of Medical Sciences, Ondo City, Ondo State, Nigeria.

Routledge African Studies

For a full list of available titles please visit:
https://www.routledge.com/African-Studies/book-series/AFRSTUD

Health Care Education in Nigeria

Evolutions and Emerging Paradigms

Joseph A. Balogun

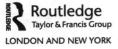
Routledge
Taylor & Francis Group

LONDON AND NEW YORK

First published 2021
by Routledge
2 Park Square, Milton Park, Abingdon, Oxon OX14 4RN

and by Routledge
52 Vanderbilt Avenue, New York, NY 10017

Routledge is an imprint of the Taylor & Francis Group, an informa business

© 2021 Joseph A. Balogun

British Library Cataloguing-in-Publication Data
A catalogue record for this book is available from the British Library

Library of Congress Cataloging-in-Publication Data
Names: Balogun, Joseph A., 1955– author.
Title: Healthcare education in Nigeria : evolutions and
emerging paradigms / Joseph A. Balogun.
Description: Abingdon, Oxon ; New York, NY : Routledge, 2021. |
Includes bibliographical references and index.
Identifiers: LCCN 2020045051 (print) | LCCN 2020045052 (ebook) |
ISBN 9780367482091 (hardback) | ISBN 9781003127529 (ebook)
Subjects: LCSH: Medical education–Nigeria. |
Health occupations schools–Nigeria. | Medical personnel–Nigeria.
Classification: LCC R824.N6 B35 2021 (print) |
LCC R824.N6 (ebook) | DDC 610.71/1669–dc23
LC record available at https://lccn.loc.gov/2020045051
LC ebook record available at https://lccn.loc.gov/2020045052

ISBN: 978-0-367-48209-1 (hbk)
ISBN: 978-0-367-65035-3 (pbk)
ISBN: 978-1-003-12752-9 (ebk)

Typeset in Bembo
by Newgen Publishing, UK

I dedicate this book to my late parents, Mr. Ezra and Mrs. Rhoda Balogun for imparting in me the virtues of hard work, and my secondary school teachers, Mr. and Mrs. Philips, for stimulating my interest in science.

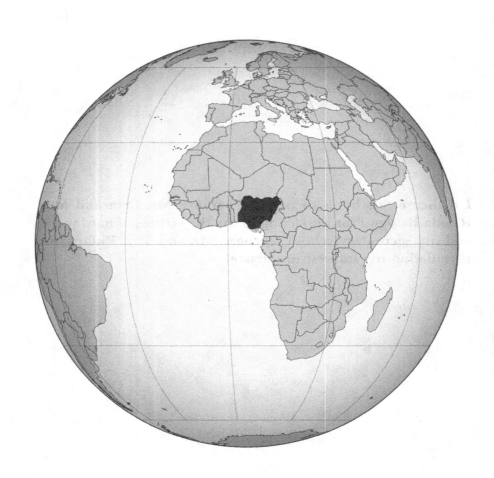

Contents

About the author

Joseph Abiodun Balogun, FAS, is a Distinguished University Professor in the College of Health Sciences at Chicago State University (CSU), USA; Emeritus Professor of Physiotherapy, and Associate Director of Research Development and Innovation at the University of Medical Sciences, Ondo City, Nigeria; and Visiting Professor/Program Consultant at the Centre of Excellence in Reproductive Health and Innovation, University of Benin, Nigeria. He is the Founder and President/CEO of Joseph Rehabilitation Center, a social service organization at Tinley Park, Illinois, USA, that provides community-integrated living arrangement services for adults with physical, developmental, and intellectual disabilities.

Professor Balogun obtained his Bachelor of Science (Honors) degree in physiotherapy in 1977 from the University of Ibadan, Nigeria. He earned a Master's degree in orthopedic and sports physical therapy (1981) and a PhD in exercise physiology (cardiac rehabilitation) with a minor in research methodology from the University of Pittsburgh (1985). He has held full-time and administrative positions at various universities around the world – Russell Sage College, Troy, New York; Obafemi Awolowo University (OAU), Ile-Ife, Nigeria; University of Florida, Gainesville; Texas Woman's University, Houston; the State University of New York Health Science Center at Brooklyn (SUNY-HSCB). He also held a visiting faculty position at Barry University, Florida, and King Saud University, Saudi Arabia. He served for 13 years (1999–2013) as dean of the College of Health Sciences at CSU, where he established seven academic programs and the HIV/AIDS Research and Policy Institute to address the disproportionate incidence and complex burdens of HIV/AIDS in minority populations. He also served for six years as chairman of the Department of Physical Therapy (1993–1999) and associate dean for student academic affairs (1994–1999) at SUNY-HSCB; consultant physiotherapist (1988–1991) and vice-dean of the Faculty of Health Sciences at OAU (1990–1991).

Professor Balogun has contributed to knowledge in physical therapy, cardiovascular epidemiology, ergonomics, and HIV behavioral research. He has authored 2 books, 17 book chapters, monographs, and technical compendia, over 150 full articles, and 24 peer-reviewed conference abstracts and proceedings. In 2015, he delivered the third Christopher Ajao's keynote address at the 55th annual conference of the Nigeria Society of Physiotherapy. In 2017, he presented the second distinguished guest lecture at the University of Medical Sciences, Ondo City, Nigeria.

Professor Balogun is the Deputy Editor of the *African Journal of Reproductive Health* and serves on the editorial board of the *International Journal of Physiotherapy Theory and Practice*, *Journal of the Nigeria Society of Physiotherapy*, *Kanem Journal of Medical Sciences*, and *International University of Sarajevo (IUS) Law Journal*. He also currently serves as an affiliate member of the Women's Health and Action Research Centre, Benin City, Nigeria. He has received over a dozen major academic and service awards, including Fellow of the Royal Society for Public Health (FRSPH), Institute of Management Consultants (FIMC), Academy of Science (FAS), Nigeria Society of Physiotherapy (FNSP), and American College of Sports Medicine (FACSM). He was awarded the Warren Perry distinguished author's award by the *Journal of Allied Health* (2003), and the distinguished decorated affiliate award of the American Health Council (2018).

Professor Balogun is married to Dr. Adetutu Olusola Balogun (Nee Olotu), an occupational therapist and entrepreneur in Tinley Park, Illinois, USA. They have four children.

Foreword

As the most populous and arguably the most culturally diverse and sophisticated nation in sub-Saharan Africa, Nigerian health and educational systems are usually of interest to anyone desirous of socioeconomic development in Africa. Professor Joseph Balogun's textbook, *Health Care Education in Nigeria: Evolutions and Emerging Paradigms*, makes significant contributions to the academy by documenting the developmental milestones of the different health care professions and contextualized the changes within health care education in Nigeria.

According to the World Health Organization, Nigeria has some of the most daunting health challenges and unfavorable health outcomes. Globally, health care has both supply and demand sides. While the demand side in Nigeria has been influenced negatively by illiteracy, poverty, religious division, socioeconomic, cultural, and ethnic differences, the supply side also has negative determinants that, if not addressed soon, will curtail the development of health. On the supply side of health care, active human resource development remains one of the most effective paradigms. The analysis provided in this book allows the readers to understand the multiple intractable problems within the country's health care education programs. It provides an excellent expository framework that will enable academics, change advocates, technocrats, and policymakers to develop strategies to tackle those challenges and improve the country's critical health care education indicators.

As eloquently presented in this book, the major challenge in Nigeria has been the insular training along professional lines, without the integrated team approach needed to create a positive work environment in academia and clinical sectors. The curriculum chasm has led to dysfunctional delivery of health services, low staff morale, and interprofessional rivalry among the health workers. Over time, the situation has caused an increased number of lockouts and industrial strikes and rising waves of migration of Nigerian health care professionals to other parts of the world. The different analyses contained in this textbook should enable academics to rethink their practice methods and instructional strategies. It also should allow clinicians and researchers to identify more scientifically proven ways and evidence-based practices based on formative and intervention research methods that promote the best principles in health care delivery.

As epitomized in the title of the book, there should be a paradigm shift in human resource development from the current approach of individualism and solo professional efforts to interprofessional education team philosophy and a unified vision for health improvement in the country. This book will be well received as it comes at a convenient time when these issues are frontline-burner topics of discussion among academics and clinicians. The publication will be useful, especially to development partners, nongovernmental organizations, multilateral and bilateral organizations, students, academics, and philanthropists interested in the development of health care education in Nigeria. A healthy Nigeria sets an excellent example for a continent that is currently epitomized by some of the most burdensome health and social challenges of our time. This publication poignantly challenges health care academics and clinicians to learn from the various examples drawn from the Northern countries.

I found the book extremely exciting and easy to read as it is expertly laced with anecdotes and examples that allow a better understanding of the subject discussed even by those who may never have visited the country. I strongly recommend the book to laypersons, policymakers in the education and health sectors, and its adoption in undergraduate and postgraduate health care core and elective courses offered in Nigerian universities.

Friday E. Okonofua
June 2020

Preface

The impetus to write this book began in 2018 after conducting a two-day workshop on "Best Practices in Academic/Clinical Department Administration and Scholarship of Discovery" at the University of Medical Sciences, Ondo City, Nigeria. To my surprise, the overwhelming majority of the academics at the workshop did not have any formal training in andragogy, and heads of departments appointed into administrative positions had no formal training on their roles and responsibilities. Sadly, there are no readily available textbooks or training institutes on teaching and academic administration in the country. Critics affirmed that these deficiencies are partly responsible for the poor quality of instruction in Nigerian universities.

In the ten chapters in this book, the term "health care education" is used instead of a discipline-specific genre to underscore the interprofessional education philosophy advocated by the author. The health disciplines presented are those offered in Nigerian universities. They include medicine, dentistry, nursing, pharmacy, optometry, physical-and-occupational therapy, speech-language pathology and audiology, prosthetics and orthotics, clinical psychology, medical laboratory science, radiography, nutrition/dietitian, biomedical engineering/technology, community health, and veterinary medicine. The terms "lecturer," "scholar," "academic," "scientist," and "faculty" are used interchangeably throughout the book.

The fundamentals of health care education are presented in Chapter 1 to thoroughly contextualize the issues discussed in the book. The subsequent chapters covered the basic principles of andragogy, and heutagogy, teaching and modeling professionalism, and administration of academic departments. The book traces the developmental journey of different health care education and the life histories and contributions of pioneer health care academicians in Nigeria. The emerging paradigms in health care education in the last decade and contemporary challenges were analyzed. The last two chapters of the book provide recommendations to reform health care education in the country and include profiles of elite Nigerian health care academics in the diaspora. The examples cited in this publication reflect contemporary and best practices drawn mostly from the United States because of its enormous achievements in education and health, and the prolonged socialization arising from my academic, professional work experience, and extended residence in the country.

Several of the issues discussed in this book and the recommendations prescribed may be controversial because they challenge the status quo and the entrenched dogma. I hope the comments will engender open and frank dialogue that will improve the quality of health care education in Nigeria. This book should be of interest to a variety of audiences interested in the Nigerian health care education system; aficionados, so to say, will find much in this book to engage them. The contents are supported by extensive references that may be of interest to specialists or even general readers who seek in-depth exploration of the numerous topics presented. These factors account for the deliberate interprofessional and transdisciplinary structure of the publication, going beyond one particular health field. Although Nigeria is the primary focus of the publication, this book contains precious resources applicable to any country. Many of the policy recommendations that are prescribed, if implemented by the Nigerian government, will no doubt improve the quality of health care education in the country.

This publication is ideal for adoption as a reference textbook in Health Care Education and Administration and Medical History courses offered in Nigerian universities. The contents are illustrated heavily by empirical data presented in tables and figures. Central titles and subtitles are liberally inserted into the appropriate sections to enhance easy retrieval of information. The book is organized and illustrated in a reader-friendly format and each chapter can be read independently. Readers may begin with any section of their choice, unconstrained by any desire to start from the beginning. Happy reading!

Acknowledgments

My employment as a faculty member and administrator at Obafemi Awolowo University (OAU), Ile-Ife, Nigeria, from 1986 to 1991 and half a dozen trips to several Nigerian universities between 2015 and 2019 informed the opinions expressed in this book. During these visits, I had the unique opportunity to deliver keynote speeches at different professional conferences and presented workshops to a diverse audience. The experiences allowed me to network with colleagues at various universities across the country – University of Medical Sciences (UNIMED), Ondo City, University of Benin, University of Ibadan, OAU, Bowen University, University of Lagos, and the University of Maiduguri. I owe the individuals with whom I met my profound gratitude and appreciation.

The writing of this book commenced during the 2017 fall semester, but it stalled for a year as other academic and domestic priorities arose. It accelerated swiftly during my sabbatical leave in 2019. I am grateful to Chicago State University (CSU) for granting me a paid educational leave after 20 years of service. The reprieve from teaching facilitated the completion of this book. I sincerely appreciate my esteemed colleague and research collaborator, Professor Philip Aka, former dean of the Faculty of Law at the International University of Sarajevo, in Bosnia and Herzegovina, for meticulously reading the initial draft of this work and provided extensive feedback. I also want to express my appreciation to my mentor Professor Eyitayo Lambo, former Nigerian Minister of Health, for meticulously reading the first draft and provided many useful references and comments used to improve the depth and clarity of this work. I owe sincere gratitude to all the authors whose work I cited and appreciate my publishers, Routledge, for working with me to meet the production deadline.

Many individuals in my family deserve noteworthy recognition here. First and foremost is my dear wife, Dr. Adetutu Balogun, and our four children for their unwavering support of my academic career spanning more than three decades. I owe my brothers-in-law, Admiral Bamidele Daji and Admiral Olumuyiwa Olotu, and sister-in-law, Dr. Feyisayo Daji, a lot of gratitude for providing transportation and security protection during my many visits to Nigeria. I want to express my sincere appreciation to Ms. Efe Mamuzo for assisting me with collecting the H-index data presented in Chapter 10 and my professional colleague, Dr. Emmanuel John, for drawing the university organogram in Chapter 4. I owe Moyo Abiona and Professor Rosalind L. Fielder-Giscombe, a ton of gratitude for painstakingly creating the index section of this book at a short notice to meet the publication deadline. And finally, colleagues in Nigeria – Professor Mathew Olaogun of Bowen University, and I acknowledge the support of my Professor Babatunde Adegoke, University of Ibadan, Temitope Oluwatayo at UNIMED, and Vivian Onoh, at the University of Benin – Col. (retired) – who provided the pictures in this book. No doubt, these pictures have added value to the information presented.

1 The fundamentals of health care education

Introduction

As a result of the shifts in demographics, developments in medical technology, and evolving academic standards and policies in the last two decades, the training of health care professionals (HCPs) have also changed significantly. Health care education is a dynamic process that begins at the undergraduate level to postgraduate training and continues throughout the professional career. The clinicians and academics acquire knowledge and clinical skills through continuing education development courses, workshops, seminars, or colloquia. The structure, content, and delivery of education continue to grow as medical technology improves and learning and instruction are better understood. For example, the entry-level education for optometrists, pharmacists, and physiotherapists in a few countries (the United States, Australia, Taiwan, Pakistan) are at the doctoral level, like physicians and dentists. But these issues are insular within professions and often not shared across disciplines. This chapter analyzes the differences, commonalities, and emerging global trends in health care education.

History of medical and dental education

Medical education's origin is contentious, but many academics consider that it began with the ancient Greeks' method of rational inquiry that introduced the practice of observation and reasoning around a disease process. Some academics posited that this training led to teaching and the formation of institutions where the Greek physicians such as Hippocrates taught in the fifth century BC and came up with the oath that became a credo for HCPs today. In the West, the Christian religion significantly influenced medical education as it favored the protection and care of the sick and the establishment of hospitals where observation, analysis, and patient discussions among physicians were encouraged. Apprenticeship training in medical education occurred in monastic infirmaries and hospitals during the early middle ages.

In the early 1900s, Sir William Osler pioneered medical education as we know it today. He posited that medical students' exposure to patients and clinical experience over time would make them become competent physicians. This point of view led to the current structure of medical training that includes clerkships and rotations through the specialties during the clinical year. Over the years, this model of instruction, Kwan, and associates opined is inefficient, inadequate, and obsolete because it has failed to prepare physicians to provide safe and complex care adequately due to the high rate of preventable medical errors. They would like to see a considerable improvement in the next generation of physicians (Kwan, Sebasky, and Muchmore, 2019). As new diseases and public health challenges emerge, academics strived to address them by providing high-quality education.

As we know it today, medical education evolved between the 9th and 11th centuries with the establishment of a school at Salerno in southern Italy. During that era, the teaching of students was by apprenticeship and systemization of knowledge and some health precepts. The Holy Roman Emperor Frederick II approved the registration of physicians to practice. In the same period, medical education flourished in Baghdad, Cairo, and Córdoba. With the increasing number of universities in Italy and later in Cracow, Prague, Paris, Oxford, and Western Europe, medical education transitioned from training in the hospitals to the university setting because of the prestige associated with the professoriate.

By 1518, the Royal College of Physicians in the United Kingdom, through the effort of Thomas Linacre, established a system that mandated medical practitioners to take a written examination. The importance of hospital experience and the students' training to use their sight, hearing, and touch in studying disease were reasserted gradually between the 17th and 18th centuries. In Europe, medical education slowly developed through the application of botany, chemistry, and human anatomy. However, it was in the mid-19th century that a systematic pattern of science-oriented teaching evolved where the students mostly listen, rather than learning, and their role is more investigative. The clinical training during that era was not well organized. It was confined primarily to charitable hospitals staffed by unpaid consultants. The enactment of the Medical Act of 1858, in the United Kingdom, charted a new direction for medical education and the establishment of the General Medical Council, which controlled admission to the medical register with considerable powers over medical examinations.

The origin of dentistry dates back to 7000 BC with the Indus valley civilization, but it was not until 5000 BC that descriptions related to dentistry and tooth decay were available. In ancient Greece, Hippocrates and Aristotle wrote about dentistry, specifically about treating decaying teeth. The first book on dentistry was not published until 1530 AD. In 1723, an influential book that defined a comprehensive system for caring for and treating teeth was published by Pierre Fauchard, a French surgeon, who is credited as the father of modern dentistry. The College of Dental Surgery in Baltimore was the first dental institution opened in 1840, and the first dental practice act was enacted in the state of Alabama in 1841. Two decades later, the American Dental Association was formed, and the first university-based dental program was established in 1867 at Harvard University (American Dental Education Association, 2015).

The establishment of Johns Hopkins medical school in 1893 greatly influenced the development of medical education in the United States. The academic program admitted only Johns Hopkins' graduates with a year of courses in the natural sciences. The clinical training offered at the institution was purposely created for teaching and research. In 1910, the Carnegie Foundation for the Advancement of Teaching issued a report that emphasized that training in health care is a unique type of education rather than a mysterious process of professional initiation or apprenticeship. The publication, authored by Abraham Flexner, laid the groundwork for the medical and dental curricula model that prevailed throughout the first half of the 20th century. A decade and a half after his proposal, Dr. Flexner observed that the new curriculum gave precedence to scientific knowledge over the social and humanistic aspects of medicine. For decades, this curriculum proposal, which was centered on the importance of scientific knowledge in place of biological understanding of social and humanistic characteristics, was a subject of fierce debate.

Between 1913 and 1929, the number of medical schools in the United States increased from financial support by the General Education Board, the Rockefeller Foundation, and some private donors. The medical schools implemented many of the recommendations contained in Abraham Flexner's report, which emphasized the need for full-time faculty in academic departments, teaching students in the hospital settings with access to laboratories, libraries, and seminar rooms (Scarborough, Turner, and Gregg, n.d.).

Global history of nursing, pharmacy, physiotherapy, and optometry education

The origins of nursing, pharmacy, physiotherapy, and optometry education closely followed that of medical and dental education, all of which evolved from the apprenticeship system to formal educational courses. The first pharmacy training program was established in the United States at the Philadelphia College of Pharmacy and Sciences in 1821. Shortly after, the United Kingdom and continental Europe established colleges of pharmacy as independent organizations or as a school within universities (Hartley and Krantz, 2020).

Globally, nursing is the largest profession, and men remain significantly underrepresented. In the United States, there are more than 2.9 million registered nurses. Before 1800, the training of nurses was not formal, but women during that era performed "nursing tasks." As far back as 250 BC, there were reports of caregivers in cathedrals and patient homes who worked to "nurse people back to health." Before 1854, physicians typically teach women menial tasks in their caretaking efforts. By 1854, Florence Nightingale, a well-educated daughter of wealthy British parents who defied social conventions and decided to become a nurse, began the first serious analysis of the nursing profession by writing memoirs and thoughts as she cared for soldiers wounded during the

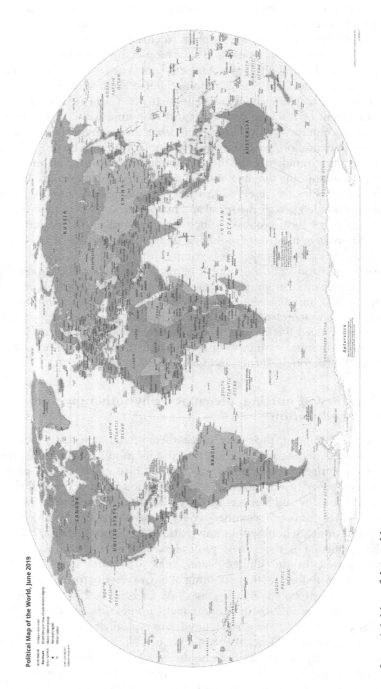

Image 1.1 Map of the world.

Crimean War. In 1859, she wrote the "Notes on Nursing," which was the first instructional manual in nursing that laid the foundation for training nurses today. And in 1860, she opened the Nightingale Training School in London. Between 1870 and 1880, other nursing schools opened in the United States in New York, Massachusetts, and Connecticut. Their curriculum followed the Nightingale model (Buhler-Wilkerson and Patricia D'Antonio, 2020; Duquesne University, 2020).

Thousands of years ago, physiotherapy modalities such as massage, hydrotherapy, and therapeutic exercises were commonly used in India, China, and Greece. Around 1000 BC, the Chinese used the *Kung fu* exercise to correct body positioning and improve breathing. Indians also used yoga and massage to treat arthritis. Around 180 BC, the Romans employed *gymnastics* to enhance physical strength, and by the second century, Galen, a famous physician, taught the use of exercises to improve the overall strength. By 460 BC, Hippocrates, an ancient Greek physician regarded as the father of medicine, also used exercise to improve physical strength. In the same year, in Greece, Hector employed hydrotherapy to treat patients. Furthermore, Aristotle recommended massage with oil to relieve tiredness. At around 500 BC, Herodicus, a Greek physician, used different types of exercise (*Ars Gymnastica*, or *The Art of Gymnastics*), including walking, weightlifting, and wrestling to strengthen weak muscles.

Between 1500 and 1700, the use of exercises was adopted widely, and various books on the modality were written. One such book is the *Libro del Excerciso*, written by Jaen and published in Spain. In 1723, Nicholas Andry, a Professor at Medical Faculty in Paris, posited that exercise could help build muscles of the arms and legs. In 1813, Per Henrik Ling, a Swedish poet, revolutionized physiotherapy by promoting *Tunia* techniques, an ancient Chinese martial art, and called it the Swedish massage. He later introduced it to the United States and Europe. In 1860, George H. Taylor also popularized these massage techniques in the United States. In 1864, Gustav Zander, a Swedish physician, invented machines to assist patients in performing their exercise. In 1894, four nurses in the United Kingdom formed the Charted Society of Physiotherapy. By 1913, the University of Otago in New Zealand established a School of Physiotherapy. A year later, Reed College opened in Portland, United States, to train "reconstitution aides."

During the first world war in 1917, Zander's machines and Ling's Swedish exercises were used to treat the injured soldiers. During that era, physiotherapy was known as "mechanotherapy," and Zander machines were widely used. In 1920, an outbreak of poliomyelitis led to higher demand for physiotherapy services. In 1921, *PT Review* published the first research paper, and Mary McMillan, known as the "mother of physical therapy" established the American Women's Physical Therapeutic Association – currently known as the American Physical Therapy Association (APTA). The importance of physiotherapy as a health discipline shot to prominence during the Second World War (1935–1945), with the establishment of clinics to treat injured soldiers. In early 1950, physiotherapy was primarily hospital-based and did not extend beyond the four walls of the hospital setting until the late 1950s. By 1974, the APTA formed the orthopedic section, and the International Federation of Orthopedic Manipulative Therapy established the same year (Sahi and Dutta, 2020).

The origin of optometry education is linked to the development of vision science, optics, and optical aids/instruments that are traced to the studies of optics and image formation by the eye. The history of optical science dates back a few thousand years BC, as evidence by the existence of lenses for decoration, found in Greece and the Netherlands. The earliest mention of spectacles was in circa 1300. Roger Bacon, in 1263, was the first to opine that lenses are "useful for those with weakness of sight." And by 1286, the first pair of glasses was created (Lasik, 2020). Peter Brown, a pilgrim to the United States in 1620, was the first to wear a pair of eyeglasses in the United States (Goss, 2003). The Optical Society was formed in 1896, followed by the American Association of Opticians founded in 1898, but changed its name to the American Optical Association in 1910. The term "optometrist" was adopted in 1904. In 1934 the Council on Optometric Education was established to accredit the optometric educational programs. Irvin M. Boris is widely considered the "father of modern optometry," for publishing a renowned textbook of optometry – *Clinical Refraction* – and for establishing several optometry programs and research institutions (American Optometric Association, 2020; Multimedia Foundation, 2019, 2020).

The Illinois College of Optometry was established in 1872, and the predecessor private schools include Northern Illinois College of Ophthalmology and Otology, Needles Institute, Northern Illinois College of Optometry, Monroe College of Optometry, and Chicago College of Optometry. The Philadelphia Optical College was the first to offer the Doctor of Optics (OD) in 1889. The private schools all awarded the OD degree, but public schools resisted. Before 1920, optometrist generally resisted using the term "doctor," but the attitude gradually changed through the 1940s (Goss, 2003). The most significant advancements in optometry were in the 20th century. The state of Minnesota, in 1901, was the first to pass a law to regulate optometry practice. The foundation university-based optometry school was established at Columbia University in 1910 but closed in 1954 (Goss, 2003). In 1915, optometry evolved from a niche field within medicine to a respected discipline with the legal backing of the Pennsylvania Supreme Court, which defined optometry as a distinct discipline and not a minor branch of medicine. By 1921, all the states recognized optometry as a separate health care discipline (Lasik, 2020).

Emerging global trends in medical and dental education

With globalization, medical and dental education continues to evolve in all its ramifications. The need to deliver quality and cost-effective educational programming became the central theme with institutions continuously modifying their curriculum to ensure the graduates produced are capable of responding to the current and future trends in the discipline. The rule of thumb for any curriculum revision is to provide optimum integration between the primary and biomedical sciences with the clinical sciences and prevent student and faculty burnout. In the last century, program accreditation has also taken center stage. The training of medical and dental students at all levels (entry-level, postgraduate /fellowship/residency, and continuing education) occur at accredited institutions of higher learning. During the training, various teaching platforms (face-to-face classroom, online, and preceptorship) and instructional methods are utilized to optimize learning. Typically, the academic programs are located in the university setting, and students receive their clinical experience in the hospitals, clinics, urban, and rural community health centers.

The duration of medical and dental education varies considerably, and the curriculum within a discipline varies from country to country. In North America, it takes about ten years (including premed, med-school, and residency) to earn the medical degree needed to practice. The Doctor of Medicine (MD) or Doctor of Osteopathy (DO) degree is conferred after satisfactory completion of the course of study in an accredited medical school. Some students opt for a dual degree research-focused MD/PhD program, which typically lasts 7–10 years. The first-year training after earning the MD or DO degree is commonly called an internship, before the residency training as a specialist called the "fellowship." In some states, the fellowship can begin immediately after the MD/DO degree. In contrast, other states require generalist (unstreamed) training for some years before starting the fellowship program (Scarborough, Turner, and Gregg, n.d.).

In the Commonwealth countries, undergraduate medical training is five years following the completion of the Advanced Level General Certificate Education (GCE) examination or four years for students with a Bachelor's degree. In some medical schools, students who opted for an intercalated BSc degree at some point after the preclinical studies take six years, after which the Bachelor of Medicine and Surgery (MBChB/MBBS/MBBCh) academic degree is conferred. Only after postgraduate study is the MD degree earned. Other countries outside the Commonwealth award similar degrees, but they are not always of the same status. After medical school, the physician in the United Kingdom completes two years of clinical (internship) training, after which they register with the General Medical Council at the end of the first year. They may pursue further years of study at the end of the second year. The Australian training system is very similar, and the graduates register with the Australian Medical Council.

The admission criteria include preparation in the arts, humanities, and social sciences, in addition to the biological and physical sciences. Students are selected based on their intellectual ability, motivation for the health discipline, previous relevant experiences, character, and integrity. Admission varies across the globe and is generally competitive as the number of applicants always exceeds the number admitted. For example, many universities in the United States accept only about 5% of its applicants. In most countries, academically gifted students enroll following completion of high school education. On the other hand, a university degree is required in the United States. Between 1913 and 1929, many countries (the United States, the United Kingdom, and the Commonwealth nations), generally limit the number of students admitted. In contrast, in Western Europe, South America, and Russia, the number of students enrolled is less restrictive. During that era, some medical schools in North America had a faculty–student ratio of 1 to 1 or 1 to 2, while in some countries, a 1 to 20 or even 100 ratio was enforced.

Medical and dental education is categorized into four phases: premedical, undergraduate, postgraduate, and continuing education. The goal is to prepare competent practitioners capable of applying contemporary scientific knowledge to promote health, prevent, and cure diseases. All physicians and dentists are accountable for their actions and have a responsibility to their profession and patients. They are expected to maintain a high ethical standard in clinical practice. Their curricula include, in addition to patient care contents, disease prevention, clinical or basic research, leadership, and management, and education contents. The educational environment also encourages learning and inquiry by providing support for faculty to acquire research skills and engage in independent or collaborative research (World Medical Association, 2017).

The preclinical phase concentrates on the study of human anatomy, histology, embryology, physiology, biochemistry, pharmacology, and biophysics. Subsequently, pathological anatomy, bacteriology, immunology, and parasitology are presented and followed by medical psychology, biostatistics, public health, biomedical engineering, emergency medicine, ethics, and elective courses. The clinical phase is offered through small group conferences and discussions, a decrease in the number of classroom lectures, and an increase in contact hours with patients in teaching hospitals and clinics. In the medical profession, the clinical training usually begins with the general medicine and surgery courses that include pathology, microbiology, hematology, immunology, clinical chemistry, epidemiology, community, and forensic medicine, followed by the clinical specialties such as obstetrics and gynecology, pediatrics, ophthalmology, otolaryngology, dermatology, and mental health. The students rotate through the hospital's outpatient, emergency, and radiology departments, diagnostic laboratories, and surgical theatres.

The cost of medical education varies around the world. In North America, the average cost of medical school education is over $300,000 at a public institution. A license is required before graduates can practice their professions/specialties after graduation from entry-level or residency programs. In the United States, the boards of licensure in each state control the process. The boards screen the credentials of applicants and conduct examinations to determine competence to practice the profession. Also, the National Board of Medical Examiners administers licensure examination, and the exam scores must be acceptable to the state boards. The Medical Council of Canada also conducts written tests before the names of the successful candidates put on the medical register. The provincial governments recognize the examination as the primary condition for licensure. In the United Kingdom, the General Medical Council registers and oversees the licensure process. In Japan and some European countries, graduation from a state-approved medical school serves as a license to practice medicine (Scarborough, Turner, and Gregg, n.d.).

An emerging trend in medical/dental education all over the world is that faculty now advocate outcome-based or competency-based training that emphasizes the attainment of skills in performing concrete critical clinical activities. But an enormous amount of effort and time is spent by clinical instructors to observe students directly, assess clinical skills, and provide feedback about progress. Unfortunately, the instructors' time and energy are often poorly compensated. Aside from the fact that hours worked may not translate to competency, excessive work hours can be detrimental to learning, as sleep-deprived students are more prone to errors and burnout.

Another new change in medical/dental education is the use of the electronic medical record (EMR), which has improved many aspects of patient care. But its application is associated with decreased time spent with patients, a rise in burnout, and a disruptive impact on student documentation. While most medical schools in the United States (64%) permit students to use the EMR, only two-thirds of the programs allow students to document electronically because of liability concerns or the fact that student notes cannot be used for medical billing (Kwan, Sebasky, and Muchmore, 2019).

Emerging global trends in nursing, pharmacy, physiotherapy, and optometry education

All over the world, entry-level education for physicians and dentists is at the doctoral level. Today, in a few countries around the world, the entry-level education for pharmacists, optometrists, and physiotherapists are at the doctoral degree level. In the United States, the Doctor of Pharmacy (PharmD), Doctor of Physiotherapy (DPT), and Doctor of Optometry (OD) are the recognized degrees needed to obtain a license to practice the professions. In Australia, Taiwan, and Pakistan, the DPT degree is the entry-level degree required to practice physical therapy. The duration to earn a DPT degree varies from country to country. It is six to seven years in the United States, five years in Australia, and six years in Taiwan. The OD degree takes eight years (four years of undergraduate and four years of professional training) to earn. The PharmD degree program is six years (two years of undergraduate and four years of clinical based education) in duration. The advanced degrees required by these professions with the legislative mandate in the respective countries allow the practitioners to consult and treat patients without physician or dentist referral. This development readily provides access to patients and a new level of autonomy and independence for the disciplines concerned.

In other countries around the world, the entry-level education for pharmacists, optometrists, and physiotherapists are still at the baccalaureate or Master's degree levels. After the completion of the entry-level degree, graduates can enroll in a postgraduate (MS or PhD) degree program in their discipline.

United Kingdom physiotherapists with appropriate continuing education training in medication administration are now allowed to prescribe medications without a physician's authorization. This landmark development, first in the world, is meant to decrease bureaucratic clinical practices, free up physicians' time, and subsequently lower health care costs (World Confederation for Physical Therapy, 2016).

Similar to the medical and dental programs, nursing, pharmacy, physiotherapy, and optometry programs also require a license to practice. They also have educational opportunities for clinical specialty training. For example, the American Board of Physical Therapy Specialties has graduated more than 24,000 clinical specialists who completed advanced training in nine specialty areas of cardiovascular and pulmonary, clinical electrophysiology, geriatrics, neurology, oncology, orthopedics, pediatrics, sports, and women's health. The Board of Pharmacy Specialties, an autonomous arm of the American Pharmacists Association, has certified more than 46,000 pharmacists across 12 specialties in pharmacy education – ambulatory care, cardiology, critical care, geriatrics, infectious diseases, nuclear, nutrition support, oncology, pediatric, pharmacotherapy, psychiatric, and compounded sterile preparations. The American Board of Certification in Medical Optometry has, as of January 2020, graduated over 400 licensed optometrists with an entry-level OD degree as specialists in medical optometry for diagnosis, and treatment of primary and secondary disorders of the eye, adnexa, and visual tracts.

The standard of entry-level education in nursing has been a subject of controversy for decades. There are varying entry-level training to become a nurse in different parts of the world. In the United States and Canada, there are three pathways. A two or three-year diploma program, a two-year associate degree in nursing (ADN), or a four-year Bachelor's (BSN) degree leading to a registered nurse (RN) designation. Those with BSN can pursue a Master of Science in Nursing (MSN) or Doctor of Nursing Practice (DNP) degree to enhance their career in clinical or administrative high-paying, and high-demand nursing jobs. In China, nursing education has developed rapidly in the past three decades with five pathways to become an RN – through technical secondary school, college, undergraduate, MSN, and PhD routes. About 95% of the RN train for three years after completing nine years of secondary education; the MSN and PhD prepared nurses are in the minority (Duquesne University, 2020). In Australia, undergraduate nursing education is the standard. Postgraduate degree programs are available, and a considerable number of nurses have MSN and doctoral degrees (Fei-FeiDeng, 2015). In the United Kingdom, RNs have an ADN or a BSN and are licensed by the state's board of nursing. Some states require that RNs pass a medication administration exam to administer medications (Research Careers, 2020). There are two routes to becoming an RN in Nigeria. After completion of secondary school education, a three-year basic general nursing certificate program, and a five-year generic BSN degree program (Chiedu, 2016).

In 2010, the United States National Academy of Medicine recommended that RNs with a BSN increased to 80% by 2020. In 2017, the American Association of Colleges of Nursing, which represents four-year and graduate nursing programs, proposed that nurses should be "minimally prepared" with the BSN or "equivalent nursing degree." The proposal reignited the debate on entry-level education in nursing. The American Association of Community Colleges and the Association of Community College Trustees were against the proposal (Smith, 2017). The National Council of State Boards of Nursing is responsible for administering the nursing licensure examination and has the final decision on the issue. Given the disparity in the education standards in nursing education around the world, nurses who meet the license criteria in one country may not be qualified to work in another. The globalization of health care, which began in the last decade, fuel the calls from academics and professional nursing organizations around the world, for standardization of nursing education. This led the World Health Organization (WHO) to support the harmonization of the entry-level nursing education to facilitate political, socioeconomic, and cultural cohesiveness. Unfortunately, the global response to the problem has been slow (Duquesne University, 2020).

The curriculum pattern of the nursing, pharmacy, physiotherapy, and optometry programs is similar to the medical and dental programs. During the pre-clinical phase, the other health professions take courses in medical psychology, biostatistics, research methods, biochemistry, physiology, anatomy, and microbiology. In the clinical stage, the students participate in small group conferences and discussions and acquire clinical experience working with patients in hospitals, clinics, and community settings. The programs hire qualified faculty with mixed clinical and research expertise to cover all the specialties in the discipline, to meet accreditation standards. The programs are mandated to have adequate infrastructures that include classrooms, faculty and staff office spaces, library and information technology, instructional and research laboratories, clinical facilities, and relaxation and study areas for students. Administrative support structure for academic records maintenance and registrar functions are made available. In addition, adequate educational and social support services, including counseling, tutoring, time management, mental health services, and academic advisors are open to the students. Above all, sufficient financial resources to educate the number of students enrolled is required.

All professional groups have standard requirements for continuing education in the form of courses and training activities lasting a few days to several months' duration, to ensure that licensed practitioners stay up to date by learning new developments within their professions/specialties. Practitioners can keep up to date by attending national and international conferences, discussion groups, and clinical meetings, or by reading journals in the disciplines. For instance, in the United States, the Accreditation Council for Continuing Medical Education, established in 1985, oversees physicians' continuing education. In many countries around the world, boards/councils appointed by the government statutorily regulate HCE. In the United Kingdom, the General Medical Council governs medical training and is controlled by individual professional councils in other countries. And in the United States, the Liaison Committee on Medical Education, and the Council on Medical Education, both affiliates of the American Medical and Osteopathic Associations, is the statutory body responsible for regulating medical training. Henceforth, health care education (HCE) will be used consistently instead of a discipline-specific education genre to underscore the interprofessional philosophy advocated in this book.

Global distribution of the health care workforce

A significant global challenge in the health care system is the unequal distribution of the workforce. Low-income countries carry over 55% of the worldwide burden of disease but have less than 15% of the global health care workforce (WHO, 2006). In contrast, many high-income countries carry a lower weight of disease but have a relatively higher workforce ratio. For instance, the United States with 10% of the global burden of disease has 25% of the worldwide health care workforce; whereas Africa, which carries 25% the global burden of disease has less than 4% of the workforce (Anyangwe and Mtonga, 2007; Kumar, 2007; John et al., 2012). The shortage of health care workforce in low-income countries is exacerbated by the migration of HCPs from inadequately resourced to richly resourced countries. This concept of movement is known as "brain drain." Quite often, HCPs in low-income countries immigrate for a variety of reasons – financial, unconducive practice environment, limited infrastructure, and political instability (Dodani and LaPorte, 2005; Eyal and Hurst, 2008).

Efforts made by the WHO and governments around the world to address health disparity and the workforce shortage have primary focus on training, retention, and recruitment in medicine, dentistry, public health, nursing, pharmacy, imaging, and medical laboratory sciences (WHO, 2006). Unfortunately, training in medical rehabilitation has not received any global attention, priority, and urgency. Consequently, many low-income countries, particularly in Africa, today are without education programs in physical-occupational and speech therapy fields. In sub-Saharan African countries, education and training of physicians and nurses have received a surge in human and material resources, funding, and partnerships with academic institutions in the United States. For instance, the US government has funded HIV/AIDS projects through the Medical Education Partnership Initiative and the Nursing Education Partnership Initiative programs of the National Institutes of Health and the President's Emergency Plan for AIDS Relief. Through the Nursing Education Partnership Initiative, several nursing education programs were upgraded in Botswana, Lesotho, Kenya, Malawi, Zambia, Brazil, India, Thailand, and the Philippines. Educational partnership projects between institutions from low-income countries and institutions in North America, through the Consortium of Universities for Global Health made up of over 50 institutions, were funded by the Bill and Melinda Gates Foundation (John et al., 2012).

Health care education instructional methods

Globally, there are three primary instructional delivery methods used in HCE; discipline-specific (noncollaborative), multidisciplinary, and interprofessional approaches. The terms multidisciplinary and interprofessional training is often used interchangeably in error. Therefore, the distinction between them needs clarification here. Multidisciplinary education combines students from two or more professions in learning a topic or offers the entire course in tandem, but no active real-life purposeful, collaborative learning among the students. Interprofessional education (IPE) is a student–centered dynamic learning approach that brings together students from two or more professions to collaborate during the learning process to break down the artificial barriers across disciplines.

The WHO defined IPE as

> the process by which a group of students or workers from the health-related occupations with different backgrounds learn together during certain periods of their education, with interaction as the important goal, to collaborate in providing promotive, preventive, curative, rehabilitative, and other health-related services.
>
> (WHO, 1988)

Of the three instructional methods, the IPE strategy is best suited to deliver efficient health care services as the students from the different disciplines take their classes in tandem as dictated by their curriculum pattern, and work together to provide service that addresses the health needs of the institution's communities.

Although the discussion of the IPE concept began to take roots during the 1960s in North America, Australia, England, Germany, Jamaica, and Mexico, its implementation is relatively contemporary. Multiple and complex forces influenced the development of IPE in different countries around the world. Today, the concept is shared globally among international organizations and task forces (Lavin et al., 2001). A landmark document titled "To Err is Human: Building a Safer Health System," published in 2001 by the Institute of Medicine in the United States, called for the implementation of interdisciplinary teams in health care to improve quality care and patient safety (Institute of Medicine of the National Academies, 2001). Two years later, in another report, the Institute echoed the nexus between interdisciplinary collaboration and health care quality and urged HCE programs to adopt interprofessional instructional methods. The report proposed five core competencies that entry-level graduates must acquire to practice effectively in the 21st-century health care system. The core competencies are discussed in greater detail in Chapter 9 of this book.

In Nigeria, the origin of multidisciplinary HCE started at the University of Ibadan in the early 1970s, later at the University of Ife (now Obafemi Awolowo University) in the 1980s and more recently in 2015 at the University of Medical Sciences, Ondo. In the three medical schools, the curriculum mandates medical, dental, physiotherapy, and nursing students to take anatomy, physiology, and biochemistry courses together. Sadly, the three universities' multidisciplinary instructional method never extended to the clinical classes and other medical schools (Balogun et al., 2017). Consequently, the full potential of IPE was never realized, but recommendations on how to actualize this dream are presented in Chapter 9.

Accreditation

Accreditation is the oldest and most pervasive process used around the world to evaluate the quality of health care organizations and validate the legitimacy of colleges and universities. It is a potent signal to potential students and the general public that they can have confidence in an academic program or health system. The stakeholders of accreditation are the faculty, enrolled students, administrators, and the general public. A review board consisting of faculty from similarly situated (peer) accredited institutions determines accreditation standards. New institutions or programs seeking accreditation are required to meet the high standards set by the peer review boards.

The accreditation process is committed to greater academic rigor by establishing more demanding standards and criteria to achieve and sustain certification and promote quality improvement requirements. Accreditation boards are committed to accountability and transparency by routinely publishing institutions' retention, transfer and graduation rates, and graduate employment data. And regularly report how effectively institutions meet accreditation standards, and any deficiencies institutions may need to address. Accreditation best practice requires institutions to submit a self-study analysis report on each of the standards and criteria. The following are examples of evaluation domains commonly contained in a self-study report:

1. Mission. The institution's mission is clearly articulated publicly and demonstrates the mission guides the institution's operations.
2. Integrity: Ethical and Responsible Conduct. The institution acts with honesty, and its conduct is ethical and responsible.
3. Instruction and Learning: Quality, Resources, and Support. The institution provides high-quality education by traditional or online modules, and faculty and students engage in research.
4. Instruction and Learning: Evaluation and Improvement. The institution regularly assesses the quality of its academic programs, learning environments, and the quality of the support services. Also, evaluate student learning and faculty performance in teaching, research, and service domains through processes designed to promote continuous improvement.

5. Institutional Effectiveness, Resources, Planning. The institution's resources, structures, and processes are adequate to meet its core mission, improve the quality of its academic programs, and respond to future challenges and opportunities. The institution has concrete strategic plans for the future.

The accreditation bodies in North America and the United Kingdom require a self-study evaluation report followed by an onsite team assessment visit. The rigorous accreditation process in these countries no doubt contributes to their university's high world ranking. Examples of institution and program accreditation self-study reports are available at the following websites:

Institutions

- www.clarke.edu/wp-content/uploads/Clarke-University-HLC-Self-Study-Report.pdf
- https://accreditation.wsu.edu/documents/2015/10/spring-2009-wsu-comprehensive-self-study-report-for-reaffirmation-of-accreditation-to-nwccu.pdf/
- www.marquette.edu/accreditation/documents/Self-StudyReport-Website.pdf
- www.csu.edu/IER/documents/HLCSelfStudy.pdf

Academic Programs (Medicine/MPH/Nursing)

- www.jhsph.edu/about/school-at-a-glance/accreditation/_docs/JHSPH-Self-Study-Report-Prepared-for-CEPH-2015-03.pdf
- https://medicine.wright.edu/sites/medicine.wright.edu/files/page/attachments/2012%20Self%20Study_0.pdf
- http://sph.berkeley.edu/sites/default/files/SPH-Accreditation-Self-Study-Final-Report-August-2015.pdf
- www.google.com/search?q=sample+self+study+report+for+college+of+medicine&oq=sample&aqs=chrome.1.69i57j69i59j69i60j69i59l2j0.4209j0j7&sourceid=chrome&ie=UTF-8
- www.med.emory.edu/about/documents/EMORY%20UNIVERSITY%20SCHOOL%20OF%20MEDICINE%20FINAL%20SELF-STUDY%20REPORT.pdf
- http://publichealth.uic.edu/sites/default/files/public/documents/about-sph/pdf/FINAL%2CMaster%2CSelf-Study_02242015.pdf
- www.uky.edu/nursing/sites/www.uky.edu.nursing/files/Total-Self-Study-2008-11-FINAL.pdf

International accreditation

Many funding agencies such as the World Bank, now require their funded academic programs to obtain international accreditation. The pertinent question, is international accreditation the future for validating quality? Across the United Arab Emirates, a growing number of universities and academic/professional programs in computer science, engineering, business, and nursing are pursuing accreditation from the United Kingdom, Germany, and the United States. The goal of the universities seeking such certification is to enhance quality, the value of the academic degrees offer, and claim prestige (Lynch, 2015).

One of the leading international accreditation agencies is the Accreditation Service for International Schools, Colleges, and Universities (ASIC) based in the United Kingdom. The ASIC assured the public, students, parents, and other stakeholders of the quality of education offered in their accredited institutions and their dedication to high standards through continuous improvement. The ASIC accreditation process evaluates the commitment of an institution seeking certification to "internationalization and, in particular, commitment to supplying exemplary services to international students." ASIC assesses institutions in eight key performance areas:

1. Premises and health and safety
2. Governance, management, and staff resources
3. Learning, teaching, and research activity
4. Quality assurance and enhancement
5. Student welfare
6. Awards and qualifications
7. Marketing and recruitment of students
8. Systems management and compliance with immigration regulations.

The ASIC accreditation does not require a self-study report but undertakes the following processes and visits. Stage one visits focus on the inspection of the institution premises, health and safety facilities, academic/department resources, mode of course delivery, student welfare, marketing of the program, and student recruitment. Stage two visit focuses on review of administrative officers and faculty qualifications. And meetings with owners and executive officers of the institution, faculty, students, and compliance with immigration requirements. Two ASIC accreditors may undertake a single visit for one to two days. The visits are arranged after the completed application form and supporting documentation and payment of £1,000 application fees, excluding inspection and annual fees are received. The ASIC evaluation process is highly prescriptive. Detailed information can be obtained from their website at www.asicuk.com/university-accreditation/

The AKKORK is another independent professional accrediting agency based in Russia. Their primary operations include the following six areas:

1. Evaluation of the quality of education offered
2. Professional education program accreditation
3. Accreditation of e-learning programs

4. Internal quality assurance system development and certification
5. Assessment of administrative and teaching staff, and
6. Seminars and training.

More detailed information about AKKORK can be obtained online at their website at www.akkork.ru/e/about/

The leading accreditation agency that oversees standard in higher education in the United Kingdom is the British Accreditation Council established in 1984 by the British Council and the Department of Education. Today, the Council accredits over 230 institutions across 17 countries around the world. More information can be obtained online at their website at www.the-bac.org/

In the United States, there are six accreditation agencies located in each region of the country. Additional information on the agencies can be obtained online from the websites associated with the following bodies:

1. Middle States Association of Colleges and Schools
2. New England Association of Schools and Colleges
3. Higher Learning Commission formerly the North Central Association of Colleges and Schools
4. Northwest Commission of Schools and Colleges
5. Western Association of Schools and Colleges
6. Southern Association of Colleges and Schools

Because of the global desire for safe and sound quality health care, there is a growing interest in international accreditation of hospitals and health care facilities. International accreditation of a hospital confers a stamp of approval of quality health care delivery. Thus, discerning patients intentionally seek out hospitals with international accreditation because of their dedication to quality, patient-centered care, innovative health care practices, and safety. Examples of reputable international hospital and health care facilities accreditation organizations are the AABB Hospital Accreditation (2020), International Healthcare Accreditation (2020), Joint Commission International (2020), Global Healthcare Accreditation (2020) and Commission on Accreditation of Rehabilitation Facilities (2020).

University and academic program accreditation in Nigeria

The National Universities Commission (NUC), located in the nation's capital, Abuja, is the body legislatively charged with the development, accreditation, and management of the university system to ensure quality and global competitiveness (NUC, 2020). The NUC is empowered to develop minimum academic standards (MAS) for universities and to accredit all degree programs. In 1989, faculty experts from 13 academic disciplines offered in Nigerian universities developed the MAS for administration, law, social sciences, social sciences, arts, education, engineering and technology, sciences, environmental sciences, agriculture, basic medical sciences, medicine and dentistry, pharmaceutical sciences, and veterinary medicine. Besides the MAS, the experts also produced:

1. A manual detailing the accreditation procedures for academic programs
2. A self-study *form* (*not a self-study report*) to list the available resources in the educational program
3. Program evaluation form
4. Accreditation panel report form
5. Accreditation revisitation form

Before 2004, the MAS served as the reference document used for program accreditation. Following another rigorous review by a new panel of experts, they produced the benchmark minimum academic standards (BMAS). The BMAS is presently used to evaluate whether the educational program meets the accreditation criteria. The Program Accreditation Division of the Commission oversees compliance to quality assurance, sustenance, and institutional services within the university system. The primary functions of the division are to:

1. Coordinate accreditation visits to universities and degree awarding institutions to evaluate undergraduate and postgraduate programs
2. Coordinate the development and periodic review of assessment instruments needed for accreditation
3. Promote a culture of quality assurance and self-analysis by encouraging universities to develop robust internal quality assurance mechanism and conduct an internal accreditation review
4. Respond to inquiries and advise the Commission on issues about the accreditation of the academic program
5. Annually ascertain the full- and part-time undergraduate, postgraduate, and online learning educational programs approved
6. Maintain a national database of professors and update the list once a year (NUC, 2020).

In addition to the accreditation of the universities carried out by the NUC, the professional statutory regulatory boards/councils also accredit academic programs. The accreditation process of the NUC and regulatory boards/councils primarily concentrates on the inspection of resources (physical, human, equipment, and lab) and evaluation of the curriculum content's adequacy. The process does not currently involve the general public and does not include a self-study evaluation report that describes the institution and academic programs conformity with the stated accreditation standards.

In addition, the accreditation process lacked public validation and no mechanism to objectively examine the strengths and weaknesses of educational programs for continuous quality improvement. Furthermore, no assessment is undertaken to show that the universities are meeting their stated mission and conducting business ethically and with integrity, as demonstrated by the number of grievances and lawsuits from stakeholders/public. Specifically, no assessment is currently undertaken to validate (1) if the universities provide high-quality education and ethically manage their funds and research operations, and (2) student learning through processes designed to promote benchmarking and continuous improvement. Recommendations on how to improve the accreditation process are presented in Chapter 9.

Gauging institutional academic quality and efficiency

Benchmarking is the process of comparing the performance of an institution of higher learning or academic program against the output of similarly situated peer institutions or programs or against the best institutions or programs in the country/world. Around the world, institutions commonly select United States universities as the gold standard against which to compare their institutional or academic program performance. By comparing an institution's performance against peers or the best institutions, it allows the institution to understand what makes "superior" performance possible and can use the information gathered from the analysis to appropriately implement reforms that will yield significant improvements in the operations of the institution.

Benchmarking allows higher learning institutions to identify deficiencies, waste, and learn from areas of good practice. The national licensing exam is the most viable metrics for benchmarking the performance of professional programs. Other relevant benchmarking indicators commonly used include analysis of student persistence and success as measured by first-year retention rates, fourth- and sixth-year graduation rates. Sociodemographic variables such as gender, age, degrees conferred, salaries, types of academic programs, admissions requirements, tuition/fees, number, and rank of faculty and employees by position are also used to identify inequities and compare institutional resources.

In the United States, the above-benchmarking key performance indicators are regularly collected by the Department of Education's National Center for Education Statistics and published online at https://nces.ed.gov/programs/coe/indicator_ctr.asp. Many institutions around the world use statistical data for cross-national comparisons to gauge the quality and efficiency of their academic programs. The NUC should collect similar data and periodically publish them online to promote the country's culture of benchmarking. The availability of the benchmarking data will spur healthy competition among academic programs at different universities nationwide.

Impact of corruption on health care education – global status

Many countries around the world, in 2015, as part of the 2030 Agenda for Sustainable Development, agreed to pursue the United Nations' 17 Sustainable

Development Goals (SDGs) – Goal number four calls for "inclusive and equitable quality education for all." Sadly, the 2017 progress report revealed that 263 million children of school age, including 61 SDGs million primary schools worldwide, were not enrolled in school. The 2018 progress report revealed that 41% of children in sub-Saharan Africa and 52% in North Africa and Western Asia attend school. Many students in school, especially in Africa and Latin America, do not acquire critical skills. Furthermore, the 2018 report showed that 58% of the 617 million youth of primary and lower secondary school age around the world are not achieving minimum proficiency in reading and mathematics. The reasons include a lack of qualified teachers and inadequate school facilities (Kirya, 2019).

Embezzlement or diversion of school funds deprives the students of needed resources. Nepotism and favoritism often lead to unqualified lecturers' appointment, while corruption in procurement results in inferior quality in laboratory equipment and school textbooks/supplies. Students who are sexually harassed for sex by lecturers can potentially drop out of school. When parents pay bribes or fraudulent fees for educational services that are supposed to be free, this unexpected spending reduce access to education for economically disadvantaged students. Such students, who potentially could become HCPs, are deprived of the opportunity because of the corrupt practices of public officers. Thus, addressing corruption at the global level is critical if SDG number four is to be achieved.

Corruption is often packaged using innuendo and code, and when bribery practices cross global borders, multiple jargon and dialects are used (Table 1.1).

In contrast, in many countries, only rogues are clandestinely involved in crime. In the United States, unaccredited and fake online institutions have become breeding grounds for the award of bogus Bachelor's, Master's, and doctoral degrees. The corruption in the Nigerian educational system is discussed further in Chapter 8 of this book.

Faculty salaries in selected countries

Remuneration is a critical component of the conditions of service needed for faculty to do their jobs efficiently. Academic salaries vary widely depending on the country, individual university, and academic rank. For comparative purposes, Table 1.2 presents what professors in all HCE disciplines, on the average, make in Europe and North America. All data are reported in the local currency and are pretax (Academic Media Group International AB, 2018).

The information presented should be digested with an abundance of caution because professors in the health care discipline in most countries are paid higher salaries. In many countries around the world, like German and France, professors are considered civil servants, and their salaries are fixed by national legislation according to the state economic health. In some countries, faculty

Table 1.1 Terminology used for bribery in Nigeria and other parts of the world

	Country	Bribery jargon (Tillen and Delman, 2010)
1	Nigeria	Igbo = *Igbuozu;* Yoruba = *Egunje;* Hausas = *Chuachua; toshiyar-baki.* Among urbanites and elites = *"Envelope"; kola; dash* (Nwaokugha, Ezeugwu 2017)
2	Argentina	*Cohecho; soborno; coima; cometa*
3	Angola	*Gaseoso*
4	Brazil	*Propina; jetto; jetinho; caixinha; graxa; troco; nota; acerto*
5	Bulgaria	*Rusvet*
6	Cambodia	*Tea money*
7	China	*Huilu; chaqian*
8	Croatia	*Mitto; podmititi (v.)*
9	East Africa	*Chai;* Kiswahili = Kutu-kidogo
10	Egypt	*Baksheesh; shay*
11	France	*Pot-de-vin; arroser (v.); graisser (v.)*
12	Gambia	*Maslaha*
13	Germany	*Shmiergeld*
14	Greece	*Bakssissi*
15	Honduras	*Pajada*
16	Hong Kong	*Hactzien*
17	Hungary	*Megvesztegetes; kezet fogni (v.); keno penz; csuszo penz; lekenyerezni; lefizetni*
18	India	Rishwat; baksheesh; ghoos; hafta; chai-pani
19	Indonesia	Suap; pungli; uang sogok
20	Iran	Roshveh
21	Italy	Tangento; omaggi; spintarella; bustarella
22	Japan	On; wairo; kuroi kiri
23	Malaysia	Suap; duit kopi
24	Mexico	Soborno; mordida; refresco; gratificaci—n; dinero por debajo de la mesa
25	Mozambique	Gaseoso
26	Pakistan	Rishvat
27	Peru	Coima
28	Philippines	Lagay; kotong; suhol;
29	Romania	Rasplata
30	Russia	Vzyatka; otkat; dat' na lapu (v.)
31	Serbia	Mitto; podmititi (v.)
32	South Korea	Noemul; gum eun don; dŸ don; chonji
33	Southeast Asia	Kumshaw
34	Spain	Untar (v.); soborno
35	Sweden	Muta
36	Syria	Rashwah; finjaan Ôahwa
37	Thailand	Sin bone; tea money
38	Turkey	Rusvet
39	Ukraine	Habar; oplata
40	United States	Bribe; kickback, payola; sweetener; backhander; hush money; grease; wet my beak
41	Zaire	Tarif de verre

Table 1.2 Global average/median annual faculty salaries (in local currency) by academic rank

	Country	Full Professor	Associate Professor	Assistant Professor	Comment	Reporting Year
1	United Kingdom (£)	82,506		43,607	Average = 79,030	2015–2016
2	Germany (€)	68,972–82,013	60,154–72,246	49,548–57,373		
3	Sweden (SEK) (Median)	729,600	534,000	480,000	Taxes are approx. 45%	2016
4	Switzerland (CHF)	149,728–171,380	125,250–158,783		163,564–210,793 professor/chair	(Highest in Europe)
5	Zurich (CHF)	209,247–275,359	178,996–245,080	148,682–214,767		
6	Denmark (DKR)	698,832	533,040	460,128	Taxes at 40–50%	
7	Netherlands (€)	64,008–112,500	57,780–84,864	41,700–64,860	Taxes around 40%	
8	France (€)	36,560–73,343	25,225–53,828	25,225–53,828		
9	Belgium (€)	40,109–68,633	34,255–58,402	29,914–47,443	Taxes around 45–52%	
10	Norway (NOK) (Median)	610,296	487,104	468,696–496,296	Taxes around 40%	
11	Finland (€)	55,872–104,184	40,080–67,608	40,080–67,608	Median = 80,760 Taxes = 25–32%	2015
12	United States (USD)	102,402	79,654	69,206		2016/2017
13	Canada ($) (Median)	124,325	97,423	77,269–71,060	Median = 98,400	2016/2017

salaries are determined by collective agreements/contracts negotiated between academic unions and the government. The wages are determined by seniority (years since the completion of a PhD and years of job experience), and academic rank (Academic Media Group International, 2018).

Conclusion

This chapter chronicles the global history of medical, dental, nursing, pharmacy, and physiotherapy education, the emerging and changing educational landscape, including instructional methods, the accreditation process, and benchmarking institutional academic quality and efficiency. It also presents the impact of corruption on HCE and faculty salaries in selected countries around the world. Although HCE is diverse, there are several similarities in their origin, curriculum pattern, resource needs/utilization, and postprofessional licensure requirements. The analysis revealed the history and curriculum pattern of pharmacy, physiotherapy, and optometry education closely followed that of medical and dental education. All health care professions require the same postprofessional requirements to ensure that licensed practitioners stay up to date by learning new developments in the discipline. The issues presented cut across regional boundaries and academic disciplines and lay the foundation for the topical issues presented in this book.

References

AABB Hospital Accreditation. (2020) [online]. Available at: www.aabb.org/sa/Documents/accreditation-international.pdf (Accessed: 25 January 2020)

Academic Media Group International. (2018) Professor salaries from around the world. [online]. Available at: https://academicpositions.com/career-advice/professor-salaries-from-around-the-world (Accessed: 25 January 2020)

American Dental Education Association. (2015) History of dentistry. [online]. Available at: www.adea.org/GoDental/Health_Professions_Advisors/History_of_Dentistry.aspx (Accessed: 25 January 2020)

American Optometric Association (2020) The history of the American Optometric Association. [online]. Available at: www.aoa.org/archives/ (Accessed: 25 January 2020)

Anyangwe, S and Mtonga C. (2007) Inequities in the global health workforce: the greatest impediment to health in sub-saharan Africa. *International Journal of Environmental Research and Public Health*, 4(2):93–100.

Balogun, JA, Aka, PC, Balogun, AO and Obajuluwa, VA. (2017) A phenomenological investigation of the first two decades of university-based physiotherapy education in Nigeria. *Cogent Medicine*, 4(1) 10.1080/2331205X. [online]. Available at: https://bit.ly/2SEF1oa (Accessed: 25 January 2020)

Buhler-Wilkerson, K and D'Antonio P. (2020) Nursing. *Encyclopædia Britannica*. [online]. Available at: www.britannica.com/science/nursing (Accessed: 25 January 2020)

Commission on Accreditation of Rehabilitation Facilities – CARF-. (2020) [online]. Available at: www.carf.org/home/ (Accessed: 25 January 2020)

Chiedu, J. (2016) Must read: Before you buy that School of Nursing admission form. *Nursing World Nigeria.* [online]. Available at: www.nursingworldnigeria.com/2016/03/must-read-before-you-buy-that-school-of-nursing-admission-form-by-jude-chiedu (Accessed: 25 January 2020)

Dodani, S and LaPorte, RE. (2005) Brain drain from developing countries: How can brain drain be converted into wisdom gain? *Journal of the Royal Society of Medicine*, 98(11):487–491.

Duquesne University. (2020) A history of modern nursing education. [online]. Available at: https://onlinenursing.duq.edu/online-dnp-program/history-modern-nursing-education/ (Accessed: 25 January 2020)

Duquesne University. (n.d.) Harmonizing nursing education worldwide. [online]. Available at: https://onlinenursing.duq.edu/blog/harmonizing-nursing-education-worldwide/ (Accessed: 25 January 2020)

Eyal, N and Hurst, SA. (2008) Physician brain drain: can nothing be done? *Public Health Ethics*, 1(2):180–192.

Fei-FeiDeng. (2015) Comparison of nursing education among different countries. *Chinese Nursing Research*, 2(4):96–98. [online]. Available at: https://nursejournal.org/articles/types-of-nursing-degrees/ (Accessed: 25 January 2020)

Global Healthcare Accreditation. (2020) [online]. Available at: www.prnewswire.com/news-releases/global-healthcare-accreditation-standards-accredited-by-isqua-300864158.html (Accessed: 25 January 2020)

Goss, DA. (2003) History of optometry. Indiana University School of Optometry.

Hartley, F and Krantz, JC. (2020) Pharmacy. *Encyclopædia Britannica.* [online]. Available at: www.britannica.com/science/pharmacy (Accessed: 25 January 2020)

Institute of Medicine of the National Academies. (2001) Educating health professionals in teams: Current reality, barriers, and related actions. *Institute of Medicine Report*, 1–10. *Issued at the 68th World Medical Association General Assembly, Chicago, USA.*

International Healthcare Accreditation. (2020) [online]. Available at: www.dnvgl.com/services/international-healthcare-accreditation-7516 (Accessed: 25 January 2020)

John, EB, Pfalzer, LA, Fry, D, Glickman L, Masaaki, S, Sabus, C, Okafor, UAC and Al-Jarrah, MD. (2012) Establishing and upgrading physical therapist education in developing countries: Four case examples of service by Japan and United States physical therapist programs to Nigeria, Suriname, Mongolia, and Jordan *Journal of Physical Therapy Education*, 26(1): 29–39. [online]. Available at:https://pdfs.semanticscholar.org/6520/aebb7b1b952616be65632ffacdc76e64e208.pdf (Accessed: 25 January 2020)

Joint Commission International. (2020) [online]. Available at: www.worldhospitalsearch.org/the-value-of-jci-accreditation/who-is-joint-commission-international/ (Accessed: 25 January 2020)

Kirya, M. (2019) Education sector corruption: How to assess it and ways to address it. *Education Public Service Delivery*, U4 Issue. [online]. Available at: www.u4.no/publications/education-sector-corruption-how-to-assess-it-and-ways-to-address-it (Accessed: 25 January 2020)

Kumar, P. (2007) Providing the providers-remedying Africa's shortage of health care workers. *N Engl J Med.* 356(25):2564–2567.

Kwan, B, Sebasky, M and Muchmore, EA. (2019) The changing landscape of medical education: A brave new world. *The Hospitalist.* [online]. Available at: www.the-hospitalist.org/hospitalist/article/206173/leadership-training/changing-landscape-medical-education (Accessed: 25 January 2020)

Lasik, MD. (2020) The evolution of optometry: A quick look at history. [online]. Available at: www.lasikmd.com/blog/evolution-optometry-quick-look-history (Accessed: 25 January 2020)

Lavin, M, Ruebling, I, Banks, R, Block, L, Counte, M, Furman, GE, Miller, P, Reese, C, Viehmann, V and Holt, J. (2001) Interdisciplinary health professional education: A historical review. *Advances in Health Sciences Education*, 6:25–47[online]. Available at: www.researchgate.net/publication/11857303_Interdisciplinary_Health_ Professional_Education_A_Historical_Review (Accessed: 25 January 2020)

Lynch, S. (2015) A growing number of Arab universities seek international accreditation. [online]. Available at: www.al-fanarmedia.org/2015/03/a-growing-number-of-arab-universities-seek-international-accreditation/ (Accessed: 25 January 2020)

Multimedia Foundation (2019) Irvin Borish. [online]. Available at: https:// en.m.wikipedia.org/wiki/Irvin_Borish (Accessed: 25 January 2020)

Multimedia Foundation (2020) Optometry. [online]. Available at: https://en.m. wikipedia.org/wiki/Optometry#History(Accessed: 25 January 2020)

National Universities Commission (NUC, 2020.) [online]. Available at: www.nuc.edu. ng/ (Accessed: 25 January 2020)

Nwaokugha, DO, and Ezeugwu, MC. (2017) Corruption in the education industry in Nigeria: Implication for national development. *European Journal of Training and Development Studies*, 4 (1): 1–17 [online]. Available at: www.eajournals.org/wp-content/uploads/Corruption-in-the-Education-Industry-in-Nigeria-Implications-for-National-Development.pdf (Accessed: 16 February 2020)

Research Careers. (2020) Payscale average registered nurse (RN) salary in United Kingdom. [online]. Available at: www.payscale.com/research/UK/Job=Registered_ Nurse_(RN)/Salary (Accessed: 25 January 2020)

Sahi, A and Dutta S. (2020) Physiotherapy history. *News-Medical.Net*. [online]. Available at: www.news-medical.net/health/Physiotherapy-History.aspx (Accessed: 25 January 2020)

Scarborough, H, Turner, EL and Gregg, A (n.d.) Medical education. [online]. Available at: www.britannica.com/science/medical-education (Accessed: 25 January 2020)

Smith, AA. (2017) Debate continues on nursing degrees. *Inside Higher Ed.* [online]. Available at: www.insidehighered.com/news/2017/12/22/battle-over-entry-level-degree-nursing-continues (Accessed: 25 January 2020)

Tillen, JG. and Delman, SM. (2010) Lost in translation: The language of bribery. *The Corporate Governance Advisor*, 12 (July/August): 12–17. [online]. Available at: www. studocu.com/en-ca/document/university-of-prince-edward-island/intercultural-management/other/lost-in-translation-bribery/882301/view (Accessed: 25 January 2020)

Todowede, BJ. (2016) Corruption and the future of Nigeria's educational system. *International Journal of Arts and Sciences*, 9(2):325–334. [online]. Available at: www.universitypublications.net/ijas/0902/pdf/M6K13.pdf (Accessed: 25 January 2020)

WHO. (1988) Learning together to work together for health. Report of a study group on multi-professional education of health personnel: The team approach. *WHO Technical Report Series*. Geneva: WHO, 769:1–72.

WHO. (2006) The World Health Report 2006: *Working Together for Health*. Geneva: WHO, 1–15.

World Confederation for Physical Therapy. (2016) Legal go-ahead for UK physiotherapists to prescribe independently. [online]. Available at: www.wcpt.org (Accessed: 25 January 2020)

World Medical Association. (2017) Statement on Medical Education. [online]. Available at: www.wma.net/policies-post/wma-statement-on-medical-education/ (Accessed: 25 January 2020)

2 The art of teaching in health care education

Introduction

The fastest-growing segment of students enrolled in health care education (HCE) programs are highly motivated, mature adults with work experience. This paradigm shift calls for a self-directed educational system where the students should have input on how learning should take place. Therefore, the utilization of heutagogy principles has become more critical and valid in HCE. The overwhelming majority of faculty in HCE does not have any formal training in teaching. Unfortunately, there are no readily available publications on this topic in many countries around the world. Many experts opined that this curriculum deficit is partly responsible for the poor quality of instruction in HCE programs around the world.

This chapter focuses on teaching techniques by discussing the primary differences between pedagogy, andragogy, and heutagogy. It also presents the effective strategies to promote self-directed learning and self-determined learning, domains and taxonomy of learning, course syllabus, the link between course objectives and program students learning objectives, curriculum mapping, application of evidence-based practice in teaching, formative and summative assessments and the relevance of online instruction in HCE.

Pedagogy, andragogy, and heutagogy

The theories and methods used in teaching children is *pedagogy*, while *andragogy* focus on the practices used to teach adults. The term pedagogy first appeared in the literature in the mid-to-late-1500s, in Middle French, and has roots in Latin and Greek. The term andragogy was coined in the 1800s by Alexander Knapp, a German educator, and popularized by Malcolm Knowles, an American educator, in the 1960s (Halupa, 2014). The word *heutagogy* was coined in 2001 by Stewart Hase and Chris Kenyon from Southern Cross University, Australia. They argued that the rapid rate of change in society, and associated information explosion, call for an educational system where the students should determine what and how learning should occur. A process they termed "self-determined learning" (Hase and Kenyon, 2001).

Andragogy and heutagogy affect faculty behaviors, professionalism, and judgments. The teaching strategies are based on the theories of learning, understandings of the students, their needs, backgrounds, and interests. They also include how the instructors' interface with students and the social and intellectual milieu the instructor seeks to establish. Training in the principles of andragogy and heutagogy is now becoming an integral part of HCE. In the United States, postgraduate medical students are increasingly required to have formal training in education. This emerging requirement has led to a rapid increase in the number of postgraduate programs in medical education training.

The campaign in the early 1990s led by Ernest Boyer – author of *Scholarship Reconsidered: Priorities of the Professoriate* and proponent of Scholarship of discovery, integration, application, and teaching – gave visibility to the call for an academician to have formal training in education. In his campaign, Professor Boyer eloquently asserted that *"a poor surgeon hurts one patient at a time, but a poor educator hurts 130. In the end, excellence in education means excellence in teaching, and if this country would give the status to first-grade teachers that we give to full professors, this one act alone would revitalize the nation's schools."* Unlike the United States, health care academics in Nigeria do not presently have formal training in education and have limited access to textbooks on this critical and consequential topic. The distinguishing characteristics of pedagogy, andragogy and heutagogy are presented in Table 2.1.

Now that the primary characteristics of pedagogy, andragogy, and heutagogy have been discussed, the strategies to improve learning will be presented next. The following are effective strategies to promote undergraduate-level learning:

Strategy 1: *State the lesson objectives clearly*: The instructor must be able to quickly and easily state what the students must learn and demonstrate at the end of a given lesson.

Strategy 2: Utilize the *"show and tell" method*: The instructor should start the class session when possible with "show and tell" imaginative narratives. Telling involves information sharing or knowledge with students while showing consists of modeling how to do something. Sharing information about your research will attract students' interest.

Strategy 3: *Regularly question students to check for learning*: The instructor should always check for understanding of information presented before moving onto the next more complex content.

Strategy 4: *Graphically summarize new learning*: The instructor can enhance learning by using graphic outlines such as flow-charts and Venn diagrams to summarize the information presented and the interrelationships between them.

Strategy 5: *Introduce plenty of practice*: The idiom, "practice makes perfection," helps students retain the skills and cognitive knowledge that they have acquired while also allowing the instructor another opportunity to check for understanding.

Table 2.1 The major attributes of pedagogy, andragogy, and heutagogy

Concept	Pedagogy	Andragogy	Heutagogy
Role of students	Dependent on the instructor to learn	Self-directed learning	Self-determined learning
Role of lecturer	Delivers knowledge to students	Facilitates knowledge	Supportive and collaborative
Experiential learning	No	Yes	Yes
Primary activities	Classroom milieu and lecture-based	Experiential instructional methods using group work, e-learning, simulations, preceptorship	Contractual: reflective journaling, action research, one on one case reviews, internship
Evaluation of learning	Multiple-choice (objective) method	Essay, term paper, practical	Negotiated assessment: Creation of product, portfolio, practical
Readiness	Students are told when they are ready	Students decide what additional knowledge they need	Experiment with real-life situations
Sequencing	Step-by-step uniform progression	Progression is based on students' skills and readiness	Using outcome of formative and summative evaluation
Learning	Facts which will only be useful later on	Process-oriented for future potential	Collaborative learning
Curriculum	Simple to complex	Competency-based or categorical	Workplace-based and flexible
Age group	Primary and secondary school level	Higher education —undergraduates	Higher education – vocational/postgraduates/fellowships
Motivation	External pressures, consequence of failure, competition for grades	Internal motivators, better quality of life, recognition, self-esteem/actualization/confidence	Solving workplace and societal challenges
Knowledge	Done without question	Students must understand why it is important	Graduate students who will work as trouble-shooters, problem solvers, and general consultants on change and improvement in the clinical setting
Readiness to learn	What is required	When content is relevant	Emphasize the provision of resources rather than content
Focus	Student-centered	Skills-centered	Life skills-focused

Strategy 6: *Provide regular feedback*: Letting students know how they have performed on a particular task and how they can improve learning and build confidence. The input must be provided timely.

Strategy 7: *Be flexible about the time it takes to learn*: The notion that given enough time, students will learn is not as revolutionary as it may sound as it underpins the way we teach every clinical skill. It is also the central premise behind the mastery learning concept.

Strategy 8: *Promote productive teamwork*: Group work among students is typical in every classroom, but productive group work among students is rare. Students often rely on the person who seems most willing and able to the task at hand – social loafing – when working in groups. This practice should be discouraged by getting students equally involved. Require students to state their contribution(s) to a group assignment. Let the students know the rationale behind that – assign group and individual grade to the assignment.

Strategy 9: *Teach strategies not just content*: The instructor should explicitly teach the students how to use problem-solving strategies and guided practice before asking them how to apply concepts independently.

Strategy 10: *Develop meta-cognition thinking*: Meta-cognition involves thinking about options, choices, and results. The students should be encouraged to think about what strategies they could use before choosing.

Heutagogy is a student-centered teaching and learning strategy where the postgraduates and fellowship students determine the learning by encouraging self-directed learning. By jettisoning the traditional rigid control of education, the instructors' role becomes one of support and a facilitator by allowing students to define their needs and learning outcomes. In this model of education, the instructor spends more time working with students individually to establish their goals, or else creating a more comprehensive range of contents from which the student can choose what to study (Schroeder, 2018). A few strategies to encourage self-directed learning include a degree of autonomy that allow the students to create their degree plan, set their completion dates for assignments and create modules that will enable them to begin with whatever interests them most. For example, faculty can provide projects that improve evidence-based practice inpatient care or improve the effectiveness of organization operations.

The heutagogy method of education contains learning contracts, flexible curriculum, student-directed questions, and flexible and negotiated assessment. The elements of the course design include reflective journaling, action research, which allows students to experiment with real-life situations, formative and summative evaluation, and collaborative learning (Hase and Kenyon, 2001). Teaching and evaluating the performance of postgraduates and fellowship students are not the same as teaching undergraduates. Assessment of learning at the undergraduate level focus quizzes on drilling the facts into student minds within Bloom's "recall/reproduction" or "remembering and understanding." On the other hand, assessment of learning at postgraduate level build more in-depth knowledge by requiring students to apply, analyze, evaluate, and create products/materials (Schroeder, 2018). Educational theorist Malcolm Knowles proposed four principles of teaching postgraduate students:

1. They should be allowed to plan and assess their instruction.
2. Experience, including mistakes, should form the basis for the learning activities.
3. Teach contents that have immediate relevance and impact on students' job or personal life.
4. The learning should be problem-centered rather than content-oriented.

The following are effective strategies to promote learning among postgraduates and fellowship students:

Strategy 1: *Development of students learning capacity*: The purpose of heutagogy is to enable students to remember how to learn and facili-tate the development of capability. Involve the faculty, students, and administration in the formulation of the learning objectives and how to achieve them. Emphasize process rather than outcome, and mean-ingful person-centered learning is enhanced.

Strategy 2: *Evaluation is ongoing and not summative*: Assessment of learning should be continuous (formative), and the program must be flexible enough to accommodate changes. Workplace-based projects can be used as an assessment method.

Strategy 3: *Emphasize resources rather than content*: The learning outcomes and assessment should be negotiated with a few signposts provided to the students who will make sense of the issues and come to their con-clusion. Student-directed questions should become the norm rather than the instructor-led answers.

Strategy 4: *Create a more active role for student input and feedback*: Learning should be cooperative and negotiated to produce a win-win process as possible. Learning experiences should be creative to allow students to ask questions that have universal practical application.

Strategy 5: *Create opportunities in the clinical environment*: Utilize less the traditional classroom instruction and the internet media but making learning an integral part of the day-to-day clinical work and find ways to harness that learning. The faculty must encourage students to design projects, within their work environment, using meaningful and measurable outcomes to assess the effectiveness of interventions. For example, students can evaluate the impact of an educational program on maternal mortality rate.

Domains of learning

Learning is categorized into three domains – *cognitive* (mental knowledge/thinking), *affective* (attitude), and *psychomotor* (manual skills). There are multiple levels of learning within each domain, and they progress from more basic, surface-level learning to more complex deeper-level learning. Cognitive taxonomy was first described in 1956 by Dr. Benjamin Bloom, and the affective in 1964 by David Krathwohl, Benjamin Bloom, and Masia, BB. The psychomotor domain was not fully defined until 1972 by Simpson EJ and refined by Anita Harrow in 1972, and Dave RH in 1975 (Hoque, 2016).

The six levels of cognitive complexity proposed by Dr. Bloom are knowledge, comprehension, application, analysis, synthesis, evaluation. As academics try to construct optimal learning experiences, a newer version of Bloom's taxonomy of learning was developed by Krathwohl in 2001. The revised version from fundamental to complex consists of remembering, understanding, applying, analyzing, evaluating, and creating (Figure 2.1).

The affective domain comprises the way we deal with things emotionally, such as feelings, values, appreciation, enthusiasms, motivations, and attitudes (see

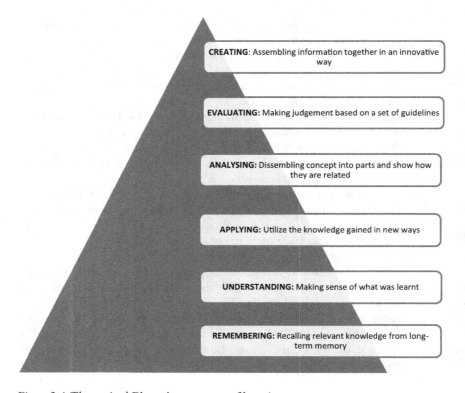

Figure 2.1 The revised Bloom's taxonomy of learning.

Table 2.2). This domain is classified into five sub-domains: receiving, responding, valuing, organization, and characterization (Hoque, 2016).

The psychomotor domain includes manual, kinesthetic, coordination, and physical skills. The development of these skills requires practice, measured in

Table 2.2 The categories and examples for each domain of learning

Cognitive Domain Categories	Examples and key words to use (verbs)
Level 1: Remembering: Recall or remember data or information	Defines, describes, identifies, knows, label, lists, matches, names, outlines, recalls, recognizes, reproduces, selects, states
Level 2: Understanding: Explain ideas or concepts. Understand the meaning, translation, interpolation, and interpretation of instructions and problems. State a problem in one's own words	Comprehends, defends, converts, distinguishes, estimates, interprets, explains, extends, generalizes, gives an example, infers, paraphrases, predicts, rewrites, summarizes, translates
Level 3: Applying: Use a concept of a new situation or unprompted use of an abstraction. Ability to apply the knowledge learned in the classroom into novel situations in the workplace. Use information in a new way	Applies, changes, computes, operates, constructs, demonstrate, discovers, solves, manipulates, modifies, predicts, prepares, produces, relates, shows, uses
Level 4: Analyzing: Distinguish between the different parts	Analyzes, breaks down, discriminates, compares, contrasts, diagrams, deconstructs, differentiates, relates, distinguishes, identifies, illustrates, infers, outlines, selects, separates
Level 5: Evaluating: Justify a stand or decision	Appraises, argues, supports, defends, judges, selects, values, evaluates
Level 6: Creating: Create new products or point of view	Assembles, formulates, constructs, creates, designs, develops
Affective domain categories	**Examples**
Level 1: Receiving phenomena: The receiving is the awareness of feelings, emotions, and the ability to utilize selected attention.	Listening attentively to someone express their views, watching a movie, listening to a lecture, watching the waves crash on the sand.
Level 2: Responding to phenomena: Responding is the active participation of the student. Participating in a group discussion	Having a group discussion, giving a presentation, complying with procedures, or following directions.
Level 3: Valuing: Valuing is the ability to see the worth of something and express it. Valuing is concerned with the quality attached to a particular object, phenomenon, behavior, or piece of information. This level ranges	Developing a plan to improve team skills, proposing ideas to increase proficiency, or informing leaders of possible issues. It is the ability to see the worth of something and express it. For example, a researcher shares his hypothesis before data collection.

(continued)

Table 2.2 Cont.

Cognitive Domain Categories	Examples and key words to use (verbs)
from simple acceptance to a more complex state of commitment. More uncomplicated recognition may include the desire for a team to improve its skills. In contrast, a more sophisticated level of involvement may consist of taking responsibility for the overall improvement of the group.	
Level 4: Organization: The ability to prioritize value over another and develop a unique value system.	An undergraduate medical student spends more time watching movies instead of studying.
Level 5: Characterization: The ability to internalize values and let them control the person's behavior	The ability of healthcare professionals to keep to themselves the private information of their patients (Krathwohl, Bloom, Masia (1964); Hoque, 2016).
Psychomotor domain categories	**Examples**
Level 1: Perception: The ability to integrate sensory information to motor activity.	A laboratory scientist adjusts the concentration of a reagent to achieve the right pH.
Level 2: Set: The readiness to perform.	An elderly patient displays motivation in completing the planned exercise.
Level 3: Guided response: The ability to reproduce a particular behavior or to utilize trial and error.	A person follows the manual in operating an equipment
Level 4: Mechanism: The ability to translate learned responses into habitual actions with confidence and proficiency.	A resident was able to perform cardiac catheterization after watching a consultant perform the procedure
Level 5: Complex overt response: the ability to skillfully perform intricate procedures or techniques.	A technician can operate the MRI machine without reading the manual for the process.
Level 6: Adaptation: The ability to modify the learned skills to meet special events.	A physiotherapist uses the *Cannabis* oil instead of the recommended gel when applying the ultrasound for the treatment of lateral epicondylitis injury.
Level 7: Origination: Creating new movement patterns for a specific situation.	A surgeon develops a new surgical procedure (Harrow 1972; Hoque, 2016)

terms of speed, precision, distance, procedures, or techniques in execution (Hoque, 2016). Examples of psychomotor skills range from manual tasks, such as a physiotherapist perform a kneading massage to more complex tasks, such as a neurosurgeon perform a craniotomy. The seven major psychomotor domain categories range from the simplest behavior such as perception, set, guided response, mechanism, complex overt response, adaptation, to the most complex such as origination (see Table 2.2).

Syllabus and course objectives

In many countries around the world, the syllabus is nothing more than a course calendar providing the dates and topics to be covered. Best practice in HCE requires more details about the course because the syllabus is an educational contract between the students and the instructor. The road map describes the intended journey, destination, and the rationale for the trip in the first place. A syllabus must articulate the conceptual framework, including the contents of the course, specific skills, and the knowledge students will demonstrate at the end of the course. A sample syllabus is presented at the end of this chapter.

The course goal is usually published in the university/college/department handbook or on the website as a "course description" on what the students need to know and understand. It is often written in broad terms and often unprecise. On the other hand, the course objectives, an essential component of the syllabus, must specify the knowledge, behaviors, and psychomotor skills that students will demonstrate to achieve mastery of the course. Each learning objective should be measurable, observable, and should target one specific aspect of student performance. The course objectives must start with the statement: At the end of the course, students will be able to:

1. Select a verb (see examples in Table 2.2) that corresponds to the specific action that students must be able to demonstrate.
2. Specify the knowledge, skills, and behaviors that the students will acquire or be able to construct.
3. State the criterion or Bloom's level of learning that the students will reach to show mastery of knowledge.

The instructor must specify the methods that will be used to assess the knowledge acquired during the course. For example, evaluating students' learning at Bloom's levels I (Remembering) and Level II (Understanding) is best achieved with multiple-choice test questions. Assessing levels V (Evaluation) and VI (Creating) require a high level of ability to respond to essay questions and term paper assignments.

The following tips are useful in writing impactful course objectives:

1. Do not list multiple verbs in one objective – since each action will be measured and assessed differently, each verb should be in a separate objective.
2. WRONG: Upon successful completion of this course, students will be able to *read and write* with a critical perspective.
3. RIGHT: Upon successful completion of this course, students will be able to read from a critical perspective
4. Do not use your assignments for your objectives. An assignment measures a student's success with the objective.

5. WRONG: Upon successful completion of this course, students will be able to write a 20-page paper.
6. RIGHT: Upon successful completion of this course, students will be able to construct a thesis statement with a clear and persuasive claim.

Program students learning outcomes

The curriculum of all HCE programs should have sound and well-articulated program objectives developed in response to the health care needs of the region and country. The program objectives should guide the curriculum content and the faculty and student assessment aligned with the accreditation standards. The curriculum should provide in-depth knowledge of the discipline, including biological and behavioral sciences, management, leadership, ethics, research methods, and supervised clinical experience in different settings.

The program students learning outcomes (SLO) must describe the learning across the curriculum in specific and measurable terms, of the knowledge, competencies, and behaviors after completing the degree program. The development of the SLOs is a reflective process that must involve every faculty member in the academic department. The SLOs must reflect the three learning domains:

1. Knowledge (cognitive) – what students must understand.
2. Competencies (psychomotor skills) – what students will be able to do.
3. Values, dispositions, or attitudes (affective) – what students care about.

Perhaps the most crucial step in the assessment process is the development of meaningful SLOs. This is crucial because, without appropriate SLOs, it is difficult, if not impossible, to collect relevant or useful information about student learning that will be used for program improvement. The SLOs should be:

1. Consistent with the program mission and goals.
2. Comprehensive – cover the primary program goals.
3. Focused on student learning (not teaching or some other aspect of the program).
4. Stated clearly and realistic to achieve (can potentially be performed by a significant percentage of students).
5. Measurable and actionable (can be used for program improvement) and must include an acceptable performance level (Bloom's).

Curriculum mapping

Curriculum mapping is the indexing on a platform system the list of curriculum courses for each year of the academic program, type of course (core or elective), performance goal (emerging, developing, or proficient) for the SLOs to identify and correct academic gaps, redundancies, and misalignments with the goal to improve the overall coherence and effectiveness of an educational program (Table 2.3).

Table 2.3 Example of program curriculum mapping with performance targets

Semester	Course	Type of Course	Program SLO #1	Program SLO #2	Program SLO #3	Program SLO #4	Program SLO #5	Program SLO #6
			Academic Program: MPH			*Class of 2020*		
1	CHSC 5110	Core	1		1			1
1	CHSC 5111	Core	1	1	1	1	1	1
1	CHSC 5112	Core	1		1	1	1	
1	CEDU 5223	Elective				1		
2	CHSC 5113	Core	2	2	2	2	2	2
2	PUBH 5126	Required	2		2	2	2	2
2	PUBH 5114	Required	2					
2	PUBH 5115	Required	2	2	2	2	2	2
3	PUBH 5116	Required						
3	PUBH 5117	Required	2	2	2	2	2	2
3	PUBH 5122	Required	2	2	2	2	2	2
3	PUBH 5118	Required	2		2	3		
4	PUBH 5120	Required	3	3	3	3	3	3
4	PUBH 5122	Required					3	
4	PUBH 5128	Required		3		3		3

Performance Goal

| Emerging (1) | Developing (2) | Proficient (3) |

Curriculum mapping was first conceptualized by Fenwick English in the 1980s and embraced by Dr. Heidi Hayes Jacobs. They added a variety of instructor-driven curriculum maps, horizontal and vertical coherence, cyclic reviews, and professional curricular dialogue. Curriculum mapping has become the hub for making decisions about teaching and learning and creating the opportunity to discuss curricula and programmatic issues (Jacobs, 2010). The primary benefit of systematic curriculum mapping is improved in four ways – horizontal, vertical, subject area, and interdisciplinary coherence.

A curriculum is horizontally coherent when its learning outcome is similar when compared to another institution's curriculum. For example, the learning outcomes for a biochemistry course at institution A are horizontally consistent when benchmarked with the learning outcomes of a biochemistry course at institution B. A curriculum is vertically coherent when it is logically sequenced. That is, one course prepares the students for what they will learn in the next class. A curriculum is coherent within a course area when students receive similar instruction and learn the same contents across related courses. For example, if there are three sessions of a particular class offered and taught by three different instructors, the learning outcomes should be the same in each of the three sessions regardless of the instructor who taught the sessions. A curriculum has interdisciplinary coherence when preclinical courses (biochemistry, anatomy, physiology, and microbiology) instructors collaborate to improve the critical cross-curricular skills that students need to succeed in the specialty clinical courses.

The curriculum mapping process allows the faculty to plan the course contents students will learn during the program's duration by building up content from that one year to the next. It follows a logical, time-progressive sequence to develop a well-rounded and comprehensive educational experience. The development is a seven-step process which includes:

Phase 1: Collection of the pertinent curriculum assessment data.
Phase 2: The review of the curriculum plan together by all the faculty to identify the corresponding performance outcome (emerging, developing, or proficient) for the program SLOs each semester.
Phase 3: In an extensive academic program, such as the medical school, the faculty should be divided into five to eight cognate departments and ask each group to review the map carefully and share opinions. In small academic programs, faculty members teaching similar courses can review the plan together.
Phase 4: All faculty members should come together again to examine the input of the smaller groups.
Phase 5: Compilation of the immediate revision points suggested and the creation of a timeline for resolution.
Phase 6: Identify other positions requiring additional research and plan for it by creating a timeline for the decision on those points.
Phase 7: Plan for the next review cycle.

The completed curriculum map helps the entire faculty keep track of what will be taught each academic semester and year.

Evidence-based practice in teaching

The best practice is a method or technique generally accepted as comparatively better than the alternatives because it produces superior results than the other options or because it has become a standard way of doing things. As an alternative to mandatory or legislated standards, best practices are used to maintain quality based on self-assessment or benchmarking. Evidence-based practice (EBP) is the integration of best research evidence with clinical expertise and patient values' which, when applied by practitioners, will ultimately lead to an improved patient outcome.

The original EBP model proposed by Sackett and associates in 1996 has three fundamental components – best practice, clinical expertise, and patient values. The best evidence is found in clinically relevant research conducted using sound methodology. Clinical expertise refers to the clinician's cumulated education, experience, and clinical skills. Patient values are the unique preferences, concerns, and expectations each patient brings to a clinical encounter. The integration of the three components defines an evidence-based clinical decision (Sackett et al., 1996). Like in clinical decision making, EBP is also relevant in teaching. Evidence-based teaching is an instruction that uses existing educational research findings and evidence collected in the classroom as the lesson unfolds (Figure 2.2). It is undertaken in the spirit of inquiry, with the enrichment of the learning experience as its goal.

For a lecturer to deliver effective teaching, the instructional strategies must be well supported by the evidence in the literature. When faculty use research evidence with fidelity, they can be confident their teaching will likely support student learning and achieve purposeful outcomes.

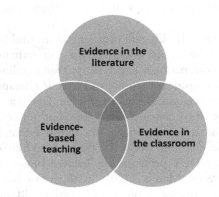

Figure 2.2 Evidence-based practice in teaching.

Formative and summative assessments

Formative and summative assessments are the two primary ways to evaluate students learning. The result of formative evaluation is used by faculty to improve teaching and to identify where students are struggling and to address the problem immediately. It also enables students to identify their weaknesses and strengths so they can concentrate on the areas needing more work. Conversely, the goal of summative evaluation is to evaluate student learning at the end of the course or instructional unit by comparing their performance scores against known published standards or benchmarks (Table 2.4).

Online instruction in health care education

Online education is the educational instruction delivered via the internet to students using their home computers. Online degree programs and courses offered via the institution's online learning platform frees the students from the usual routines of on-campus degree programs – including planning their schedule around classes, driving, and physically present on campus for each sequence of their coursework. A high-quality degree offered through online platforms should fundamentally not differ from the traditional campus-based offerings.

Every year, over half of the 1.5 million Nigerian high school students fail to gain admission into local universities. Still, only a few universities in the country have approved online degree programs to meet the domestic demand. To the surprise of many Nigerians, the National Universities Commission (NUC) in 2016 announced that it would no longer recognize online degrees from foreign universities and recommended that employers and universities not accept such degrees (Kazeem, 2016). At the time, the decision was condemned widely as unrealistic and unprogressive. The criticisms led to a reversal in policy as the federal government reinvigorated the National Open University of Nigeria, created in 2002. The NUC no longer ban online degrees from foreign universities but now only "disapproves of the patronage of an unaccredited online degree."

Online education has provided access to health care professionals in middle and low-income countries who otherwise would not have had postgraduate education. There are now models of international partnerships using online instruction to offer short term courses, transitional Doctor of Physical Therapy (t-DPT), and PhD degree programs in Nigeria, Suriname, Jordan, Japan, and Mongolia. For example, the University of Michigan-Flint (UM-Flint), in collaboration with the Nigeria Physiotherapy Network in the United States, developed a memorandum of understanding between Nnamdi Azikiwe University and UM-Flint to offer the t-DPT program for licensed Nigerian physiotherapists (John et al., 2012). As of March 2020, 27 Nigerians have completed the t-DPT program. Many interested physiotherapists could no longer afford the program because of the increase in educational expenses and

Table 2.4 Differences between formative and summative assessments

	Construct	Formative Assessment	Summative Assessment
1	When does the assessment take place?	Ongoing activity; several times during the learning process	Takes place at the end of the course or unit's completion
2	Assessment strategies	Instructor monitors the learning process to determine whether students are doing well or need help	Instructor assign grading scores. Grades will reflect whether the students achieved the learning goal or not
3	Purpose of assessment	Assessment is to improve student's learning. Instructor must give meaningful feedback	To evaluate students' overall achievements
4	Size of the evaluation packages	Includes little content areas assessed	Includes complete chapters or content areas. The lesson material package is more extensive and comprehensive
5	Role of instructor	Evaluation is a process. Instructors can observe students develop and can steer those not learning in the right direction	Impossible to steer the students in the right direction because the evaluation is already completed. Evaluations considered a "product"
6	Stakes	Low point value	High point value. Outcome information can be used formatively to guide students' efforts and activities in the following semester
7	Examples	Ask students to: (1) draw a concept map during the class session to represent their knowledge of a topic, (2) summarize the main point of a lecture, and (3) turn in an outline of a research proposal for feedback	Midterm exam, final exam, term paper, capstone project

plummeting of the Nigerian economy. When the program started a decade ago, the tuition was $18,000, and the Nigerian currency (₦) was at an exchange rate of ₦240 to the US dollar. In 2020, the fees have increased to $23,0000, and the exchange rate rose to ₦380. Under this circumstance, only one or two students a year have enrolled.

Most universities in Nigeria are presently not able to fully utilize e-learning technology, and this situation has hindered most academics in using innovative teaching strategies in the presentation of their lectures. Online education is still few and far between. At present, the approved online universities offer bachelor's and master's degree programs in management, law, humanities, psychology, social sciences, and HCE. However, only few universities offer online programs in HCE. The University of Lagos offers an online program in dental sciences. And Obafemi Awolowo University provides a professional diploma program in oral health, a degree program in nursing science, and a master's degree in public health. Online education in the country has a major challenge because of the low technology and constant interruption of the power supply. Many of the universities install a camera connected to a computer with internet access. Other universities use "Skype" and "Join Me" to facilitate student monitoring during the exam. The primary challenges associated with the implementation of e-learning in Nigeria include unreliable WiFi connectivity, inadequate computers, limited digital technology, unavailability of instructional software due to cost, and limited opportunities for human capacity development in e-learning (Odutola, 2015; Eze, Chinedu-Eze and Bello, 2018).

The COVID-19 pandemic took a sledgehammer to the fundamental structure and norms of university education globally, leading to the near-total closures of schools, universities, and colleges. As of 27 April 2020, about 1.73 billion learners worldwide were affected due to school closures in response to the pandemic. According to UNICEF, 186 countries, including Nigeria, implemented nationwide school closures, and eight countries implemented local closures, impacting about 98.5% of the world's student population. School closures not only negatively impacted students, faculty, and families, but have far-reaching economic and societal consequences. To address the undesirable impact, UNESCO recommended the use of e-learning platforms to reach students remotely and limit the disruption of education (Multimedia Foundation, Inc., 2020; Snyder, 2020).

In response to the closure of the universities in many countries, the World Bank worked actively to support government efforts to transition educational instruction to the e-learning platform. Over 50 countries worldwide participated in the project. In Nigeria, a Coordination Taskforce Team was set up by the Federal Ministry of Education to provide information, guidance, and resources that will enable the students to continue their education and individualize their learning at home (World Bank, 2020).

In the United States, course offering through the web began in 1994, since then, online education has steadily grown in popularity. In 2010, 33% of college students in the United States took at least one course online. During the last decade, online course offerings have become popular alternatives to acquire education for a wide range of nontraditional students. Particularly, students who are working full-time or raising families. Online learning is usually delivered using several modes or platforms. Online degree programs are standard in humanities, arts, education, business, and law. The most extensive offering of such academic programs in the United States is the University of Phoenix, Walden University, Kaplan University, and Purdue University Global. This mode of online program delivery is not feasible in many entry-level

HCE, such as medicine, dentistry, pharmacy and, physiotherapy, because of the need for "hands-on" skill acquisition in the laboratory and clinical settings.

Blended/hybrid courses and flipped classroom combines face-to-face with online instruction. The flipped classroom model moves the traditional lecture away from the face-to-face classroom offering into online delivery. Synchronous e-learning involves real-time (live) virtual classroom online learning via chat and video conferencing that allows students to ask questions, and the instructors respond instantly. Students easily interact with fellow students and the instructor during the course. Asynchronous e-learning involves coursework delivered via the web, email, and message boards posted on online forums. Students complete the course independently at their own pace; learning occurs while the student is offline.

The top ten e-learning delivery systems/platforms are:

1. Blackboard dominates the Learning Management System market, reaching into both the academic and professional sectors: www.blackboard.com/index.html
2. Pearson Ecollege: www.ecollege.com/
3. Moodle: http://moodle.org
4. Sakai: www.sakaiproject.org/
5. Lore: http://lore.com/
6. Myedu: www.myedu.com/
7. Goingon.com: www.goingon.com/
8. Instructure Canvas: www.instructure.com/
9. Ace Distance Delivery: www.acedistancedelivery.ca/
10. Webstudy.com: http://webstudy.com/

Online e-learning is on the rise but teaching remotely is still a relatively novel concept. Teaching online requires patience and empathy on the part of the instructor. Students often assume that because they are learning remotely, they are absolved of their professional obligations of appropriate classroom behaviors. The professional behavior expectations must be clarified during the first session. Because students are in their home environment, they tend to move back and forth engaged in different activities, with background noise and telephone interruptions during lectures; these unexpected behaviors can be unnerving to the lecturer and the other students.

Teaching online requires specific technical skills and familiarity with the platform to help the lecturer make the classroom the best it can be. The lecturer must keep the work environment free of distractions such as television, household chores, or family members. It takes time and experience for the lecturer to adjust to the new medium of instruction. Planning is critical for an online classroom environment, as students' needs are different from classroom teaching. The lecturer must make sure the syllabus and content materials are laid out clearly before class starts to inform students on the deadlines and other course requirements. The lecturer must avoid surprises at all costs.

The lecturer must innovate and stimulate ongoing weekly discussions through chat rooms or discussion fora in response to an assigned reading or question. The lecturer must maintain a consistent online presence and respond to students' questions and concerns timely. Motivation plays a critical part in the learning process, and the lecturer must think of ways to motivate all the students. The motivation may include giving extra points for online discussions or optional assignments. Periodically ask students and colleagues for feedback on the positives and negatives of the overall e-learning experience (Hardy, 2016; Phillips, 2016).

Conclusion

The COVID-19 crisis exposes the Nigerian education system's fragility as instruction in the universities came to a standstill and lecturers were unable to transition to the e-learning platform like other low-income countries around the world. This embarrassing situation is because only a few lecturers have the technical knowledge and skills needed to develop and teach online courses. As a matter of urgency, the NUC should provide funding to acquire an e-learning delivery platform in each university and embark on training of lecturers to use the system. Implementation of this recommendation will enable Nigerian academics to use innovative teaching strategies to present their lectures and undertake rigorous operational research.

References

Anderson, LW and Krathwohl, D. (2000) *A Taxonomy for Learning, Teaching, and Assessing: A Revision of Bloom's Taxonomy of Educational Objectives.* New York: Longman Publishing.

Dave, R.H. (1975) *Developing and Writing Behavioral Objectives* (pp. 67–89). (RJ Armstrong, ed.) Tucson, AZ: Educational Innovators Press.

Eze, SC, Chinedu-Eze, VC and Bello, AO. (2018) The utilization of e-learning facilities in the educational delivery system of Nigeria: a study of M-University. *International Journal of Educational Technology in Higher Education*, 15 (34). [online]. Available at: https://educationaltechnologyjournal.springeropen.com/articles/10.1186/s41239-018-0116-z (Accessed: 29 April 2020)

Halupa, CP. (2014) Pedagogy, andragogy, and heutagogy. In book: Transformative curriculum design in health sciences education [online]. Available at: www.researchgate.net/publication/297767648_Pedagogy_Andragogy_and_Heutagogy (Accessed: 24 January 2020)

Hardy, L. (2016) 5 skills that online teachers are constantly developing. [online]. Available at: https://elearningindustry.com/10-best-practices-effective-online-teacher (Accessed: 24 January 2020).

Harrow, A.J. (1972) *A Taxonomy of the Psychomotor Domain.* New York: David McKay Co.

Hase, S and Kenyon, C. (2001) Moving from andragogy to heutagogy in vocational education: Implications for VET, AVETRA [online]. Available at: https://epubs.scu.edu.au/cgi/viewcontent.cgi?article=1147&context=gcm_pubs(Accessed: 24 January 2020)

Hoque, ME. (2016) Three domains of learning: Cognitive, affective and psychomotor. *The Journal of EFL Education and Research*, 2(2) [online]. Available at: www.researchgate. net/publication/330811334_Three_Domains_of_Learning_Cognitive_Affective_ and_Psychomotor (Accessed: 24 January 2020)

Jacobs, HH. (2010) Curriculum 21: Essential education for a changing world. Alexandria, VA: Association for Supervision and Curriculum Development [online]. Available at: www.usd320.com/vimages/shared/vnews/stories/5a1448f5d101a/ What%20is%20curriculum%20mapping%20article.pdf (Accessed: 24 January 2020)

John, EB., Pfalzer, LA., Fry, D, Glickman L, Masaaki, S, Sabus, C, Okafor, UAC and Al-Jarrah, MD. (2012) Establishing and upgrading physical therapist education in developing countries: Four case examples of service by Japan and United States physical therapist programs to Nigeria, Suriname, Mongolia, and Jordan-39. [online]. *Journal of Physical Therapy Education*, 26(1): 29 Available at: https:// pdfs.semanticscholar.org/6520/aebb7b1b952616be65632ffacdc76e64e208.pdf (Accessed: 24 January 2020)

Kazeem, Y. (2016) Online degrees are "unacceptable" in Nigeria even though they could plug an education gap [online]. Available at: https://qz.com/africa/784761/ online-degrees-are-not-acceptable-in-nigeria-even-though-it-could-plug-a-hole-in-university-education/ (Accessed: 24 January 2020)

Krathwohl, DR, Bloom, BS and Masia, BB. (1964) *Taxonomy of Educational Objectives: The Classification of Educational Goals. Handbook II: Affective domain.* New York: David McKay Co.

Multimedia Foundation, Inc. (2020) Impact of the COVID-19 pandemic on education. [online]. Available at: https://en.m.wikipedia.org/wiki/Impact_of_the_COVID-19_pandemic_on_education (Accessed: 16 February 2020)

Odutola, A.T. (2015) Challenges of e-learning technologies in Nigerian university education. *Journal of Educational and Social Research*, 5(1). [online]. Available at: www.researchgate.net/publication/322851272_Challenges_of_E-Learning_ Technologies_in_Nigerian_University_Education (Accessed: 24 January 2020)

Phillips, J. (2016) 7 tips on how to prepare for teaching online. [online]. Available at: https://elearningindustry.com/5-skills-online-teachers-developing (Accessed: 24 January 2020).

Sackett, DL, Rosenberg, WMC., Gray, JAM, Haynes, RB and Richardson. WS. (1996) Evidence based medicine: what it is and what it isn't. *British Medical Journal* 312:71–2. [online]. Available at: www.physiopedia.com/Evidence_Based_Practice_(EBP) (Accessed: 24 January 2020)

Schroeder, R. (2018) Pedagogy, andragogy, and now heutagogy. [online]. Available at: https://upcea.edu/pedagogy-andragogy-and-now-heutagogy/ (Accessed: 24 January 2020)

Snyder, JA. (2020) Higher Education in the age of coronavirus. *Boston Review*. [online]. Available at:http://bostonreview.net/forum/jeffrey-aaron-snyder-higher-education-age-coronavirus (Accessed: 16 February 2020)

World Bank (2020) How countries are using edtech (including online learning, radio, television, texting) to support access to remote learning during the COVID-19 pandemic. [online]. Available at: www.worldbank.org/en/topic/edtech/brief/ how-countries-are-using-edtech-to-support-remote-learning-during-the-covid-19-pandemic (Accessed: 24 January 2020).

SAMPLE COURSE SYLLABUS

Chicago State University
College of Health Sciences

Course Number/Title:	PUBH 5111-Biostatistics and Computer Applications
Semester Hours/Term:	3 Credits/Fall 2019
Day/ Time/Class Venue:	Thursday; 5:00 pm–7:50 pm; BHS 507
Instructor:	Name
	Contact Email
	Contact Telephone
	Office Location:
	Office hours:

Course description

This course will enable the students acquire advanced understanding and skills in statistical concepts; descriptive and inferential statistical analyses; linear, multiple, and stepwise regression analyses; data plotting and analysis using the SPSS software; and interpretation of health data.

Prerequisite: College Math or Basic Statistics Course

Course objectives

At the end of this course, the student will be able to:

1. Apply fundamental concepts in the research process: population, sample selection, normal distribution, dependent/independent variables, hypothesis testing, descriptive and inferential statistics, confidence interval concept, levels of measurement and implication for statistical methods and be able to identify the use of inappropriate statistical methods in published public health research, policy or practice (Bloom's Taxonomy Level 3 – Application).
2. Code raw data into an SPSS template; test for normality and homogeneity of variance (Bloom's Taxonomy Level 6 – Creating).
3. Construct frequency tables, scatterplots, pie, bar, and histograms graphs using the Microsoft word and SPSS software (Bloom's Taxonomy Level 6 – Creating).
4. Analyze coded data using a parametric test such as one sample, paired and unpaired t-tests, ANOVA to test the stated research hypothesis, and interpret the SPSS print outputs (Bloom's Taxonomy Level 6 – Creating).
5. Analyze coded data using a nonparametric test such as Chi-Square, Wilcoxon rank, Mann Whitney U, Sign test, Kruskal-Wallis to test the stated research hypothesis in health care research, policy or practice and interpret the SPSS print outputs (Bloom's Taxonomy Level 6 – Creating).

6. Analyze coded data using correlation, linear, multiple, stepwise, and logistic regression statistics in public health research, policy, or practice and interpret the SPSS print outputs (Bloom's Taxonomy Level 6 – Creating).

7. Analyze and classify transcription from qualitative data sources such as focus group discussion, in-depth interview, or phenomenological interviews into themes to capture as fully as possible the convergent opinions of the respondents. Students will be introduced to the NVIVO software for analyzing qualitative data (Bloom's Taxonomy Level 4 – Analysis).

Course Objectives	Assessment Method(s)
#1	Midterm and final written examinations
	Research Publication and Presentation Assignments
#2	Homework Assignments # 1
#3	Homework Assignment # 2
#4	Homework Assignment # 3
#5	Homework Assignment # 4a
#6	Homework Assignment # 4b
#7	Final written examination. Research Publication and Presentation Assignments

Assessment of student learning

Program students learning outcomes

Following the completion of the Master of Public Health (MPH) program, the graduates will be able to:

---

1. Apply knowledge of major risk factors for morbidity and mortality to analyze causal influences and health disparities in specific population segments (Bloom's Taxonomy level 3- Application).
2. Assess key issues associated with health disparities and their relevance to the design of culturally appropriate interventions (Bloom's Taxonomy level 5 – Evaluating).
3. Evaluate knowledge gaps in health promotion and disease prevention research (Bloom's Taxonomy level 5 – Evaluating).
4. Implement evidence-based health promotion and disease prevention programs among at-risk populations (Bloom's Taxonomy level 6 – Creating).
5. Evaluate the effectiveness of evidence-based interventions to prevent disease and/or promote health (Bloom's Taxonomy level 5 – Evaluating).

Course objectives and program students learning outcome link:

This course satisfied the MPH competencies #3 and 5 for the Health Promotion and Disease Prevention concentration

Required textbook.

List

Supplemental textbook.

List

Video resource materials

List

Accommodations for students with disabilities/ Americans with Disabilities Act (ADA)

Students with disabilities who require reasonable accommodation to participate in this course fully should register with the Abilities Office of Disabled Student Services, SUB 190 (773) 995–4401. The Abilities Office provides services and accommodations for qualified students with verified disabilities per provisions of Section 504 of the Rehabilitation Act and the Americans with Disabilities Act (ADA).

Emergency evacuation plan

Emergency Evacuations: All emergencies occurring on campus, life-threatening and non–life-threatening, should be reported to the campus police by calling ext. 2111 from any campus phone and either 911 or (773) 995-2111 from a cell phone. Evacuate a building when the fire alarm sounds, you smell gas or smoke, see fire, or instructed to do so by staff or emergency personnel. You may also receive instructions over the university's public address system and RAVE, the emergency notification system.

Course format and requirements

This course will be taught as a "hands-on, real-world applied" biostatistics course. The theoretical concepts and mathematical models/computations will be discussed, and fundamental skills on how to analyze and interpret research data output from the SPSS software will be covered.

Relevant course information will be presented during class lectures, and opportunities will be provided for hands-on experience on computers working on-class exercises.

- Students are expected to attend class regularly and to participate in classroom exercises. Integrated learning tasks will include small group exercises.
- Students are expected to read all assigned material.

In order to successfully complete the course, a student must complete all required assignments, group exercises, and exams.

Criteria for grading

Grades for examinations will be assigned according to the following grading policy:

A = 100–90
B = 80–89
C = 75–79
D = 65–74
F = 64 & below

Grading components and weightings

Homework Assignment 1: Central Tendency and Graphing	10%
Homework Assignment 2: T-tests	10%
Homework Assignment 3: ANOVA	10%
Homework Assignment 4: Scatter plot/Correlation/Regression	10%
Midterm Exam	15%
Research publication critique and presentation assignments	20%
Final Exam	20%
Class Participation/Attendance/Class behavior	5%
Total	100%

Homework assignments and course examinations

Students are required to complete four homework assignments designed to assess knowledge of the statistical concepts and procedures discussed in class. Each assignment will comprise 10% of the final grade for the course.

Two examinations (a midterm and a final exam) will be given during the semester to assess the understanding of the course material. The exams will consist of a combination of multiple-choice, short-answer, and computational questions. No date is specified on the Course Schedule for the midterm exam. At least one-week notice will be provided in class or via email before the examination is administered.

Class participation/attendance/class behavior

It is expected that students will conduct themselves in a professional manner. This includes, but is not limited to, arriving to class in a timely manner, participating in class exercises and refraining from disruptive behavior (e.g., cross-talking, talking to classmates). Moreover, students are prohibited from using cell phones or pagers while in class. Failure to conduct oneself in a professional manner while in the classroom will result in a reduction of the class participation grade.

Late work

Hard copies of all assignments must be submitted on or before the scheduled due date. *No email submission of the assignment will be accepted.* Late work or missed assignments will not be accepted without penalty. The penalty will be a 10% deduction for every day the assignment is late. This will include weekends. A *serious* medical emergency or death in the family (need to provide medical documentation) is permissible reasons for a late submission. The following situations are not considered acceptable reasons for turning in a late assignment:

- My computer crashed
- My files are corrupted
- A busy week of exams, papers
- A busy work schedule
- Going out of town for personal or family business
- Job or graduate school interviews
- Doctor or dentist appointment

It is the student responsibility to plan to prevent late submission of assignments. www.owlnet.rice.edu/~bios311/bios311/latework.html

Course requirements and academic policies

Students enrolled in the College of Health Sciences courses are expected to:

1. Complete assigned readings before class.
2. Meet assignment, task, and schedule deadlines.
3. Attend all classes and off-campus visits and trips.

4. Be punctual to all classes and off-campus visits and trips.
5. Contribute positively to classroom discussions and activities.
6. Maintain positive nonverbal demeanor in class.
7. Interact with peers and instructors respectfully and professionally.
8. Exhibit appropriate habits of self-care, hygiene, and grooming.
9. Dress appropriately and decently to class. Tank tops, cutoff shorts, and "see-through" dresses are not permitted.
10. Dress professionally (semiformal or formal dress) for presentations and all arranged off-campus visits and trips.
11. All cell phones must be silenced or set to vibrate during class time. If you make or accept a telephone call during class time, you must leave the classroom for the duration of the call. During testing, all electronic devices, such as cell phones, PDAs, palm pilots, etc. must be put away in your bag and not used. If an electronic device is found with you during testing, you will not be allowed to complete the test. Similarly, if you leave the classroom during an exam without permission and supervision by the instructor, you will not be allowed to complete the test. Any violation of this policy on the use of electronic devices will affect your grade and standing in the program according to course, department, college, and university regulations and guidelines.
12. Abide with the University, College, and Department policies, procedures, and code of conduct. Refer to the University catalog and Department Student Handbook Manual for details.

Research publication and presentation assignments

Students will apply the concepts learn in this course toward answering questions from a published manuscript. Each student will select a manuscript of interest published in a peer-referenced journal and obtain my approval. The instructor must approve the manuscript selected. It must be an empirically based research study. The student will submit a written response in an easy format to the following questions:

1. What is the purpose of the study? (5 points)
2. What type of hypothesis (null or alternate) was stated in the manuscript? State one if there is none and specify the type of hypothesis. (5 points)
3. What are the independent variables? (5 points)
4. What are the dependent variables? (5 points)
5. What are the scales of measurement for each independent variable? (5 points)
6. What are the scales of measurement for each dependent variable? (5 points)
7. What type of statistical program/software was used in this study? (5 points)
8. What type of descriptive statistics was reported in the study and for what variables? (5 points)
9. What sampling method was used for data collection? (5 points)
10. What type(s) of inferential statistics was used in the study? (5 points)
11. Are the inferential statistics used parametric or nonparametric and why? (5 points)
12. What is the alpha level used for the hypothesis testing? (5 points)
13. Did the researchers use appropriate statistical methods for their data analysis? (5 points)
14. Where the findings logically and sequentially presented? (5 points)

15. What are the major salient findings in this study? State in your own words (10 points)
16. Present samples of graphical representation that you would have used to better convey the findings in this study. (20 points)

In responding to each question, the page and corresponding paragraph from the published manuscript must be cited. All responses must be in your own words. The writing assignment term paper will be 10%, and Presentation will be 10% of the course grade. See Class Schedule on deadline date.

Class presentation

Toward the end of the semester, each student will present their written response during a class session using multimedia resources such as power point slides, poster, etc. The grading rubric for the presentation will be posted on the Moodle course management system.

1. Each presentation will last 15–20 min., with 5 min. discussion time.
2. A grading rubric posted on Moodle course management system will be used to evaluate the class presentation.
3. Presentation should provide detailed review of all the components of the published manuscript to educate the audience and follow up with answering all the questions required in the writing assignment.
4. Review the grading rubric carefully to ensure you cover all the parts.

Course Calendar and Schedule

Week	Topic	Readings	Assignment	Important university timeline
Week 1	Course Orientation/ Syllabus			August 20 – 30: Add/Drop/ Change of Schedule period for registered students only
Week 2	Fundamental Biostatistics concepts; statistical terms; Variables; Null/ Alternate hypothesis Differences between population vs. sample	Chapters 1		
Week nth	Scales of Measurement and influence on inferential statistics Normal Distribution; Central Tendency; Skewness and Kutosis;	Chapters 1 and 3		September 9: Last day to completely withdraw from the Regular (16-weeks)
Week 16	Final Exam			

Educational contract

I have received the course syllabus for PUBH 5111-Biostatistics and Computer Applications. The study objectives, grading policy, attendance policy, and assignment requirements were explained by the instructor. I attest that I have met the prerequisite for this course.

I will obey all the rules and follow the grading policy specified in the syllabus.

I agree to respect the instructor and my classmates by being punctual to class and ready to participate.

I also understand that it is reasonable to have to spend two hours doing homework for each hour of actual class time.

Tutoring is available at the Student Services Center (Phone#: 773995xxxx). The instructor may recommend you seek such additional help, but it is your responsibility to schedule the appointment.

_____   _____   _____
Name – Please print   Email Address   Phone Number

_____   _____
Signature   Date

3 Teaching and modeling professionalism in health professions

Introduction

Have you wondered why many health care professionals (HCPs) engage in unethical and aberrant behaviors? The unexpected behavior is because professionalism as a concept is rarely taught in some health care disciplines. Hence, the need for this chapter. Health care education (HCE) has witnessed several dynamic shifts in the didactic knowledge and clinical practice in response to the knowledge explosion in science and technology. The society at large expects HCPs to be kind, polite, ethical, trustworthy, and competent. Also, they expect them to present a positive image/attitude, speak and dress appropriately, always punctual, and fully prepared to work. Failure to meet these legitimate expectations will undoubtedly negatively impact the way HCPs are perceived, and the respect and esteem they command in the society will decline. Luckily, many HCE programs now address professionalism in their curriculum, although the strategies utilized to teach it may not always be adequate. The concept of professionalism remains very vague and unclear to most students and even some practitioners. Given this situation, HCE students must learn appropriate behaviors at the early phase of their professional education and understand the repercussions of failure to meet these obligations.

To adequately contextualize the concepts discussed in this chapter, it is necessary first consider the following salient questions.

1. Some people say that unprofessionalism is contagious. Do you agree? Why or why not?
2. What effects could acting "unprofessionally" have on the way people view health professions?
3. Would you still go to see a health care professional if they behaved "unprofessionally" even though they did their job, right?
4. How does the attitude between coworkers influence a patient's overall feeling of the hospital or clinic?
5. Why is the use of appropriate personal protective equipment (PPE) an essential component of professionalism, particularly in the COVID-19 era?

The core values of professionalism must be delivered explicitly at the beginning of the academic program and repeatedly reinforced with more complex case scenarios introduced during the educational process. Unfortunately, the teaching of professionalism formally in the HCE curriculum has only recently begun in many countries around the world. Formal instruction in professional values and the need to uphold professionalism are increasingly emphasized in HCE curricula globally. But developing a curriculum about professionalism is a challenge, and only a few published resources are available to guide academics.

This chapter examines the characteristics and attributes of professionalism, relevance in HCE, and behavioral expectations for HCPs. It also presents how to teach professionalism in an HCE program and strategies for managing "hidden curriculum" behaviors. Finally, the chapter apprises the methods, and psychometric inventories used to assess professionalism and the core components of the ethical code of conduct within the health professions.

Characteristics of professionalism

By the way, what is professionalism? The term "professionalism," derived from the Latin word "profesus," means "to have declared publicly" (Haidet, 2008). Sir William Osler, in 1903, argued that

> the practice of medicine is not a business and can never be one … our fellow creatures cannot be dealt with as a man deals in corn and coal; the human heart by which we live must control our professional relations.

Professionalism is a multidimensional social construct with no universally accepted definition. It is simple to recognize professionalism, but it is not straightforward to measure it because it is kaleidoscopic (Salam et al., 2012; Cruess and Cruess, 2010). Professionalism is the behavior or qualities that represent a profession or an individual and encompasses different characteristics and attributes. The Registered Nurses Association of Ontario (RNAO) considers professionalism as the consistent demonstration of behaviors that exemplify altruism, clinical competence, autonomy, advocacy, innovation and visionary, a spirit of inquiry, caring, ethics, respect, communication and accountability, and collaboration with the other members of the health care team to achieve optimal health and wellness in individuals and communities.

Professionalism brings HCPs together and helps them get along with one another while rendering efficient service to the patients. Appropriate professional behaviors keep patients satisfied and happy with their health care providers. The understanding of professionalism has evolved over the years; it entails a continuum of behaviors, attitudes, and beliefs that are at one end of the spectrum is as fundamental or generic as "doing the right thing" to the highly sophisticated and altruistic genre at the other end of the spectrum (Nath, 2006).

Attributes of professionalism

Often, professionalism is associated with traits, such as altruism, accountability, excellence, duty, honor and integrity, and respect for patients and their families, peers, and stakeholders (Mueller, 2015) (Figure 3.1).

Professionalism is an internalized professional obligation and role behaviors about individual clients and society as a whole. It may be collective (practiced by profession as a whole) or individual. Personal professionalism refers to the member's attributes, interactions, attitudes, values, and role behaviors, and individual professionalism is called "professional role concept" (Figure 3.2).

Relevance of professionalism in health care education

Professionalism is often associated with increased patient satisfaction, adherence to treatment plans, trust, fewer patient complaints, and reduced risk of litigation (Mueller, 2015). With the ongoing competitive changes and the outcomes-oriented clinical environment globally, HCPs and students must have a clear understanding of professionalism and be able to model behaviors that are appropriate to every particular clinical situation. With professionalism, everything matters from clinical competence to overall appearance and use of PPE. As students transition from undergraduate to postgraduate training, not all transformations are positive. Mahood (2011) noted that "often students move from being open-minded to being closed-minded, from being intellectually curious to narrowly focusing on facts, from empathy to emotional detachment,

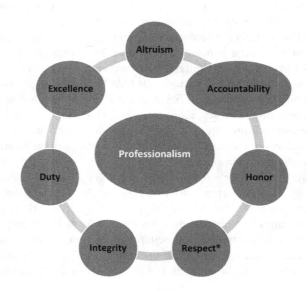

Figure 3.1 Attributes of professionalism.

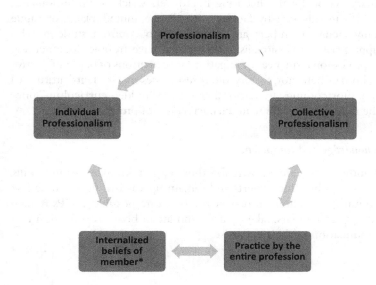

Figure 3.2 Individual vs. collective professionalism.

from idealism to cynicism; and often from civility and caring to arrogance and irritability."

While most formal curriculum teaches the virtues of interdisciplinary practice, collegiality, and patient-centered care, but interpersonal tensions among the students can subvert the formal instruction. Similarly, an off-the-cuff ridicule of patients' weight, poverty, or ethnicity can undermine the teaching on cultural sensitivity and competence. A faculty teaching "the importance of family dynamics" is undercut by leaving the ward round before families can ask questions. The hidden curriculum occurs, for example, when a consultant derides other HCPs as "dumb" and violate patient's confidentiality, ignore rules, use inappropriate language, or demonstrate an inability to work effectively with others.

For students, what constitutes professionalism can be confused with getting along socially with peers, not rocking the boat, being subservient, or remaining "flexible." Often, showing up timely, finishing the workload promptly, and covering up minor mistakes may get more recognition than abiding with avowed professional values or patient-centered care. New graduates can become ethical chameleons, slowly redefining themselves as primary technicians, narrowing professional identity, and discarding explicit professionalism for emotional detachment.

Undoubtedly, professionalism is an essential competence that must be acquired during the educational process. The most detrimental actions and behaviors involve deficiencies in professionalism, cognitive knowledge, and clinical skill. Inappropriate behavior during training is often carried over and later associated with disciplinary action by the licensing board. Yet, a lack of professionalism among students is usually met by faculty with silence, muted, bland, or vague feedback. Many faculty members are intimidated to confront students who displayed inappropriate professionalism, and several have trouble documenting inappropriate professionalism. Fear of litigation or accusations of being subjective in measuring human behavior, faculty often resist assessing students' attitudinal behavior. These shortcomings are responsible for the "hidden curriculum" phenomenon. The following are the main characteristics of professionalism.

Specialized knowledge and competency

Most importantly, HCPs are known for their expert knowledge and skills. They always strive to become experts and remain up-to-date in the discipline through continuing education. To deliver the best care possible, HCPs remain current by attending seminars, take courses, and attain board certification that serves as the foundation of their expertise.

Image

HCPs look the part of a clinician by dressing appropriately for work and maintaining a "clean-cut" neat appearance. Even if the clinical facility in which you work adopts the casual protocol, strive for snappy relaxed rather than showing up for work sloppily dressed, with unkempt hair. It is essential to earn a good reputation in the workplace. Such individuals are considered first for promotions, awarded valuable projects, and are often more successful in their careers. But professionalism is more than clinical expertise and image. It also includes the behaviors and attitudes of the HCPs toward their jobs, and the respect that they show toward the other members of the health care team.

Ethics and integrity

HCPs exhibit honesty, integrity, and are required to adhere to a strict code of ethics. Also, they find a way to get the job done by providing care to patients promptly, following through on promises and commitments immediately, without compromising their values, and do the right thing, even though it may mean taking a harder road. If a referral falls outside their scope of clinical expertise, professionals are not afraid to admit this, but immediately seek help from other sources. Professionals do not typically make excuses, but they focus on finding solutions.

Genuine respect

HCPs show genuine respect for their colleagues and patients, no matter the condition of the clinical environment. They exhibit a high degree of professionalism by appropriately responding to the emotional needs of the patients, and not allow a bad day affects how they interact with colleagues, patients, and families.

Humble and confident

HCPs are humble and exude confidence but not cocky. They are polite and well-spoken when discussing with patients, supervisors, or coworkers.

Accountability

HCPs are accountable for their actions and take full responsibility for their mistakes by not blaming it on a colleague but promptly work to resolve the issue. This personal action is closely related to honesty and integrity and an essential component of professionalism.

Self-regulation

HCPs stay calm and poise under pressure, even during tense situations. For example, when faced with an angry patient who behaves in a belligerent manner, instead of getting upset or angry in return, genuine professionals will be calm, maintain a business-like demeanor, and do everything humanly possible to make the situation right. Since body language communicates volumes, professionals must always convey the appropriate facial expression to their colleagues, patients, and their families.

Communication must strike the right tone

Face-to-face discussion and phone etiquette is a critical element of professional behavior. When making or answering a telephone, it is crucial to identify self by full name, title, and facility name. Listen attentively to the other party and not dominate the conversation. Timely return all calls and follow-up on any needed action or promises made. All written correspondence and email messages must be formal and polite.

Be structured and organized

A HCP's work area should be neat and orderly to allow quick and easy identification of what is needed. A hopelessly cluttered, messy work area convey unprofessionalism (Porcupile, 2015; Joseph and Thompson, 2019).

Behavioral expectations for health care professionals

Lecturers are expected to model appropriate behavior by matching their words with actions and practice what they preach. The following are examples of behaviors that HCPs must emulate or avoid while working in the clinical environment. The following behaviors must be taught early in the program and regularly emphasized during the educational process.

Proper grooming

Proper grooming and healthy personal habits can ward off illnesses and improve self-esteem. It is prudent to brush teeth in the morning and evening to prevent gum disease (gingivitis), and shower daily to get rid of dirt, sweat, and germs, and use face cleanser. Because the face is more sensitive than other parts of the body, hypoallergenic products with less harsh chemicals should be used. It is also necessary to use deodorant to control excessive sweat and unpleasant odor and wash clothes after wearing them. Following every use, the shirts must be washed while pants and shorts may be worn a few times. Hair should be kept neat, and fingernails and toenails clipped regularly. Men should have a clean shave, and every 4–8 weeks should have a haircut (WikiHow, 2019).

HCPs should wear a laboratory coat or other apparel mandated by the facility. In the absence of a lab coat, men should wear a suit and women should wear a two-piece skirt or pantsuit with a blouse. Avoid dangling earrings, especially when working with the pediatric population, as they are likely to pull on the pendant. The use of jewelry in the clinical setting should be limited to a watch and a ring. Shoes should hold a shine.

Prudent hand hygiene includes diligently cleaning and trimming of fingernails, which often trap dirt and germs and contributes to the spread of some infections, such as pinworms. Longer fingernails harbor more dirt and bacteria than short nails and potentially contribute to the spread of disease. Fingernails or toenails infection is indicated by swelling and pain in the surrounding area and thickening of the nail. In some cases, these infections may be severe and need to be treated by a physician (CDC, 2001).

The following necessary precautions should be taken to prevent the spread of germs and nail infections. Nails should be kept short, and the undersides cleaned frequently with soap, water, and clean nail grooming materials before using them. Thoroughly scrub the bottom of nails with soap and water (or a nail brush) every time you wash your hands. When nail tools are shared among several people, as is the case in commercial nail salons, the materials must be sterilized before using them. Biting or chewing nails and cutting cuticles must be avoided as they act as barriers to prevent infection. Never rip or bite a hangnail but clip it with a sanitized nail trimmer.

Wear personal protective equipment

HCPs are required to wear appropriate personal protective equipment (PPE) as dictated by the employer to prevent infection. PPEs consist of protective clothing, helmets, gloves, face shields, goggles, facemasks, and respirators, or other equipment designed to insulate clinicians from injury or the spread of infection or illness. They function as a barrier between infectious materials such as viral and bacterial contaminants from blood, body fluids, or respiratory secretions and the HCP's skin, mouth, nose, and the mucous membranes of the eyes. Also, PPEs postsurgery, protect patients with a compromised autoimmune system at high risk for contracting infections or those with a medical condition, from exposure to substances or potentially infectious material brought in by visitors and clinicians. When PPEs are used in conjunction with handwashing with alcohol-based hand sanitizers, the spread of infection in the clinical setting is minimized (US Food and Drug Administration, 2018).

Avoid sky-high-heel shoes

Sky-high-heel shoes are associated with falls and sprained ankles as the foot is forced into an unstable position. Prolonged use of high heels cause permanent physiological damage to the knees, hips, back, and tendons leading to joint pain, shortened Achilles tendon, low back pain, and osteoarthritis of the joints. Low-heel shoes (sneakers and flat shoes) create stability, comfort, and ideal wear in the clinical setting. Each human foot has 33 joints, 26 bones, 19 muscles, 107 ligaments, and about 200,000 nerve endings, and countless blood vessels. Pointy or wrong-sized shoes and arch-less flip-flops cause callus formation, bunions, deformed toes, ingrown toenails, hallux valgus, inflamed nerves, or bones, torn or overstretched ligaments, even hairline fractures (BlackDoctor+org, 2019).

Avoid artificial eyelids

Fake eyelids attract dirt and bacteria and can cause an eye infection. Some individuals have allergic reactions to the glue and can cause alopecia areata (loss of eyelashes). The adhesives used for the fake eyelids contain formaldehyde, which can have detrimental health effects such as blindness when used regularly. It can also cause the darkening of the iris, which can permanently change the amount of brown pigmentation in the iris PositiveMed (2013).

Avoid artificial nails

Fake acrylic nails can contribute to the transmission of pathogens, and its use should be discouraged. HCPs with acrylic nails are more likely to harbor gram-negative pathogens on their fingertips than are those who have natural nails, even after hand washing. Since artificial nails can act as a breeding milieu for pathogenic microorganisms, the World Health Organization in 2009 recommended that HCPs must keep natural nails not more than 0.5 cm long. Also, clinical facilities and hospitals must provide clean running water for handwashing and wall mounted soap dispensers installed close to the sink in every patient's room. In the COVID-19 era, these recommendations are imperative to reduce pathogenic microorganisms' transmission to patients and HCPs.

A prospective study revealed that about 86% of HCPs with artificial nails had staphylococcus aureus, or yeast under their nails, compared with 35% of a control group without fake fingernails. After washing their hands with soap or gel, 68% of HCPs with artificial nails still carried pathogens compared to 28% of the control HCPs. Staphylococcus aureus and yeast can cause infections, inflammation, or blood poisoning (McNeil, 2001).

Jansen and associates investigated the effects of fingernail length on grip strength and the manipulation speed, the number of words typed, and the active range of motion of the fingers. In the study, measurements were taken under four testing conditions: (1) with no fingernails attached, (2) with nails extending beyond the tip of the finger by 2 cm, (3) by 1 cm, and (4) by 0.5 cm. The result revealed (1) decreased grip strength with fingernails of all extended length testing conditions, and (2) decreased active range of motion, grip strength, and finger manipulation speed with nails 1 cm and 2 cm in length testing conditions. Reduced typing speed also observed with the fingernails in the 2 cm length testing condition. Furthermore, long fingernails testing conditions limit flexion of the finger joints, which restrict the excursion of long flexors and extensors in patients. Cutting nails to a length of 0.5 cm is necessary to achieve optimal functional outcomes in the clinical setting (Jansen et al., 2000).

Cover tattoos and avoid body piercing

Tattooing and body piercing are often wrongly associated with gang membership and prisoners. The procedure, in the hand of a quack, can be fatal. It can cause tetanus, TB, hepatitis B, and C and the potential for HIV infection. The ink used for tattoos contain ingredients such as mercury, cadmium, and cobalt is associated with delayed hypersensitivity reactions. High levels of iron oxide are in some dye, with potential for burns or distortions of the tattoo caused by magnetic hysteresis during magnetic resonance imaging. A few cases of anaphylaxis are associated with tattooing. The health issues related to body piercings and tattoos include mild irritations, an infection caused by staphylococcus aureus, methicillin-resistant staphylococcus aureus, or pseudomonas aeruginosa. Given these hazards, it is prudent that HCPs avoid body piercings and tattoos (Nahvi, 2011).

Teaching and modeling professionalism

All faculty members in an academic department must participate in the teaching of professionalism and must model appropriate and ethical behaviors. Modeling appropriate behaviors means proper grooming, wearing PPE when indicated, avoid wearing sky-high-heel shoes, artificial eyelids, and fake nails, and cover tattoos and avoid body piercing.

The road map in teaching professionalism involves the following steps: First, set clear expectations, perform baseline and ongoing professionalism assessments, and prevent, remediate inappropriate behaviors, and implement a cultural change. Second, the teaching process and expected actions should be defined by the stakeholders – faculty, the institution, and its affiliates. Third, the faculty must develop policies stating the due processes, including reporting channels, remediation processes, and the follow-up channels. The students and faculty should receive a list of expected behaviors for which they will be held accountable, including an explanation of the consequences of misbehaving. Lastly, all levels of the educational program should include the teaching of professionalism, and additional training provided on the history of the HCE discipline including the origin, characteristics, relevance and behavioral expectations, code of ethics, "hidden curriculum" agenda, conflict resolution, management skills, and program assessment.

The instructions on professionalism can be delivered using the lecture format by providing frameworks, definitions, and include learning activities that stimulate students' curiosity. Other teaching methods consist of small-group discussion sessions to explore personal interpretations and biases, problem-based learning, or collaborative learning formats. These instructional strategies can be reinforced by having the students participate in service-learning projects that emphasize professional responsibilities.

It is critical to combine the cognitive instruction with noncognitive contents that emphasize the development of appropriate communication (language, empathy, integrity) skills, collaboration (responsibility, respect, duty) capacity, and continuous improvement (recognition of limitations and motivation to improve) skills. The student must have the opportunity to experience real or simulated clinical situations in a small-group setting using case vignettes, video clips, narratives, role-plays, or other enliven and animate educational methods. What students see and experience in everyday practice is what makes the most durable impression rather than what the faculty says in the classroom.

The way other faculty members, senior students act as role models both intentionally and unintentionally, shapes the attitudes and hardening

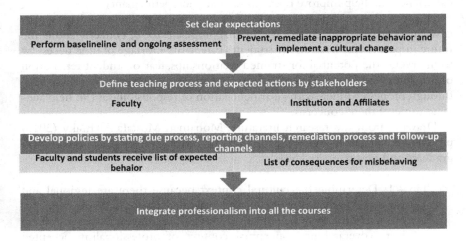

Figure 3.3 Teaching and modeling of professionalism.

perceptions about the profession's real expectations. Role models play a vital part in the teaching of professionalism, and they must be able to reflect appropriate behaviors. Sadly, negative role models exist, partly because they are partly responsible for the cynicism that can develop in some students.

Another obstacle to teaching professionalism includes the "hidden curriculum" such as routines, rituals, symbols, institutional slang, control systems, and power structures. Faculty must improve positive behavior by acknowledging in a meaningful way when a student displays an extraordinary act of professionalism. The faculty can provide the reinforcement by directly praising the student, or reflect the positive comment on the student evaluation, or sending an email to the preceptor, or sending a praise card for exemplary behavior.

Lapses in professionalism occur frequently. Altirkawi (2014) classified professionalism related failures into four categories and asserted that the classification scheme could help determine the best course for a remediation plan. The lapses may be (1) behavior-related (e.g., lack of respect for patients), (2) performance-based (e.g., inability to concentrate on tasks at hand), (3) attitude-related (e.g., arrogance), or (4) due to a lack of accountability (e.g., frequent tardiness). Categorizing lapses this way helps determine the best course for remediation. Altirkawi argued that a fair and reliable assessment and remediation plan should consider the contexts in which the mistake occurred, the conflicts that led to the failure, and the reasons behind the student's choice to resolve the disputes. Following identification of the unacceptable behavior, a meeting with the student should be scheduled immediately to explain what acceptable behavior is and how to correct the inappropriate behavior and the consequences of not improving also clearly stated. The faculty must conduct frequent follow-up and praise the student when improvement is observed and discuss ways the student can continue to grow. Of utmost importance is the need to develop a supportive institutional culture and opportunities for the students to interact outside the institution – the experience can help improve both attitudes and job performance.

It is critical to recognize that many factors may impair the remediation process. Such factors include the use of inappropriate tools, concern about the future impact it may have on the student's career, the shortage of time necessary to intervene, the potential for strained relationships, fear of student retribution or litigation, and lack of skills to address the issues. Communicating these fears through proper channels with clear delineation of responsibilities can help alleviate some of these concerns.

Drawing from the research literature, Mohamed Mostafa Al-Eraky (2015) provided 12 practical suggestions for teaching professionalism at both undergraduate and postgraduate levels.

> Tip #1: Determine the cultural context because there are regional and variances and similarities in understanding professionalism concepts, most of which can be explained by cultural differences because there is no overarching conceptual context of professionalism accepted universally.

Tip #2: Ensure the institution agrees on the "cognitive base" of professionalism by defining its nature, components, the expectation of students, and priorities of what will be taught and evaluated.

Tip #3: Seek institutional support by advocating the value of teaching professionalism to university administrators, faculty members, and students.

Tip #4: Promote the professional milieu to ensure professionalism is not taught and learned in a vacuum but integrated into the curriculum.

Tip #5: Foster positive role-modeling using faculty and senior students to shape the students' professional attitudes

Tip #6: Train other faculty members to teach professionalism at all levels of the curriculum. Design continuing development programs to empower faculty members with teaching tools to address professionalism in their courses and also supplement professionalism education in different dimensions.

Tip #7: Ensure expectations are observable, measurable, and not threatening but can be operationalized easily rather than a set of abstract attributes and values

Tip #8: Provide learning opportunities appropriate to the level of the students and professionalism contents infused throughout the curriculum.

Tip #9: Allow structured time for guided students' reflection to create a greater understanding of self and situations by analyzing, questioning, and reframing (real or simulated) experiences to make an assessment of it for learning (reflective learning) and to improve practice (reflective practice).

Tip #10: Evaluate the outcome, provide ongoing feedback, and recommend appropriate remediation plans.

Tip #11: Share the teaching experience in your specialties with peers from other departments. This experience will create "communities of learning and practice." Communicate what teaching strategies worked and what did not work and why and explore better approaches for future practice.

Tip #12: Consider the use of digital (electronic) – social media, including Facebook, Twitter, and YouTube – aspects of professionalism in defining, teaching, and role-modeling.

Birden and associates (n.d.) conducted a systematic review to identify the best evidence for how professionalism should be taught in the medical curriculum. The findings revealed that role-modeling and personal reflections, guided by faculty, are the crucial elements and the most effective techniques for developing professionalism. The results also showed that, in general, faculty agree that professionalism should be part of the medical curriculum. However, the specifics of sequence, depth, detail, and the nature of how it should be integrated with other curriculum elements remain matters of evolving controversy.

Managing "hidden curriculum" phenomenon

The "hidden curriculum" phenomenon is the obscure socialization and behaviors associated with the transfer of knowledge and skills during the educational process and the norms and values transmitted to students. It consists of what is implicit but unknowingly taught from day to day, but not explicitly stated. Standardized evaluation inventories and accreditation guidelines can facilitate the "hidden curriculum" if they encourage faculty members to avoid confronting inappropriate behaviors to please other students or colleagues. The changes observed in student behavior requires an organizational change by way of institutional policies and resources supporting the "hidden curriculum." The allocation of resources reflects an institution's real value in identifying problems and instituting appropriate role-modeling standards on the part of the faculty members.

Faculty members must break peer silence and challenge behaviors that do not meet professional standards and ethical expectations. The "hidden curriculum" and its messages can be a topic of explicit discussion at faculty meetings. Topics can include analysis of medical errors and how to minimize it, fragmentation of care, interprofessional disrespect, truth-telling, racism and prejudice, and power dynamics and hierarchy of professions. Faculty development courses that model professionalism and ways to assess it in action, including practical educational approaches, should be pursued.

Collectively, adding "above all be not silent" (*Primum non tacere*) and "first do no harm" to the modus operandi of the academic department will go a long way to build resistance to the hidden curriculum. It will also allow faculty to reclaim their authenticity as trusted professionals whose knowledge is attached to the collective values to uphold, model, and reproduce (Mahood, 2011).

Assessment of professionalism

In response to the knowledge explosion in science and technology, HCPs have described the behaviors and attitudes that typify professionalism differently (Figure 3.4). The term *"attributes of professionalism"* is often used in the nursing literature (RNAO, 2007; Fantahun et al., 2014), *"fundamental elements of professionalism"* in medicine (Kim and Choi, 2015; Al-Sudani et al., 2013; Salam et al., 2013), *attitudinal/behavioral professionalism* in pharmacy (Kelly et al., 2011) and *professionalism core values* in physical therapy (American Physical Therapy Association – APTA, 2003). Several psychometric instruments and methods are utilized in the literature to measure the behaviors of HCPs (Balogun et al., 2017).

Evaluating students' professionalism, using formative assessment strategies helps to ensure the fundamental values, etiquette, attitudes, and behaviors expected from HCPs are front and center. The assessment process should align with the objectives and methods used for teaching and learning. The

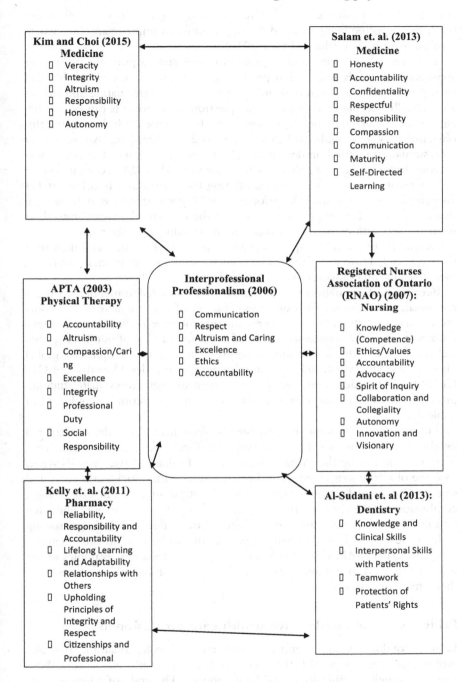

Figure 3.4 Fundamental elements and core values associated with professionalism.

assessment and feedback provided in the early stages help to develop and teach the expected behaviors and the opportunity to improve and internalize professionalism (Shwetha and Gali, 2016).

To foster an understanding of professionalism and to promote its broader application in HCE and clinical practice, it is necessary to have reliable and valid psychometric tools to measure it. Given the subjective nature and lack of a universally acceptable definition, the question of whether it can be reliably assessed is concerning. Luckily, a growing body of evidence indicates that this objective is quite feasible, and there are several tools available. Assessment of professionalism focused on determining if students have learned its core competency and what kind of deficiency they need to address. Moreover, unless we hold students accountable for demonstrating these attributes in a high-stakes assessment, they are unlikely to prioritize the accepted standards. It is essential that faculty members explicitly incorporate the expected behaviors into their formative and summative evaluations. Ongoing feedback on observable positive behavioral change would help to improve students' performance and their final review as well. However, if the students fail to show growth in their behaviors, then a follow-up evaluation will be needed.

Because professionalism is multidimensional, it is recommended to use a combination of assessment tools. Nine clusters of assessment tools are commonly used in the literature. They include observed clinical encounters, collated views of coworkers, records of incidents of unprofessionalism, critical incident reports, simulations, paper-based tests, patients' opinions, global views of the supervisor, and self-administered rating scales. Shwetha and Gali (2016) recommended using multiple assessment strategies to evaluate students' professionalism, depending on the defined learning outcome, as reflected in Table 3.1.

The strategies commonly used to assess professionalism include: standardized psychometric inventories, direct observation by faculty, peers and patient surveys, staff evaluation using the Professionalism Mini-Evaluation Exercise (P-MEX) tool, the objective structured clinical examination, critical incident reports, and students maintained professional portfolios. Multiple-source evaluation using a combination of the above methods is preferred to a single assessment conducted by the direct supervisor. Judging a student's knowledge and decision-making abilities are essential but knowing how the student behaves in other settings is equally crucial (Altirkawi, 2014). Figure 3.4 provides a few examples of the instruments used in different health fields for professional self-assessment and their attribute/trait subscales.

Ethical code of conduct for health care professionals

Ethical conduct is an essential component of professionalism. Typically, professions do declare publicly that their members will act ethically and that those who fail to behave ethically would be disciplined. The code of ethics governs the acts and moral obligations of members. The professional organizations and

Table 3.1 Assessment of professionalism by linking professional values with behaviors and learning outcomes

Values	Appropriate student behavior	Learning outcome: The students must be able to:	Teaching strategies	Assessment method
1 Responsibility/ Accountability	Carry work out tasks effectively and punctual.	Demonstrate commitment toward duties timely.	Logbook, Role play	Faculty, Peer survey, P-MEX
2 Honors and integrity	Accept blame for mistakes. Do not make inappropriate request. Not abusive or disorderly working under stress. Well groom and dress professionally at work.	Demonstrate respect and modesty. Demonstrate honesty.	Videos, observing role models at work.	
3 Altruism	Going beyond the call of duty in caring for patients.	Attitude: places patient welfare before self.	Standardized patients.	Patient feedback, P-MEX

the regulatory boards expect their members to display high ethical standards concerning the services they deliver to the public, and in dealing with their colleagues. Across the health care professions, the moral standard is similar, and they include language that requires their members to:

1. Interact with patients and others without discriminating by religion, ethnicity, gender, educational, or socioeconomic status.
2. Treat patients without discrimination, regardless of religious beliefs, socioeconomic status, gender, and national origin.
3. Recognize the impact of religion and culture on health and disease and respect such cultures and religions.
4. Be free from any conduct or actions that show preference or disdain for religion, ethnicity, gender, or socioeconomic status of patients, relations, or staff.
5. Demonstrate positive work habits, including punctuality, dependability, and professional appearance.
6. Be honest, reliable, and trustworthy.
7. Dress professionally at all times in a way that inspires confidence in patients and friends.
8. Be responsive to the needs of patients and society that supersedes self-interest.

9. Sacrifice personal comfort or convenience to achieve positive patient outcomes.
10. Always see self as the servant of the community.
11. Consistently preserve the confidentiality of all information transmitted both during and outside of a patient encounter.
12. Be knowledgeable about the regulatory issues relating to the practice of the profession, including biomedical research, regulations, registrations, licensing, and renewal, and applicable state laws.
13. Be knowledgeable as to when to seek informed consent and how to go about it.
14. Be appreciative of the need to work within the bounds of the laws of the country.
15. Embrace excellence and ongoing professional development, including postgraduate studies.

Conclusion

Several professionalism related behaviors that are sine qua non in health professions may be less of an issue in other fields. For example, practices such as wearing PPE, length of fingernails, artificial eyelashes may not be a concern in non-health related professions. Because professionalism shapes the public perception of HCPs, the related behavior expectations discussed in this chapter apply to both "professionals" and "occupational" workers. The benefits of professionalism include (1) increase inpatient and community trust in the health care system, (2) improved health care quality, patient safety, and (3) enhanced organizational performance. It also includes an increased sense of meaning and purpose on the part of the HCPs, which can lead to increased staff morale, well-being, and overall productivity. Infusion of professionalism in the curriculum of HCPs at the undergraduate and postgraduate levels is critical and it should be part of the continuing education requirement for licensure renewal.

The findings from existing literature revealed that role-modeling and personal reflections, guided by faculty, are the crucial elements and the most effective techniques for developing professionalism. Although faculty agreed that professionalism should be part of the curriculum, the specifics of sequence, depth, detail, and the nature of how it should be integrated with other curriculum elements remain matters of evolving controversy.

References

Al-Sudani, D, Al-Abbas, F, Al-Bannawi, Z and Al-Ramadhanb A. (2013) Professional attitudes and behaviors acquired during undergraduate education in the College of Dentistry, King Saud University. *Saudi Dental Journal*, 25(2): 69–74.

Altirkawi, K. (2014) Teaching professionalism in medicine: what, why and how? *Sudan J Paediatr.* 2014; 14(1): 31–38. [online]. Available at: www.ncbi.nlm.nih.gov/pmc/articles/PMC4949913/ (Accessed: February 3, 2020)

Anderson, DK and Irwin, KE. (2013) Self-assessment of professionalism in physical therapy education. *Work,* 44(3):275–81. [online]. Available at:http://europepmc. org/abstract/med/23324679 (Accessed: February 3, 2020)

APTA. (2003) Professionalism in physical therapy: core values. American Physical Therapy Association, Alexandria, VA. [online]. Available at:www.apta.org/ Professionalism/ (Accessed: February 3, 2020)

Balogun, JA, Mbada, E, Balogun, A and Okafor, UAC. (2017) Development and evaluation of the readability, stability and internal consistency of a psychometric instrument designed to assess physiotherapists' knowledge and attributes of professionalism. International Journal of Medical and Health Sciences Research, 4(6): 102–117. [online].Available at: www.researchgate.net/publication/319552123_Development_ and_Evaluation_of_the_Readability_Stability_and_Internal_Consistency_of_a_ Psychometric_Instrument_Designed_to_Assess_Physiotherapists_Knowledge_and_ Attributes_of_Professionalism (Accessed: February 3, 2020)

Birden, H, Glass, N, Wilson, I, Harrison, M, Usherwood, T and Nass, D. (n.d.) Teaching professionalism in medical education: A best evidence in medical Education (BEME) systematic review. [online]. Available at: https://bemecollaboration.org/downloads/ 1387/Birden-SR-web.pdf(Accessed: February 3, 2020)

BlackDoctor+org. (2019) The health dangers of "cute" shoes. [online]. Available at: https://blackdoctor.org/185463/health-dangers-of-high-heels/(Accessed: February 3, 2020)

CDC. (2001) CDC nails nurses. U.S. Department of Health and Human Services. [online]. Available at: www.infectioncontroltoday.com/hand-hygiene/cdc-nails-nurses (Accessed: February 3, 2020)

CDC. (2002) Hand hygiene in healthcare settings – core. [online]. Available at: www. cdc.gov/handhygiene (Accessed: February 3, 2020)

Cruess, RL and Cruess, SR. (2010) Teaching professionalism: why, what and how. [online]. Available at: www.ncbi.nlm.nih.gov/pmc/articles/PMC3987476/ (Accessed: February 3, 2020)

Davis, DS. (2009) Teaching professionalism: a survey of physical therapy educators. *Journal of Allied Health,* 38(2):74–80.

Fantahun, A, Demessie, A, Gebrekirstos, K, Zemene, A and Yetayeh G. (2014) A cross sectional study on factors influencing professionalism in nursing among nurses in Mekelle Public Hospitals, North Ethiopia. *BMC Nursing,* 13:10. [online].Available at: www. cdc.gov/healthywater/hygiene/hand/nail_hygiene.html (Accessed: February 3, 2020)

Haidet, P. (2008) Where we "re headed: A new wave of scholarship on educating medical professionalism," *Journal of General Internal Medicine,* 23, 1118–1119.

Jansen, CWS, Patterson, R and Viegas, SF. (2000) Effects of fingernail length on finger and hand performance. *Journal of Hand Therapy,* 13(3):211–7. [online]. Available at: www.researchgate.net/publication/12356229_Effects_of_fingernail_length_on_ finger_and_hand_performance (Accessed: February 3, 2020)

Joseph, C and Thompson, J. (2019) Ten characteristics of professionalism. [online]. Available at: https://smallbusiness.chron.com/10-characteristics-professionalism-708.html (Accessed: February 3, 2020)

Kelly, A, Stanke, LD, Rabi, SM, Kuba, SE and Janke, KK. (2011) Cross-validation of an instrument for measuring professionalism behaviors. *American Journal of Pharmaceutical Education,* 75, 1–10.

Kim, S and Choi, S. (2015) The medical professionalism of Korean physicians: Present and future. *BMC Medical Ethics,* 16, 56. [online]. Available at: https://bmcmedethics. biomedcentral.com/articles/10.1186/s12910-015-0051-7 (Accessed: February 3, 2020)

Mahood, SC. (2011) Medical education: Beware the hidden curriculum. *Can Fam Physician,* 57(9): 983–985. [online]. Available at: www.ncbi.nlm.nih.gov/pmc/articles/PMC3173411/ (Accessed: February 3, 2020)

McNeil, SA, Foster, CL, Hedderwick, SA and Kauffman, CA. (2001) Effect of hand cleansing with antimicrobial soap or alcohol-based gel on microbial colonization of artificial fingernails worn by healthcare workers. *Clinical Infectious Diseases,* 32 (3), 1: 367–372. [online]. Available at: https://academic.oup.com/cid/article/32/3/367/282937(Accessed: February 3, 2020)

Mostafa Al-Eraky, M. (2015) Twelve tips for teaching medical professionalism at all levels of medical education. *Medical Teacher,* 37: 1018–1025. [online]. Available at: www.uky.edu/chs/sites/chs.uky.edu/files/Article-%2012%20tips%20for%20teaching%20medical%20professionalism%20at%20all%20levels%20of%20education.pdf (Accessed: February 3, 2020)

Mueller, PS. (2015) Teaching and assessing professionalism in medical learners and practicing physicians. *Rambam Maimonides, Med J.* 6(2): e0011. [online]. Available at: www.ncbi.nlm.nih.gov/pmc/articles/PMC4422450/ (Accessed: February 3, 2020)

Nahvi, FA. (2011) How safe is that tattoo? [online]. Available at: www.clinicalcorrelations.org/2011/04/27/how-safe-is-that-tatoo/ (Accessed: February 3, 2020)

Nath, C, Schmidt, R and Gunel, E. (2006). Perception of professionalism varies most with educational rank and age. *Journal of Dental Education,* 70(8), 825–834.

Porcupile, DW. (2015) What is professionalism? What does professionalism mean to you? [online]. Available at: http://graduate.auburn.edu/wp-content/uploads/2016/08/What-is-PROFESSIONALISM.pdf (Accessed: February 3, 2020)

PositiveMed (2013). Ten dangers of fake eyelash. [online]. Available at: www.positivemed.com/2013/ 10/ 25/ 10- dangers- fake- eyelashes/ (Accessed: February 3, 2020)

RNAO. (2007) Professionalism in nursing: Healthy work environments best practice guidelines. [online]. Available at: http://rnao.ca/sites/rnao-ca/files/Professionalism_in_Nursing.pdf (Accessed: February 3, 2020)

Salam, A, Yousuf, R, Islam, MZ, Yesmin, F, Helali, A, Alattraqchi, A, Rao, U and Haque, M. (2013) Professionalism of future medical professionals in Universiti Sultan Zainal Abidin, Malaysia. *Bangladesh Journal of Pharmacology,* 8(2), 124–130. doi:10.3329/bjp.v8i2.14158.

Shwetha, KM and Gali, S. (2016) Professionalism in healthcare education. *Journal of Dental and Oro-Facial Research,* 12 (1): 14–18. [online]. Available at: www.researchgate.net/publication/302959443_Professionalism_in_health_care_education (Accessed: February 3, 2020)

US Food and Drug Administration. (2018) Personal protective equipment for infection control. . [online]. Available at: www.fda.gov/medical-devices/general-hospital-devices-and-supplies/personal-protective-equipment-infection-control (Accessed: February 3, 2020)

Vicarelli, G and Spina, E. (2015) Professionalization and professionalism: The case of Italian dentistry. *Professions and Professionalism,* 5 (3):1–16. [online]. Available at: https://journals.hioa.no/index.php/pp/article/view/1324 (Accessed: February 3, 2020)

WikiHow. (2019) How to be hygienic. [online]. Available at: www.wikihow.com/Be-Hygienic (Accessed: February 3, 2020)

William, O. (1903) William Osler papers father of modern medicine: The Johns Hopkins School of Medicine, 1889–1905. [online]. Available at: https://profiles.nlm.nih.gov/spotlight/gf/feature/biographical (Accessed: February 3, 2020)

World Health Organization. (2009) WHO guidelines on hand hygiene in healthcare: First global patient safety challenge clean care is safer care. Printed in France. WHO/IER/PSP. [online]. Available at: https://apps.who.int/iris/bitstream/handle/10665/44102/9789241597906_eng.pdf;jsessionid=7178C541A4517379F94B0F6CA3DC13DF?sequence=1 (Accessed: February 3, 2020)

4 Administration of health care education departments

Introduction

An academic administrator is responsible for overseeing the daily operation of a university, college, or department. The role of an administrator is separate from the faculty, although, in some institutions, some personnel may have joint responsibilities. In Nigeria, some different administrative structure exists at almost all academic institutions. Many senior administrators who have advanced degrees serve in faculty roles (Babatola, 2017; Briggs, 2013; Itakpe, 2012). In many countries around the world, including Nigeria, department chairs or heads of departments (HODs) are appointed into the management position without any administrative instruction or formal training on their roles and responsibilities.

This chapter is the quintessential source of information for such academic administrators as it describes the university organization structure, opportunities, and challenges in the administration of health care education (HCE) programs. It also discusses the roles and responsibilities of the HODs in program assessment, evaluation of faculty performance in the teaching, scholarship of discovery, and service domains. The chapter provides sample program assessment tools (course evaluation, HODs, and peer evaluation of teaching performance forms, student exit, alumni, and employers' satisfaction survey questionnaires), and offers pertinent administrative recommendations for newly appointed HODs.

University organizational structure

The universities in Nigeria functions through the "visitor" (chancellor), pro-chancellor, governing council, vice-chancellor (VC), and other principal officers, senate, congregation and convocation committees and the colleges/schools/faculties/departments. In federal universities, the "visitor" is the president of the country, and in-state universities, the governor is the "visitor" and the proprietors for private universities (Briggs, 2013). The chief executive officer of the university, depending on the country is called the VC (in commonwealth countries), or the president/pro-chancellor/chancellor (in the United States), and the principal (in Scotland and Canada), or rector (in

Europe, Russia, Asia, the Middle East, and South America). The administrative executive officer in charge of a college/faculty within a university is the dean. The VC reports to the university council (a term used in commonwealth countries) or board of trustees (the United States). Typically, the office of the VC oversees undergraduate and graduates academic programs, student affairs, athletics, sponsored research, graduate admissions, public relations, marketing, international programs, works, and maintenance.

In many of the "first-generation" universities in Nigeria, there are usually two DVCs: one for academic affairs and the other for administration. The office of the DVC or the office of academic affairs (in the United States) is responsible for academic planning and accreditation of educational programs, support services, faculty, and student matters. The registrar and DVC report to the VC and they both keep the VC informed of all university matters within their purview. The registrar oversees specific divisions/units (council and general administration, academic affairs, and personnel) and program secretaries and faculty officers in the institutional arms (colleges, faculties, schools, directorates and academic programs of the university) and serves as the secretary of the university council, congregation and convocation committees. Administratively, the deans of the colleges report to the provost and the HODs report to the dean (Babatola, 2017).

The internal audit unit evaluates the effectiveness of the university internal control system and ensures effective implementation of management policies consistent with existing rules and regulations. The bursary department is responsible for the accurate and timely reporting of the university finances based on principles of transparency, efficiency, and accountability. The dean of students oversees the academic, personal, and overall well-being of the students. The office informs students about counseling and leadership opportunities, scholarship and loan announcements, university status (leaves of absence, or withdrawals).

The critical administrative responsibilities of the VC and DVC includes providing oversight over the departments/unit in charge of the admission of students, supervision of hiring, promotion, tenure, and evaluation (with faculty input where appropriate), maintenance of university records, and audit of financial records, and construction of campus buildings (physical plant), campus grounds, safety and security of personnel and property on the campus, installation and supervision of the campus computers and network (information technology), fundraising from private individuals and foundations, research administration (including grants and contract administration, institutional compliance with federal/state regulations), public affairs (including media relations, community), and student services, including disability services and career counseling.

All the "first-generation" universities at Ibadan, Lagos, Ife, Nsukka, and Zaria established colleges/faculties of medicine/health sciences and university teaching hospitals located off-campus as a mini-campus. In addition to medicine and dentistry, other HCE programs (nursing, physiotherapy, occupational

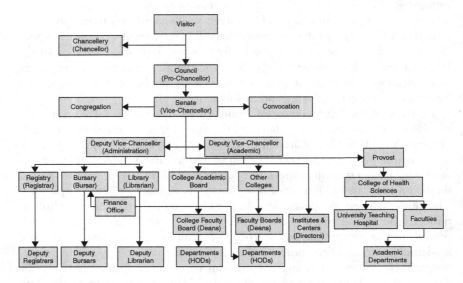

Figure 4.1 The organogram for a conventional university.

therapy, medical laboratory science, optometry, etc.) are offered within the colleges/faculties. Pharmacy is usually a full-fledged standalone entity, not affiliated to the colleges/faculties of medicine/health sciences. The organizational structure created at the University of Ibadan (UI) in 1948 became the model for the other conventional universities in the country (Figure 4.1).

Responsibilities of the provost and deans

In all the colleges/faculties of medicine/health sciences established in the country, the provost is the chief academic officer and provides leadership and vision for the mini-campus. The deans oversee the administrative functions of academic programs and support faculty research, teaching, and service (Babatola, 2017). From inception, administrators of HCE programs in Nigeria advocated for a high degree of autonomy separate from the other faculties/schools within the university. The advocacy resulted in the evolution from "school" or "faculty" systems to the adoption of the "collegiate" system. Sadly, the transition to the "collegiate" system did not provide the desired autonomy and independence (Itakpe, 2012; Babatola, 2017). This issue is discussed further in Chapter 7.

The university system in democratic high-income countries is undergirded by academic freedom and independence. Unfortunately, Nigerian universities lack academic freedom and autonomy because governmental bodies exert undue influence on the VC and often determine the major policies and direct the research activities of the universities. In many cases, faculty and support staff are employed by the state or federal government instead of the individual institutions. The Minister of Education confers with the president to appoint VCs in federal universities. Only the university council/board of trustees select or terminate VCs and grant tenure to faculty in the United Kingdom and the United States.

Responsibilities of the heads of departments

The HODs are the administrative officer of the academic unit, and they manage its daily operations, including the evaluation of faculty and nonacademic staff performance and coordination of program accreditation process. The roles and responsibilities of the HODs are in three broad areas.

Leadership

The HODs facilitate the long-range unit development plan to ensure it aligns with the university vision, mission, and values. They collaborate with the faculty to ensure that the unit's evolution reflects changes in the accreditation standards and changes within the university. The HODs maintain contact with other colleagues within the university and professional disciplines to facilitate relevance, coherency, and interdisciplinary integration of the academic programs and curriculum.

Furthermore, the HODs expedite the development and implementation of the unit strategic plan to ensure a clear direction corresponding with the university strategic plan and advance the development of the academic programs by building upon the faculty and students' quality. They provide leadership in personnel hiring and educational development, including working to create and assess faculty and nonacademic staff development plans.

Management

The HODs promote the administrative operations of the academic unit by overseeing the daily progress towards achieving the teaching, research, and service missions of the department strategic plan. They play a critical role in preparing the class schedules, budget, including estimates of resources needed to carry out the instructional functions.

Development and institutional support

The overall success and effectiveness of the HODs depend on the support received from the dean and provost. The HODs seek the opportunity to benchmark the department's performance with similarly situated units within and outside the university and attend internal and external meetings that allow interaction with colleagues in the disciplines to provide comparative practice perspectives within the university and at other institutions. Such meetings enable the HODs to discuss common operational issues, policies, practices, accountability, and strategies that peers have used in resolving problems. Ongoing regular meetings and an annual formal meeting with the dean/provost are needed to discuss the progress and challenge smooth communication between the parties. The provost and dean typically offer a yearly orientation for new HODs. The primary roles and responsibilities of the HODs are to:

1. Convey faculty input to the administration through the Dean, after consultation with the peers on all university recommended policy and administrative changes
2. Prepare the department's annual report and budget
3. Submit the yearly personnel needs
4. Monitor compliance with university and professional discipline academic policies
5. Facilitate academic program curriculum revisions and implementation
6. Develop class schedules and teaching assignments
7. Schedule and preside over department meetings
8. Serve as the primary contact with the university advancement, recruitment, and retention offices
9. Provide the lead on faculty hiring committees
10. Promote a team effort within the department to resolve departmental and university issues
11. Facilitate the curriculum revision policies needed on the web sites/catalog copy
12. Work to promote civility, camaraderie, and respect among faculty, faculty/students, and faculty/university offices
13. Mediate conflicts between departmental faculty formally and informally
14. Manage student grade appeal/complaints

Program assessments

One of the questions that HODs are often asked: Is the productivity of your department better than other departments? Collecting appropriate evidence data on key performance indicators will provide the HODs the empirically based information needed to answer the question. One of the primary functions of the HODs is coordinating program assessment and fostering continuous quality improvement. Program assessment is an ongoing process that occurs at the university department level, and it involves the evaluation of students learning, faculty teaching effectiveness and overall department effectiveness (Figure 4.2). The process provides evidence for decision-making in determining whether or not the academic department goals are met.

Program assessment forces faculty to ask tough programmatic related questions such as: What are the local, state, and regional professional needs? Is each faculty member teaching what is expected of them, and are the students learning what they are supposed to know? Is there a better way to teach a

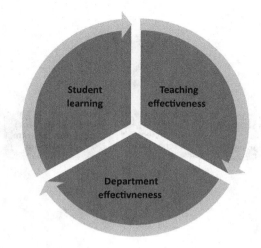

Figure 4.2 The program assessment trifecta.

subject matter and promote better learning? Are the program graduates contributing significantly to the development of their community, state, and nation? Are the program graduates meeting the needs in the health care system? Are the program graduates professional and ethical in their practices?

After answering the above questions, the faculty can develop the program's student learning objectives (SLOs) and create the curriculum plan by identifying the corresponding performance outcome (emerging, developing, or proficient) for each semester. The curriculum mapping process was discussed more comprehensively in Chapter 3 of this book. Subsequently, the faculty must collect the relevant critical performance indicator data and use the assessment results for program improvement (Figure 4.3).

The faculty should benchmark the students' outcomes to other similarly situated academic programs and use the findings during the program review to improve learning. Repeat the entire process to produce a continuous improvement loop cycle (Figure 4.4). Subsequently, appropriate programmatic decisions can be made based on the evidence accrued.

Assessment of students learning

Student learning is one of the tripartite components of program assessment that takes place at the department level and coordinated by the HODs. Direct and indirect methods evaluate students' learning. The direct process consists of faculty made nonstandardized tests and standardized tests. Faculty constructed tests are fraught with questionable readability, often lack item discrimination analysis, reliability, and validity – the conditions for administering, scoring,

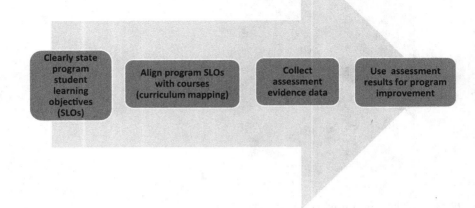

Figure 4.3 Implementation of the program assessment process.

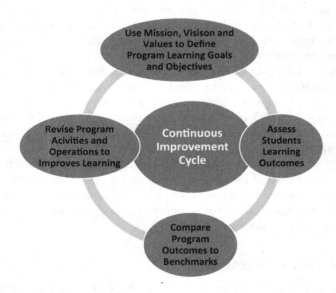

Figure 4.4 Continuous improvement loop.

and interpreting both tests consistently. The results from faculty made tests are confined to the individual schools and are not externally valid for other programs.

Currently, the use of standardized tests, which is the preferred method for gauging student learning, are presently nonexistent in Nigeria. Standardized tests are badly needed to compare students' performance in each program across the nation. Examples of standardized tests for licensing exams in most disciplines are available at the following web address: www.practicequiz.com/.

The graduates of HCE programs in Nigeria are not subjected to standardized testing during training and after the internship program. Without *benchmarking*, it is not possible to know whether graduates of program A is better than those of program B. The use of standardized tests will spur competition among programs and will be an informed basis for curriculum revision.

The indirect method of measuring student learning includes the use of formative and summative (students exit, alumni, and employers) satisfaction survey questionnaires (Sample Document #4.1 to 4.4).

Also, focus group discussion approach can be used by asking the students the following questions:

1. How do you feel now that you are about to complete the first year of the _____ curriculum? (For formative evaluation)
2. How do you think now that you are about to graduate with a _____ _____ degree? (For summative assessment)

The students' responses during the focus group discussion session recorded and analyzed qualitatively to identify significant themes about program strengths and weaknesses. The outcomes are used as a basis for program refinement.

Evaluation of faculty effectiveness

The HODs are responsible for evaluating faculty performance in the three assessment domains: teaching, scholarship, and service. Assessment of teaching performance is undertaken every semester by peers and HODs. On separate occasions, they visit the classroom to observe the faculty while teaching and communicate their observation and grading on the *Classroom Evaluation of Teaching Effectiveness Form* (Sample Document #4.5). Students are instructed to complete the *Course Evaluation Form* (Sample Document #4.6) for all courses offered at the end of the semester. Because the students complete their assessment online, confidentiality and anonymity are protected. The assessment data are tallied, including the comments, and reviewed both by the faculty and HODs to identify areas of instructional strengths and weaknesses. The outcomes are used to improve faculty teaching effectiveness within the department, and the institution considers the findings as part of the requirements for promotion and tenure.

Faculty performance in the scholarship of discovery domain is by monitored using the following ten indicators:

1. The number of publications in high impact journals
2. The number of books or chapters authored
3. The number of software programs developed
4. The number of presentations in scientific conferences
5. Keynote addresses presented at major scientific conferences
6. Number of grants received and dollar amount
7. The faculty bibliometric metrics such as H-index and number of citations. The H-index and its variants are the most robust indicators to gauge the quantity (number of publications) and quality (impact of the research work) of academics
8. The number of "reads" of faculty publications
9. Appointment on Scientific Review Panels/Advisory Committees at the national level
10. Editorship or Editorial Board member on an indexed peer-reviewed journal

Faculty performance in the service domain is assessed from their roles on committees at department, college, and university levels. Examples are serving as chair of the program accreditation committee, coordinator of the accreditation self-study, and program review self-study. Other service activities include community engagement at the local level or service on professional organization committees at state, national or international levels.

Evaluation of department effectiveness

Typically, department effectiveness is annually assessed using the following 16 key performance indicators:

1. Number of faculty and their educational profile
2. Faculty teaching workload
3. Number of students enrolled each year
4. The faculty/student ratio
5. Number of students retained at the end of the year
6. Number of students who graduated at the end of the fourth year of enrollment
7. Number of students who graduated at the end of the sixth year of enrollment
8. Number of postgraduate students (Master's and PhD) produced each year
9. Graduate performance on standardized tests, including license exam
10. Number of student scholarship awards

11. Number and types of faculty awards
12. Alumni satisfaction of program graduates
13. Budget and physical resources for research and instructional instrumentation
14. Amount of endowment fund generated
15. Graduates job placement
16. Amount of community collaborations

The HOD must analyze the above data collected to identify patterns and to benchmark the findings against similar data obtained from peer academic departments within the university. Also, compare data with national norms from other peer institutions across the country. In the United States, norm data for preprimary, elementary, and secondary education and postsecondary institutions are published on the United States Department of Education, National Center for Education Statistics website at https://nces.ed.gov/programs/coe/indicator_ctr.asp.

At the beginning of the academic year, HODs in most institutions set goals for their department. The following are examples of measurable goal-setting statements:

1. Increase by 5% the number of new students enrolled; effective _____ semester
2. Increase by 5% the number of graduates produced; effective from _____ semester
3. Increase by 5% the number of refereed publications by faculty and staff; effective _____ semester
4. Increase by 5% the number of graduate students majoring in _____ who are providing service in the community; effective _____ semester
5. Increase by 10% graduate satisfaction
6. Increase by 10% employee satisfaction
7. Increase faculty research output by 5%

Recommendations for newly appointed department administrator

The finest hour is on the day the appointment as HOD is announced. You will never have more friends than you have on that date. As HOD, you must have the ability to leverage team strengths and lead by example and be a role model for junior faculty. All stakeholders, faculty, students, and staff must believe in their leader and credibility. Hence, persuasion ability is essential to be a successful and effective leader.

Furthermore, HODs must be confident and believe in self-abilities. If not, no one will. Having the courage to say "I don't know" is a powerful skill. You must have a strong focus on the department's strategic plan and stay the course, even when the going is rough at the beginning. HODs must be flexible and realize that not everything goes as planned but have a passion for what you do.

The heart of the job involves mentoring junior faculty members, coordinating grants, working with the development office to explain long-term plans for fundraising, and other executive functions. To enhance scholarship within the department, HODs must conduct grant writing workshops and provide grant announcements and mentor junior faculty in grant writing. Furthermore, HODs mentor junior faculty on how to teach and offer instructional tools to improve the creative and teaching skills.

Be humble and never, ever say, "I am the HOD, you know." When you are humble and trusted, you are likely to get faculty and staff support and vote the way you desire because they all want to have a leader who can get things done. Please do the job once you take responsibility. If you cannot, do the right thing and resign. If you do not leave, do your job and do not get distracted by minutiae. Do *not* play favorites and treat all subordinates the same.

The HOD must be honest at all times. Your colleagues will feel like they know where they stand with you. It would be best if you worked hard to create a fair and rewards meritocracy and not mediocrity. It would be best if you cultivated an atmosphere in which contributions to the collective good are honored with prizes awards. Send out birthday cards to faculty and staff – small gestures like that boost morale and cooperation.

An urgent matter is not always an important one. Make time for issues that are important but not urgent. Use your discretion to delegate things that are urgent but unimportant. Always prioritize your time by structuring your day to accomplish many small things and at least one significant thing every day.

HODs must be supportive, compassionate, and caring when making vital decisions. You must realize it is not always just about the work but about the people in it and the people impacted by it. Ask questions and listen to the answers. After you hear the response, ask, "What one thing could I do to make your work better and your life easier?"

Conflict resolution is an essential attribute of successful leaders as disagreement is unavoidable in the workplace. Remain calm in the face of criticism and run meetings fairly and transparently. When unfairly attacked, don't get trapped into an angry rage, by giving a poorly conceived email response. You will regret it two minutes after you hit the send key. Only a few people will say in the open the horrible things they can say in an email message. Extinguish email flame wars. When conflict becomes unbearable and destructive to team cohesion, that might mean recommending for termination or transfer of the toxic staff or faculty who knows all the rules and continuously makes everyone miserable.

The HODs are often bombarded by visitors, letters, and calls all the time. They all will request the same thing: "You must care about this matter that I care about!" The burden of having to care will build-up, like histamines in the bloodstream. If this situation persists, the HOD will quickly burn out and infect the subordinates and colleagues. Hence, it would be best if the HOD found an outlet to reduce stress by creating room for fun and allow employees to recharge their batteries. It would be best if they found time to mingle with

Table 4.1 Health education programs offered in Nigerian universities

Academic discipline	Entry-level degree awarded	Years of training	Available postgraduate degree	Name of professional association	Name of professional regulatory boards
1 Medicine	MBBS/MB ChB/DO	7†	FNPMCN, FWACP/S; MD	Nigerian Medical Association	Medical and Dental Council of Nigeria
2 Dentistry	BDS/B ChB	7†	FNPMCN, FWACP/S; MD	Nigerian Dental Association	Medical and Dental Council of Nigeria
3 Physiotherapy	BPT/BMR (PT) – DPT effective 2020	5/6	MS; PhD	Nigeria Society of Physiotherapy	Medical Rehabilitation Therapists (Registration) Board of Nigeria
4 Occupational Therapy	BMR (OT)	5		Occupational Therapists Association of Nigeria	Medical Rehabilitation Therapists (Registration) Board of Nigeria
5 Pharmacy	B.Pharm Pharm.D effective 2016	5/6	MS; PhD	Pharmaceutical Society of Nigeria	Pharmacists Council of Nigeria
6 Optometry	BS – DO effective 2018	5/6		Nigerian Optometric Association	Optometrists and Dispensing Opticians Registration Board of Nigeria
7 Clinical Psychology	BS, MS, PhD	4–8	MS; PhD	Nigerian Psychological Association	None
8 Nursing and Midwifery†	Certificate/Diploma	3	MS; PhD	The National Association of Nigeria Nurses and Midwives	Nursing and Midwifery Council of Nigeria
9 Medical Laboratory Science/Science Laboratory Technology	BS	4	MS; PhD	Association of Medical Laboratory Scientists of Nigeria /Association of Science Laboratory Technologists of Nigeria	Medical Laboratory Science Council of Nigeria/Nigeria Institute of Science Laboratory Technology

(continued)

Table 4.1 Cont.

	Academic discipline	Entry-level degree awarded	Years of training	Available postgraduate degree	Name of professional association	Name of professional regulatory boards
10	Radiography	BS	4	MS; PhD	Association of Radiographers of Nigeria	Radiographers Registration Board of Nigeria
11	Nutrition/ Dietitian	BS	4	MS; PhD	Nutrition Society of Nigeria; Nigerian Dietetic Association/ Dietitians Association of Nigeria	None Approval of Dietitians Registration Council is pending
12	Prosthetics and Orthotics	BS	4		Nigerian Prosthetic, Orthotic and Orthopedic Technology Society	Medical Rehabilitation Therapists (Registration) Board of Nigeria
13	Biomedical Engineering/ Technology	BS	4	MS; PhD	Association of Biomedical Engineers and Technologists of Nigeria	College of Biomedical Engineering and Technology
14	Community Health	BS	4		The National Association of Community Health Practitioners of Nigeria	The Community Health Practitioners Registration Board of Nigeria
15	Veterinary Medicine	DVM	6	MS; PhD	Nigerian Veterinary Medical Association	The Veterinary Council of Nigeria

Source: www.medicalworldnigeria.com/2015/08/nigeria-has-only-39-orthodontists-says-nao/#.WQTmq9Lytdg/

Note: †Midwifery is not offered at the university level

the stakeholders by having an extended one on one time or lunch with every faculty and staff yearly; even those who may not like you.

The HODs must promote accountability in the management of the limited institutional budget to enhance efficiency and prevent corruption. Must promote scholarship culture by holding weekly seminars/colloquium, invite external researchers to further foster interdisciplinary collaboration, and encourage innovation and entrepreneurship by developing faculty clinical practice and consultancy services. Funds generated can be used to support faculty development activities.

Conclusion

The role of the HOD is challenging because it is a middle level administrative position and they often do not have the financial wherewithal to actualize their vision. To be successful, the HOD must develop a cordial relationship with the dean and provost who have the authority to allocate resources. While the rest of the world was developing in science and technology, Nigerian universities seem left behind in the 20th century. Reforming the university system will have to start at the department level. The HODs must fight corruption, remain pragmatic, promote meritocracy, and committed to high-quality education.

References

Babatola, JT. (2017) *Collegiate System and University Administration in Nigeria: A case study of Ekiti State University.* [online]. Available at: www.researchgate.net/publication/315046480 (Accessed: 4 February 2020)

Briggs, N. (2013) An overview of university education and administration in Nigeria. Guest lecture at the University of Port Harcourt [online]. Available at: www.nimibriggs.org/an-overview-of-university-education-and-administration-in-nigeria/ (Accessed: 4 February 2020)

Itakpe, MA. (2012) Evaluation of the effectiveness of the collegiate system of administration in Colleges of Medicine in Nigerian federal universities [online]. Available at: http://80.240.30.238/handle/123456789/729 (Accessed: 4 February 2020)

SAMPLE DOCUMENTS

Sample Document #4.1: Sample formative student survey questionnaire

The purpose of this survey is to obtain your opinions on the instructional and physical resources in the department. Your feedback is important to us as we aspire to improve our services and curriculum and goals. Your response is valuable to us and will be used in our educational planning purposes. If you have questions, please do not hesitate to contact the department by phone at 802-334-XXXX or by email at_____. Thank you for your participation.

INSTRUCTIONS

Do not put your name or ID on this survey!!! Please answer all questions as honestly as possible. All information collected will be kept confidential by the department. Please tick the option in the rectangular space provided. Please do not guess; instead please tick "Not Applicable." Thank you for your help.

For Official Use Only *(Please leave blank)*   CODE: __ __ __ __

Term: _____   Date: _____

Adequacy of Curriculum	Excellent (4)	Very Good (3)	Good (2)	Fair (1)	Poor (0)	Not Applicable
Critical thinking						
Communication						
Therapeutic interventions						
Leadership concepts						
Research concepts						
Health policy concepts						
Prevention concepts						
Health care ethics concepts						
Writing papers						
Socialization into the profession						
Publicized department policy changes						
Clinical sites provided adequate opportunities in all specialties						

Adequacy of Curriculum	Excellent (4)	Very Good (3)	Good (2)	Fair (1)	Poor (0)	Not Applicable
"Hands-on" instructions in the laboratory						
Clinical preparation for practice						
Caring for culturally diverse clients						
Conflict resolution						
Work collaboratively in groups						

Total score: _____

Faculty	Excellent (4)	Very Good (3)	Good (2)	Fair (1)	Poor (0)	Not applicable
Faculty Teaching						
Faculty mentoring						
Faculty caring						
Instructional resources (audiovisual aids, clinical sites)						

Total score: _____

Adequacy of resources and services	Excellent (4)	Very Good (3)	Good (2)	Fair (1)	Poor (0)	Not Applicable
Availability of computers						
Availability of audiovisual aids in the lab						
Clinical supplies in the lab						
Availability of lab to practice clinical skills						
Availability of a staff in the lab to assist						
Library						

Adequacy of resources and services	Excellent (4)	Very Good (3)	Good (2)	Fair (1)	Poor (0)	Not Applicable
Academic advisor						
Tutoring						
Financial aid						
Career development services						
Counseling services						

Total score: _____

Scoring of survey

Add together the options indicated for each subsection

Interpretation

Adequacy of curriculum

A total maximum score of 64 and a minimum score of 0 are possible. The overall rating on the questionnaire for each survey participant reflects their level of satisfaction with the curriculum. The higher the score the more satisfied.

Faculty

A total maximum score of 12 and a minimum score of 0 are possible. The overall rating on the questionnaire for each survey participant reflects their level of satisfaction with the faculty. The higher the score the more satisfied.

Adequacy of resources and services

A total maximum score of 44 and a minimum score of 0 are possible. The overall rating on the questionnaire for each survey participant reflects their level of satisfaction with the resources and services provided by the educational program. The higher the score the more satisfied.

Sample Document #4.2: Sample graduating student exit survey instrument

_____University

Department of _____

Congratulations on your impending graduation from _____ University! The purpose of this survey is to obtain your views as a graduating student. Your feedback is important to us as we aspire to improve our services and curriculum and goals. Your response will be used in our planning purposes. If you have questions, please do not hesitate to contact the department by phone at 802-334-XXXX or by email at_____. Thank you for your participation.

INSTRUCTIONS

Do not put your name or ID on this survey!!! Please answer all questions as honestly as possible. All information collected will be kept confidential by the department. Please tick the option in the rectangular space provided. Please do not guess; instead please tick "Not Applicable." Thank you for your help.

For <u>Official Use Only</u> *(Please leave blank)*   CODE: __ __ __ __

Directions: For each question, select or mark the most appropriate response. Return the completed survey to the _____,

1. What is your ethnicity or race?
   a. Black – non-Hispanic
   b. Asia/Pacific Islander
   c. White – non-Hispanic
   d. Native American/Alaskan
   e. Hispanic
   f. Unknown
2. What is your gender?
   a. Male
   b. Female
3. What is your major?
   a. Community Health
   b. Pre–Physical Therapy
   c. Nursing
   d. Occupational Therapy
4. Do you currently have a job offer?
   a. Yes, Full-time
   b. Yes, Part-time
   c. No, Is seeking
   d. No, Not seeking

5. Do you currently have admission to a graduate school?
   a. Yes, Full-time
   b. Yes, Part-time
   c. No, Is seeking
   d. No, Not seeking
6. How closely related is your current job or graduate schoolwork to your Bachelor's degree major?
   a. Closely related
   b. Related
   c. Unrelated by choice
   d. Unrelated not by choice
7. In general, how well did your Bachelor's degree prepare you for your present job or graduate school?
   a. Very well
   b. Well
   c. Adequately
   d. Inadequately
   e. Poorly
   f. Very poorly
8. What is your present attitude towards the _____ University?
   a. Strongly positive
   b. Positive
   c. Somewhat positive
   d. Somewhat negative
   e. Negative
   f. Strongly negative
9. What is your present attitude towards your Bachelor's degree major?
   a. Strongly positive
   b. Positive
   c. Somewhat positive
   d. Somewhat negative
   e. Negative
   f. Strongly negative
10. In my major degree program, lecturers were accessible outside of class?
    a. Very often
    b. Often
    c. Sometimes
    d. Infrequently
    e. Never
11. In my major degree program, I was expected or required to work cooperatively with other students on projects, homework, and assignments.
    a. Very often
    b. Often
    c. Sometimes
    d. Infrequently
    e. Never

12. In my major degree program, lecturers used appropriate teaching activities to help me learn.
    a. Very often
    b. Often
    c. Sometimes
    d. Infrequently
    e. Never
13. In my major degree program, lecturers' expectation for the quality of student work were high.
    a. Very often
    b. Often
    c. Sometimes
    d. Infrequently
    e. Never
14. In my major degree program, lecturers provided me with timely feedback on my performance.
    a. Very often
    b. Often
    c. Sometimes
    d. Infrequently
    e. Never
15. Please tick the option in the rectangular space provided. Please do not guess; instead, please tick "Not Applicable." On a scale of 1 (very little) to 5 (very much) what extent has your experience at _____ University contributed to your knowledge, skills and personal development in the following areas:

	1 Very much	2 Little	3 Neutral	4 Much	5 Very much
Acquiring a broad general education	☐	☐	☐	☐	☐
Writing clearly and effectively	☐	☐	☐	☐	☐
Speaking clearly and effectively	☐	☐	☐	☐	☐
Thinking critically and analytically	☐	☐	☐	☐	☐
Analyzing quantitative problems	☐	☐	☐	☐	☐
Using computing and information technology	☐	☐	☐	☐	☐
Understanding people of other racial and ethnic background	☐	☐	☐	☐	☐
Solving complex real-world problems	☐	☐	☐	☐	☐
Developing personal code of values and ethics	☐	☐	☐	☐	☐

	1	2	3	4	5
	Very much	Little	Neutral	Much	Very much
Developing a deepened sense of spiritually	☐	☐	☐	☐	☐
Contributing to the welfare of your community	☐	☐	☐	☐	☐

Total score: _____

Scoring of survey

Add together the options indicated for the 11 questions.

Interpretation

A total maximum score of 55 and a minimum score of 0 are possible. The overall rating on the questionnaire for each survey participant reflects their level of knowledge, skills, and personal development. The higher the score, the more knowledgeable.

Sample Document #4.3: Sample alumni survey questionnaire

_____ University

Department of_____

The purpose of this survey is to obtain your views as an alumnus of_____
__ University. Thanks for your willingness to provide us with useful information. Your response will not be revealed to anyone, but the data will be compiled, and aggregate data will be obtained and used for planning purposes and curriculum revision. If you have questions, please do not hesitate to contact the department by phone at 802-334-xxx or by email at smithd125@.edu. Thank you for your participation.

INSTRUCTIONS

Do not put your name or ID on this survey!!! Please answer all questions as honestly as possible. All information collected will be kept confidential by the department. Please tick the option in the rectangular space provided. Please do not guess; instead please tick "Not Applicable." Thank you for your help

---

For Official Use Only *(Please leave blank)* CODE: __ __ __ __

Directions: For each question, select or mark the most appropriate response.

What is your ethnicity or race?
- a.   Black – non-Hispanic
- b.   Asia/Pacific Islander
- c.   White – non-Hispanic
- d.   Native American/Alaskan
- e.   Hispanic
- f.   Unknown

What is your gender?
- a.   Male
- b.   Female

What is your major?
- a.   Community Health
- b.   Pre–Physical Therapy
- c.   Nursing
- d.   Occupational Therapy

Are you currently employed?
- a.   Yes, Full-time
- b.   Yes, Part-time
- c.   No, Is seeking
- d.   No, Not seeking

Are you currently in graduate school?
    a.   Yes, Full-time
    b.   Yes, Part-time
    c.   No, Is seeking
    d.   No, Not seeking

How satisfied are you with your current job or graduate education?
    a.   Very satisfied
    b.   Satisfied
    c.   Somewhat satisfied
    d.   Somewhat dissatisfied
    e.   Dissatisfied
    f.   Very Dissatisfied
    g.   No response or not applicable

How closely related is your current job or graduate program to your Bachelor's degree major?
    a.   Closely related
    b.   Related
    c.   Unrelated by choice
    d.   Unrelated not by choice

When did you secure your first job following receipt of your Bachelor's degree?
    a.   Had the same job while enrolled
    b.   Secured job by the time of graduation
    c.   Secured job after graduation

Have you enrolled in a college or university since earning your Bachelor's degree?
    a.   Yes, Full-time
    b.   Yes, Part-time
    c.   No

In general, how well did your Bachelor's degree prepare you for your job or graduate school?
    a.   Very well
    b.   Adequately
    c.   Inadequately
    d.   Poorly
    e.   Very Poorly

What is your present attitude toward Chicago State University?
    a.   Strongly positive
    b.   Positive
    c.   Somewhat positive
    d.   Somewhat negative
    e.   Negative
    f.   Strongly negative

In my major degree, professors encouraged me to challenge my own ideas, the ideas of other students and those presented in readings and other course materials.

    a.   Very often
    b.   Often
    c.   Sometimes
    d.   Infrequently
    e.   Never

In my major degree program, professors emphasized that studying and planning was important to my academic success.

    a.   Very often
    b.   Often
    c.   Sometimes
    d.   Infrequently
    e.   Never

Thanks for your willingness to provide us with useful information

Sample Document #4.4: Sample employer satisfaction survey questionnaire

_____ University

Department of _____

Instructions

This survey is sent to you in your capacity as an employer of _____ University graduate. The purpose of this survey is to find out how satisfied you are with our graduates or alumni. Your feedback will allow us to know how well prepared our graduate is for the job, their ability to work with others, attitudes and engagement, and the quality of work. We appreciate your kind participation in this survey. Please provide answers to the following questions:

How well did our graduate meet your expectations in the following areas?

	Exceeds Expectation (3)	*Meets Expectation (2)*	*Nearly Meets Expectation (1)*	*Does Not Meet Expectation (0)*
Mastery of knowledge in the field				
Ability to perform technical skills of the profession				
Ability to communicate effectively with co-workers and/or customers				
Relevancy of graduates' skill and/or knowledge base in relationship to real-world applications within the industry				
Mastery of science, technology, engineering or math skills needed in the field				
Overall preparedness for employment at your company				

Total score: _____

Scoring of survey

Add together the options indicated for the five questions

Interpretation

A total maximum score of 15 and a minimum score of 0 are possible. The overall rating on the questionnaire for each survey participant reflects their overall preparation for the job, ability to work with others, attitudes, engagement and the quality of work. The higher the score, the more competent.

1. How satisfied are you with _____ graduates' performance on the job?
   a. Very Satisfied
   b. Satisfied
   c. Unsatisfied
   d. Very Unsatisfied
2. Would you recommend _____ graduates to another employer?
   a. Yes
   b. Maybe
   c. No
3. Would you hire a _____ graduate again?
   a. Yes
   b. Maybe
   c. No
4. How important are CSU graduates to the overall success of your business?
   a. Very Important
   b. Important
   c. Somewhat Important
   d. Not Important
5. How do _____ University graduates compare to other employees from other institution?
   a. Superior
   b. Same
   c. Less engaged or competent

Sample Document #4.5: Classroom evaluation of teaching effectiveness form

_____ University

College of Health Sciences, Department of Health Studies
Classroom Visitation Form

Evaluation Purpose: Retention   Tenure   Promotion to rank of

Evaluator: Peer   Chairperson   **Course:**

Directions: Please check your response to each criterion. Phrases in parentheses are guidelines for use in evaluating each criterion.

Criteria	Excellent (3)	Good (2)	Satisfactory (1)	Unsatisfactory (0)	NA	Comments
Organization of Class Material (begins and ends on time; follows outline. Introductory and closing statements; theme development; logical sequences, etc.)						
Knowledge of Subject Matter						
Verbal Communication Skills/Skill in Expression (articulation; pronunciation; variation in pitch rate; effective use of pauses; extemporaneous delivery, etc.)						
Nonverbal Communication (eye contact; body and facial expressions, etc.)						
Objectives for the Class (Delineated at the outset of class; met)						

Criteria	Excellent (3)	Good (2)	Satisfactory (1)	Unsatisfactory (0)	NA	Comments
Classroom Climate (Atmosphere; arrangement of room, etc.)						
Use of Media						
Instructor Response to Students (flexibility of instructor; response to questions; encourages student participation, etc.)						

Additional Comments: Score: /24 (maximum possible score)

_____   _____

Name of Peer/Chair Evaluator   Date

Sample Document #4.6: Course evaluation form

You are invited to participate in a survey to determine your experience in the HSC 3445 _____ course that you just recently completed. The survey will take 5–10 mins of your time. Your participation is voluntary, and you have the right to withdraw at any time. We appreciate your kind participation in this survey.

INSTRUCTIONS

Do not put your name or ID on this survey!!! Please answer all questions as honestly as possible. All information collected will be kept confidential by the department. Please tick the option in the rectangular space provided. Please do not guess; instead please tick "Not Applicable." Thank you for your help.

For Official Use Only *(Please leave blank)* CODE: __ __ __ __

Please tick the option in the rectangular space provided. Please do not guess; instead, please tick on a scale of Strongly disagree (1) to Strongly agree (5)

		Strongly disagree (1)	Disagree (2)	Neither (3)	Agree (4)	Strongly agree (5)
1	This course challenged me to learn and developed new skills					
2	This class provided a positive learning environment					
3	I have become more competent/ knowledgeable in this area since taking this course					
4	The lecturer was well prepared to teach his course					
5	The lecturer was genuinely interested in the students' progress					
6	Overall, this lecturer was effective					

Total score: _____

Scoring of survey

Add together the options indicated for the six questions.

Interpretation

A total maximum score of 30 and a minimum score of 0 are possible. The overall rating on the questionnaire for each survey participant reflects the overall teaching effectiveness of the lecturer. The higher the score, the more effective is the lecturer.

5 The evolution of health care education in Nigeria

Introduction

Before 1472, African traditional medicine, which includes herbalists, bonesetters, spiritualists, and surgeons, was the only health care delivery system in Nigeria. The history of medical education in Nigeria began in the 19th century and has continued to evolve. Evolution is "change," and it is one of the most predictable phenomena of life. Change means to alter, to vary, to substitute, and to mutate. Change is a mark of the complexity of life and one fundamental element that binds "evolutionist" and "creationist." The core theory of evolution, "survival of the fittest," typifies "change." The fittest survived because they have undergone a change called "mutation," which confers on them reproductive superiority in a continually changing environment. Therefore, the "fittest" has a "selective advantage" to deal with a changing environment.

There was a time when lecturers would teach how they had learned, with little regard to the students' needs. The world changed when educators like Howard Gardner and others turned education on its head by advocating that educators should adapt how they taught to meet students' varying needs (Robinson, 2020). The third revolution is upon us, disrupting the existing teaching methods by empowering the learner not just through style but also through access. The modus operandi of education has evolved and differs slightly depending on whether you take the view of society, the educator, or the parents.

In the United States, parents initially used education as a child care center as they go to the farm or into the industrial work environment. Educators used to work on set principles that imposed standards and behaviors on children. The future of education now is to inspire students to learn and use their talents. Similarly, society has also influenced the evolution of education. Initially, religious interests drove the school, eventually, it became more about government or political importance; now, it is about competition, ensuring students on the world stage have an advantage. There is no single shaping force that the parents, the educators, and the policymakers are on the same page as to the primary function of the school. This chapter sets out to assess the origin and evolution of the major health care education (HCE) programs in Nigeria.

Methodology

An exhaustive search of the literature on PubMed, CINAHL (Cumulative Index to Nursing and Allied Health Literature), and PsychInfo databases were conducted to shed light on the origin and developmental milestones of the major HCE programs in Nigeria. The search used the keywords "Nigeria," combined with "health care education," "medical education," and "developmental milestones." The searches produced only three "hits," but only one of the three studies was relevant to the stated objectives in this chapter (Balogun and Aka, 2018). Information on the developmental milestones of each profession was obtained from various open access sources to construct the origin and educational activities of each profession presented below.

Results

Medicine and dentistry

The origin of Western medicine in Nigeria occurred after 1914. Medicine and dentistry were the first health occupations to become entranced into the country by the Portuguese allopathic physicians. The history of medical education in Nigeria began in 1862 when Rev. Henry Venn of the Church Missionary Society (CMS) of the United Kingdom conceived the idea of a medical school to train Africans. Subsequently, the same year, Dr. O. Harrison established the first medical school in Abeokuta, but the school was short-lived and closed.

The debut of medical education in Nigeria was at Yaba Higher College in 1934. The College was established to provide two years of premedical and three-year clinical training courses for medical officers (Adeniyi et al., 1998). In 1948, the medical program at Yaba relocated to the University of Ibadan (UI) and affiliated with London University. The first facilities provided at Ibadan within Adeoyo Hospital and the Government Hospital at Jericho were inadequate. Thus, the pioneering medical students completed their clinical education at London University. The federal government constructed a 500-bed at the University College Hospital (UCH) at Ibadan that was completed in 1957. After that, the medical students completed their preclinical and clinical training at UI. The first cohort of UI students graduated in 1960.

By 1955, the eastern region government established the University of Nigeria, Nsukka (UNN), through a legislation enacted by the parliament. The Ford Foundation and Dr. John Hannah, president of Michigan State University (1940–1968), provided the much-needed assistance to the regional government of Dr. Nnamdi Azikiwe to create the first-ever "land-grant" university in Africa. The UNN began classes in 1960, but its medical school did not start until 1970. The first two Vice-Chancellors (VC) for the UNN came from Michigan State University. And before the civil war in 1967, more than 100 Michigan State University personnel were working at UNN at any given semester (Obiorah, 2019).

Subsequently, in 1960, the federal government set up the Ashby commission to evaluate the country's need for higher education. Following its deliberation, the commission recommended the establishment of more universities and medical schools. Also established in 1962 was the College of Medicine at the University of Lagos (CMUL). This development opened the floodgate for the establishment of more medical schools by the regional governments. First, Ahmadu Bello University, Zaria (ABU) was established in 1967, followed by the University of Ife (now OAU) in 1972 and the University of Benin (UNIBEN) in 1973. The five medical programs were referred to as the "first-generation" medical schools. Following the breakup of Nigeria into 12 states in 1967, seven new medical schools, called "second-generation" medical schools, were established at the federal universities located at Jos, Maiduguri, Kano, Sokoto, Ilorin, Calabar, and Port Harcourt. The "third-generation" federal universities of technology, located in Owerri, Makurdi, Yola, Akure, and Bauchi, commenced between the 1980s and early 1990s. Subsequently, other state universities were established in Imo, Ondo, Lagos, Akwa Ibom, Oyo, and Cross River. The "fourth-generation" universities were established between 1991 to date, and they include more state universities and private universities (Ekundayo and Ajayi, 2009).

Postgraduate training in medicine and dentistry

The establishment of the West African College of Surgeons in the early 1960s facilitated collaboration with the Royal College of Surgeons to enroll talented and eager Nigerian physicians/dentists in a structured postgraduate residency training program (Irune, 2018). The majority of the physicians/dentists trained in the United Kingdom returned to Nigeria to complete their higher level of surgical education as consultants. At the time, consultants in all medical specialties were in high demand in the health and education systems.

By the early 1980s, the standards of medical training in Nigeria were considered high enough for new graduates following their junior internship year to transition and work within the British health care system as trainees. This unique opportunity was contingent on a valid certification and satisfactory references. By the mid-1990s, these very advantageous offers were replaced by the mandatory Professional and Linguistic Assessments Board Examinations that evaluate medical knowledge and written English competency before trainees can work within the United Kingdom health care system.

Pharmacy

The first community chemist outlet in the area that later became Nigeria was opened in 1887 by Dr. Richard Zachaeus Bailey along Balogun street in Lagos. It catered primarily for European and few African elites. Other retail pharmacies were established later in the 1920s. They include the West African Drug Company Ltd. established in 1924, Chief S. T. Hunponu-Wusu, and Mr. Robert

Olatunji Adebowale's commercial medicine stores. The Phillips medicine stores (owned by Thomas King Ekundayo Phillips) opened in Lagos in the 1940s.

Following a lull, several retail pharmacies developed in several towns in the western, eastern, and northern regions of the country. By the end of 1960, there were 542 registered pharmacists employed in the 150 community pharmacy shops in the country. Industrial pharmacy evolved with the arrival of May and Baker in 1944 and Glaxo and Pfizer in 1954 – both pharmaceutical companies focused on the importation and marketing of pharmaceuticals. Large-scale drug production began in the 1960s by government agencies, multinational companies, and private entrepreneurs. Presently, there are more than 115 registered pharmaceutical companies in the country.

The history of pharmacy education in Nigeria evolved through six developmental phases. Phases one and two were the training of dispensers through apprenticeship (1887–1923), and through the established Schools of Pharmacy at Yaba and Zaria, respectively. Phase three was the training of chemists and druggists (1927–1972) at the Schools of Pharmacy at Yaba, and Zaria and at the Nigerian College of Arts, Science, and Technology, Ibadan. Phase five was the training of pharmacists at the BSc degree level (1963 to date), and phase six is the pharmacists' training at the doctoral degree (Pharm.D), which started first in 2016 at the UNIBEN. The first Nigerian pharmacist, Mr. Emmanuel Caulcrick, was registered on September 1, 1902, followed in 1919 by Mrs. Ore Green, recorded as the first female pharmacist. Subsequently, as a dispenser, the Timi of Ede registered as a pharmacist and became a physician in 1914. Additionally, Chief Hunponu-Wusu also received his pharmacy diploma in 1922.

From the late 19th century to the early part of the 20th century, pharmacy education in Nigeria started with the training in dispensing through apprenticeship. During that era (i.e., the 1920's), it became apparent that the apprenticeship program could no longer meet the need for pharmacy services. Consequently, through legislation, a School of Pharmacy was established at Yaba, Lagos, in 1925. The majority of the "pharmacists" were "dispensers," and they worked under the medical officers' supervision in the dispensaries and hospitals. As of 1900, there were only four hospitals in the country at Lagos, Asaba, Abeokuta, and Calabar. The government-owned three of the hospitals, and one, a mission (Catholic) hospital, was used as a joint hospital formulary. There were also some mission operated medical "clinics" in some coastal towns. Between 1900 and 1960, there was a steady growth in the number of hospitals owned by the government and mission (Pharmapproach, 2019).

Between 1925 and 1927, a Medical College was founded in Lagos, comprising the Schools of Pharmacy and Medicine under the auspices of Dr. Gordon Taylor, a physician, and one Mr. Arthur, a pharmacist. In 1930, another School of Pharmacy opened up in Zaria. The program graduates earned the chemists and druggists diploma modeled after the British educational system. The admission requirement into the diploma program was the postsecondary certificate obtained from the Nigerian College of Arts, Science and Technology (NCAST), Ibadan, and credits in the relevant science subjects in the Ordinary Level General Certificate of Education (GCE) examination for a five-year course instead of a three-year course.

In 1957, the School of Pharmacy in Lagos was moved to Ibadan as a department in the former NCAST, Ibadan. The NCAST pharmacy program was taken over by OAU in 1962 and continued to award the chemists and druggists diploma and the diploma in pharmacy until June 1965. A degree program in pharmacy commenced at OAU in September 1963 to replace the diploma program, and the first indigenously trained pharmacists with Bachelor of Pharmacy (BPharm. classified) degree graduated in 1966.

The School of Pharmacy in Zaria was also taken over by ABU in 1968 as a three-year BSc in pharmacy. ABU also produced its first cohort of graduate pharmacist in 1973. Subsequently, in 1967, another pharmacy program was established at the UNN and effectively took off in 1970. Also, in 1970, the UNIBEN initiated a degree program in pharmacy. In the 1980s, pharmacy programs were established at the UI, CMUL, and the Federal University of Technology, Makurdi. In 2017, the pharmacy program at the UI closed down for failure to meet the NUC accreditation standards. The Makurdi program was later moved to the University of Jos when the Federal University of Technology changed to the Federal University of Agriculture (Ogaji and Ojabo, 2014). Presently, there are 21 pharmacy programs in the country, and the entry-level education for pharmacists has transitioned to the doctoral level (Pharm.D).

Tracking and overlapping these momentous events were the formation of the Pharmaceutical Society of Nigeria in 1927. After this, a significant lull in activity appeared to have occurred in the field until 1992 when the Pharmacists Council of Nigeria (PCN) was established. This law was Act 91, now reenacted as Act CAP 17, Law of the Federation of Nigeria, 2004. The Council is vested with the responsibility for regulating and controlling all aspects of the profession, including the regulation of pharmacy technicians, patent and proprietary medicine. The Medical and Dental Council of Nigeria (MDCN) and the PCN are continually feuding. For fear of domination, instead of a spirit of collaboration, pharmacy education has, from inception, been implemented as an independent faculty not located within CMUL, ABU, UNN, UNIBEN, and much later at the UI. The first academic pharmacist in Nigeria and black Africa is Professor Cletus Nzebunwa Aguwa.

Physiotherapy

A seminal and insightful address presented in 1999 by Dr. Abayomi Oshin, chronicled the history of physiotherapy in Nigeria (Oshin,1999). The profession was imported to Nigeria in 1945 by two British chartered physiotherapists, Miss Mansfield, and Mr. Williams. They were charged to treat wounded and disabled Nigerian soldiers who returned home from Burma and World War II and to start a training program in physiotherapy. A three-year diploma training program commenced at the Royal (now National) Orthopedic Hospital, Igbobi. The graduates of the program were appointed in the civil service as assistant physiotherapists, and they were supervised by the chartered physiotherapists trained in England. Several of the Igbobi program graduates later proceeded to the United Kingdom for further studies to become chartered physiotherapists. Eventually, the training program at Igbobi was discontinued (Balogun et al., 2017).

In 1966, the first BSc degree program in physiotherapy was established at the UI. Because the program was university-based, Mr. (Dr). Richards, a British orthopedic surgeon at the UCH, was appointed the academic head of the new physiotherapy program instead of Mr. Oshin. At the time, the latter only had a diploma (MCSP) credential. Only one student, Godwin Eni, was admitted into the program in 1966, and he graduated in 1969. The first-degree was awarded to Godwin Eni, and his certificate was issued on June 28, 1969, and was signed by the VC, Professor T. Adeoye Lambo. The following year, in 1970, Alani Egbedeyi graduated, and three other students (Benjamin Akinrolabu, Patrick Ajayi, and E.M. Obasuyi) also graduated in 1971 (Eni, 2011).

In 1971, a diploma program was commenced at the CMUL, and headed by Mr. Gabriel Odia. Due to external pressure from the Nigeria Society of Physiotherapy (NSP), the diploma program was upgraded to a degree program in 1977. In the same year, a BMR-PT degree program was also established at OAU. The UCH/UI and CMUL curricula were patterned after the British model of education. Between 1966 and 1997, the BSc degree programs in physiotherapy were four years in duration. In 1998, the length of training was extended to five years, and replaced by a professional Bachelor of Physiotherapy (BPT) or a BMR-PT degree. Also, a one-year clinical internship was mandated before graduates are licensed to practice.

The "second-generation" physiotherapy education programs were developed between 1985 and 2004 at the UNN; Bayero University, Kano; the University of Maiduguri; and Nnamdi Azikiwe University, Akwa. And between 2013 and 2020, the "third-generation" physiotherapy education programs commenced at the UNIBEN; University of Ilorin (UNILORIN); Bowen University, Iwo; Federal University, Dutse; University of Medical Sciences (UNIMED), Ondo City, and Kaduna State University – the newest program established in 2019. There are currently 13 physiotherapy education programs in Nigeria (Balogun et al., 2018).

The first Master's degree program in physiotherapy was initiated at OAU in 1985, and the only enrolled student was Mrs. Mabogunje. She completed the degree's requirements in 1987. The first PhD degree program in physiotherapy was launched at the UI in 1997. Currently, 6 of the 13 universities offering physiotherapy education programs provide postprofessional (MS and PhD) degrees (Balogun et al., 2016 a & b).

Another significant milestone came in 1988 when the federal government established a regulatory board for medical rehabilitation practitioners.

The regulatory body, christened the Medical Rehabilitation Therapists' Board of Nigeria (MRTBN), was not constituted until 1992. It was constituted as an amalgam of several professions - physiotherapy, chiropractic, occupational therapy, osteopathy, and speech therapy - to the dismay and disappointment of many physiotherapists in Nigeria and in the diaspora, who expected a regulatory board solely for physiotherapy.

In 2012, the NSP inaugurated the National Postgraduate Physiotherapy College of Nigeria (NPPCN) to train clinical specialists in eight domains of physiotherapy. In 2016, the Nigerian National Assembly considered a bill to create and fully fund the operations of the College, but the bill did not pass (Balogun, 2016). The entry-level education for physiotherapy practice is in the transition to a doctoral degree level. The yearning for entry-level doctoral training in physiotherapy was realized in 2018 when the NUC granted its approval. The first Doctor of Physiotherapy (DPT) program in the country was established in 2020 at Kaduna State University, College of Medicine.

Occupational therapy

Occupational therapy was imported into Nigeria by two British chartered occupational therapists in the early 1950s at the UCH, Ibadan, and in 1965 the Nigerian Association of Occupational Therapists was formed. The aftermath effect of the Nigerian civil war from 1967–1970 brought about an increase in demand for occupational therapy services. The need was met by an increased inflow of occupational therapists into the country from around the world to provide services in the military clinics and a few civilian hospitals.

Before the debut of an occupational therapy training program, the few Nigerians who obtained their credentials abroad returned home to form the Nigerian Association of Occupational Therapists and registered the organization with the Occupational Therapy African Regional Group and World Federation of Occupational Therapy in 2001 and 1992, respectively. In 2002, OAU established the first BMR in occupational therapy, and a year later, in 2003, the Federal School of Occupational Therapy at Oshodi, Lagos, was launched to train occupational therapy assistants. Within 12 years, OAU produced 20 occupational therapists, and the Federal School of Occupational Therapy graduated 109 occupational therapist assistants (Olaoye et al., 2016). In 2017, the UNIMED Senate approved a BSc degree program in occupational therapy, and two years later, the first cohort of students enrolled. To date, OAU and UNIMED are the only universities in sub-Sahara Africa (excluding South Africa) offering a degree program in occupational therapy.

Between 1952 and 1999, Nigerians health care professionals who trained abroad, formed professional associations, and contributed to the development of HCE programs. In 1958, a professional association was established for radiographers, followed by nutritionists in 1963, prosthetics and orthopedic technologists in 1967, optometry in 1968, biomedical engineers/technologists in 1999, and dietitians in 2009.

Speech therapy (speech-language pathology and audiology)

Professor Clement Ayodele Bakare of the Department of Special Education at the UI in 1987 established the Speech Pathologists and Audiologists Association in Nigeria (SPAAN). The Association maintains oversight on the educational programs and ensuring ethical standards in the practice of speech pathology and audiology. Membership is open to academics and clinicians in Ear, Nose, and Throat departments in private or governmental institutions. The Association is the Nigerian equivalent of the Worldwide Association of Professionals in Speech and Hearing Rehabilitation. The Association is registered under the Nigerian Corporate Affairs Commission, and the Federal Ministry of Health, and is an affiliate of the MRTBN.

The qualification required for full membership of SPAAN is a Master's degree or equivalent in speech pathology and audiology, and one-year internship experience in an approved hospital/clinic and pass the requisite clinical competence examination. Associate members have a BSc degree in other allied professions with related practice experience in speech/language and hearing such as psychology, otolaryngology, counselors, social workers (Speech Pathologists and Audiologists Association in Nigeria, 2020). Although the MRTBN legally recognizes speech pathology and audiology, there is currently limited relevant information on hearing health care in the country. Presently, there is only one audiologist to one million Nigerians (Oyiborhoro, 1988; Wikimedia Foundation, 2019).

Radiography

The first School of Radiography started in Lagos, and it instructed x-ray assistants for the whole country. By 1957, it has graduated a total of ten radiographers: five from the west, three from the east, and two from the northern regions of the country. In 1957, the Orthopedic Hospital in Igbobi, Lagos, trained six assistant physiotherapists.

The Association of Radiographers of Nigeria (ARN) was formed in 1958 at the Adeoyo Hospital, Ibadan, and became a foundation member of the International Society of Radiographers and Radiological Technologists in 1961. It was not until 1987 that the federal government approved the establishment of the Radiographers Registration Board of Nigeria (RRBN) to regulate the profession's practice. The first-degree program in radiography was established in 1982 at the University of Calabar, followed by the UNN in 1983 (Sule, 2017; Radiographers Registration Board of Nigeria, 2017).

Medical laboratory science

In the early 1950s, Lagos Hospital and Kano Hospital were the only centers that trained laboratory technicians. By 1954, 29 had graduated from Lagos and two from Kano. In July 1971, the late Mr. AY Eke, then Federal Commissioner of Education, proposed establishing a professional association for Science Laboratory Technologists. His proposal materialized on March 25, 1972, as the Nigerian Institute of Science Technology based in Ibadan, the forerunner of the present regulatory body, Nigeria Institute of Science Laboratory Technology, which was enacted in 2003 to regulate the practice of science laboratory. The Council for the new Institute was formally inaugurated on May 27, 2004 and charged with the core mandate to advance the science laboratory technology profession.

A legislation was enacted by the federal government on June 23, 2003, to repeal the laws that established the Institute of Medical Laboratory Technology Act, Cap. 114 of the Federation of Nigeria. The Act also created the Medical Laboratory Science Council of Nigeria. The Council is empowered to regulate the education for persons seeking to become medical laboratory scientists ("scientists"), medical laboratory technicians ("technicians"), and medical laboratory assistants ("assistants") in this legislation (LawNigeria.Com, 2017b). Presently, the Nigerian Institute of Science Laboratory Technology as a professional regulatory agency of government ensures that all persons practicing or aspiring to become practitioners of the science laboratory technology profession are registered and licensed by the Institute after the acquisition of the relevant skills, including the appropriate level of exposure to equipment, and practical experience (Association of Science Laboratory Technologists of Nigeria, 2012).

Veterinary medicine

Veterinary medicine has its origin in France with the establishment of the first veterinary school at Lyon in 1762. The occupation was imported into Nigeria in 1901 by the British colonial government with the appointment of the first veterinary officer. In 1913 a Veterinary Department was established in Zaria, and by 1924 the Federal Department of Veterinary Research (now National Veterinary Research Institute) was established at Vom to combat the devastating death of livestock. Until 1954, the Federal Department of Veterinary Research provided only veterinary services in Nigeria, and it became the responsibilities of the regional governments (Garba et al., 2011).

The Agricultural Research Institute Decree of 1975 changed the name of the Federal Department of Veterinary Research to National Veterinary Research Institute. The establishment of the Nigerian Veterinary Department in 1913 was later backed up by the diseases of Animal Ordinance in 1917, Veterinary Ordinance of 1952, Veterinary Council of Nigeria Professional Regulatory Board in 1958, Veterinary Surgeons Act (Decree 37) of 1969, Veterinary Ethics (first edition) in 1985, Veterinary Surgeons Amendment Act (Decree 40) of 1987 and the Animal Diseases Decree (No. 10) of 1988. In between these laws, various veterinary related laws exist, which were promulgated by the then Central/Regional governments.

By 1927 only 11 veterinary officers were in Nigeria, all British nationals, and employed mainly in the northern province. Capt. WW Henderson was the acting chief veterinary officer. The only Nigerian in government service at the time was Mr. SA Shonekan, a laboratory storekeeper. By 1928, the veterinary officers in charge of immunization camps trained "native administration veterinary Malams" to diagnose animal diseases and inoculate livestock.

The first veterinary school was established in Kano in 1934 to train veterinary assistants. By 1941 another school was launched at Vom to offer a three-year assistant veterinary officers' program with ten students. The first-degree awarding veterinary school was at the UI in 1963, followed by ABU in 1964, the UNN in 1970, and the University of Maiduguri in 1980. Subsequently, in 1984, Usman Dan Fodio University, Sokoto, was opened, followed by the University of Agriculture, Makurdi, in 2001 and the University of Agriculture, Abeokuta, in 2004. Additional educational programs were subsequently developed (Garba et al., 2011).

The Veterinary Council of Nigeria was enacted in 1952 and amended in 1958 to constitute a board of examiners to regulate professional qualifications and training. The first meeting of the Council was held on April 9, 1953, and chaired by Mr. RS Marshall with Mr. SG Wilson as the Governors nominee. Others in attendance were Mr. FD Jakeway, Mr. JKA Wilde, and Dr. HD Hill, from UCH. At this inaugural meeting, Mr. GHV Blyth was appointed the first registrar of the Council (Garba et al., 2011).

The Nigerian Veterinary Medical Association (NVMA) was formed in 1967 as a follow up to the biannual conference held by the predominantly British veterinary officers, and licentiates started as far back as 1932. The Association represents all veterinary surgeons registered with the Veterinary Council of Nigeria. It is a corporate body registered with the Corporate Affairs Commission of Nigeria in 1996. The officers are vested with responsibility for the day-to-day running of the Association ((NVMA, 2018).

Presently, 12 veterinary schools are offering the entry-level Doctor of Veterinary Medicine (DVM) degree program and have trained veterinarians for the country and other neighboring African countries, such as Cameroun, Niger, and Chad. The DVM program is presently offered at the UI, ABU, UNN, the University of Maiduguri, Usman Dan Fodio University, University of Agriculture, Makurdi, University of Agriculture, Abeokuta, Michael Okpara University of Agriculture, Umudike, University of Abuja, Federal University Agriculture, Abeokuta, Federal University of Agriculture, Makurdi; and UNILORIN (NVMA, 2018).

There are educational opportunities in the country for postgraduate (MS and PhD) degrees in the various specialties of veterinary medicine - Veterinary Anatomy, Veterinary Medicine, Veterinary Microbiology, Veterinary Pathology, Veterinary Parasitology and Entomology, Veterinary Pharmacology and Toxicology, Veterinary Surgery and Radiology, Veterinary Physiology and Biochemistry, Veterinary Public Health and Preventive Medicine. Both the NUC and the Veterinary Council of Nigeria regulates the undergraduate and graduate academic programs.

Optometry

In 1968, the Association of Optical Practitioners was formed by Nigerians who trained abroad. The organization's name was changed later to the Nigerian Optometric Association. The members lobbied for a regulatory body, and the federal government granted it in 1989 (Decree No 34 for Optometry and Dispensing Optics). The board was signed into law by the military regime under General Ibrahim Babangida administration when Prince Bola Ajibola was Attorney General/Minister of Justice and Professor Olikoye Ransome-Kuti, the Minister of Health. Before the decree, the profession was practiced by self-styled practitioners, charlatans (indigenous and foreign), in conjunction with individuals with credible credentials obtained from international and Nigerian universities.

The regulatory body for optometry and dispensing optics was announced in 1989, but the board was not formed until October 16, 1992. For three years, there was no organ of government to operate the provisions of the law. A physician chaired the first appointed board with 14 other members in attendance - Dr. Efe Odjimogho (orthoptist), Dr. Sam Ntem (optometrist), Dr. Frank Kio (optometrist), Dr. Solo Adeniyi (dispensing optician), Dr. B Nworah (ophthalmologist), Dr. Eric Bassey (optometrist), Dr. Joe Owie (Optometrist), Dr. MA Awe (represented Federal Ministry of Health - FMH), Dr. Goodluck Achoja (optometrist), Professor Adenike Abiose (ophthalmologist), Professor M. Majekodunmi (ophthalmologist), Mr. Ben Nwokedi (representing public interest), Dr. ED Ikonne (optometrist), and Dr. Ronald Eyime (optometrist, Registrar and Secretary to the Board).

The appointment of a physician to chair the first board (instead of a qualified optometrist) was a source of anger and dissatisfaction among optometrists. Many expressed no confidence in the board. The decision, in a way, undermined the credibility and fairness of the health minister. No one would better represent the interest of optometrists than optometrists themselves. That board was short-lived, barely existing for two years before the military adventurism of General Abacha, who dissolved all government boards and appointed sole administrators who served for seven long years until the return to civilian rule in 1999. On December 18, 2000, a new committee was inaugurated and chaired by Professor Paul Oghuehi, an optometrist.

Nursing and midwifery

A few years following the establishment of the Nursing Council of Nigeria in 1947, three Schools of Nursing opened in Lagos, Kano, and Aba. The nursing Preliminary Training School in Lagos later transferred to Ibadan. The Schools of Nursing in the south (Ibadan and Aba) had only a 6-month training program. In contrast, the school in the north (Kano) had two types of training programs: one training program admitted students with lesser qualifications and lasted for one year. The other training program lasted six months and opened for students with higher requisite education. By 1954, 23 trainees, all of them men, graduated from the Kano School - 40 (16 women and 24 men) graduated from Aba, and 71 (42 women and 29 men) graduated from Ibadan (Scott-Emuakpor, 2010).

The duration of training for nurses was extended to three years to increase their knowledge base and clinical skills. Several schools of nursing at designated government hospitals were established: seven in the north, six in the east, and eight in the west. Also, the Nursing Council approved 17 private (church-related) Schools of Nursing to train full-fledged and part-time nurses. By 1955, 100 female student nurses enrolled in the British-type nursing education at the UCH, Ibadan.

During that era, there were two cadres of midwifery schools - Grade I and Grade II. Grade II has a lower entry qualification requirement and shorter duration of training. Grade I midwives trained in designated government centers. By 1954, 12 women graduated from the School of Midwifery in Kaduna, 23 from the School of Midwifery in Aba, ten women from the School of Midwifery in Calabar, and 20 women from both the School of Midwifery in Lagos and Adeoyo Hospital, Ibadan. Grade II midwives trained in the private-owned (church-related) hospitals or native authority (equivalent of the present-day local government area) facilities. The midwives were employed primarily in rural areas.

By 1954, five Grade II midwives trained in Kaduna, 21 in Aba and Calabar, and 103 in Lagos and Ibadan (Scott-Emuakpor, 2010). Nurses who are interested in training as clinical specialists can now obtain fellowship by examination through the West African College of Nursing. There are five major specialty areas in nursing. First is the medical-surgical nursing, with three options (critical nursing – accident and emergency – intensive care, perioperative nursing, special care babies nursing; palliative nursing option (terminally ill–HIV/AIDS, cancers, etc.), and the rehabilitation, and adult nursing (noncommunicable diseases) options. The second and third nursing specialties are reproductive health and mental health/psychiatric, respectively. The fourth specialty is community health Nursing, and the fifth is administration, management, and education (West African College of Nursing, 2008). The National Association of Nigeria Nurses and Midwives has urged the federal government to establish the National Post Graduate College of Nursing to enhance the training of the high-level workforce in the nursing profession (Makinde, 2016).

Several universities in Nigeria now offer postgraduate (Master's and PhD) degree programs in nursing. They include the University of Calabar, UNN, UNIBEN, Niger Delta University, Nnamdi Azikiwe University, UI, OAU, Babcock University, and ABU. It is pertinent to note that not all these universities offer all the nursing specialties (Nurses Arena Forum, 2016).

Medical records

In Nigeria, there are two categories of medical/health records education (certificate and the diploma) offered in the School of Health Technology. The certificate program, which is a two-year, full-time study track, is designed for West Africa School Certificate (WASC) holders without the qualifications required for the diploma program. The National Diploma (ND) option in medical record/health record/health information is a two-year, full-time program designed for WASC holders with credit passes in English language, mathematics, biology, and two other subjects.

There are many entry-level qualifications accepted for registration with the Health Record Officers Registration Board of Nigeria: diploma of the Health Records Officers' Registration Board of Nigeria, a degree, Higher National Diploma (HND) or diploma in health studies, diploma in medical records, a certificate in medical records from the United Kingdom, or diploma in health statistics. The Health Record Officers Registration Board of Nigeria tasked with the responsibility of monitoring the standards of knowledge also conducts examinations in health records management, and award certificates or diplomas to successful candidates.

Nutrition

The Nutrition Society of Nigeria, a nonprofit and nongovernmental organization founded in 1963 at the UI, is the sole and largest stakeholder for the nutrition profession in Nigeria. Membership in the association is diverse and represents several disciplines such as nutrition, agriculture, physiology, medicine, food science and technology, social science, home economics, and education. The Society is a member of the International Union of Nutritional Sciences and strives to integrate nutrition science into practical solutions for healthy living. The College of Education at the UI offers graduate (MS and PhD) degree programs in nutrition (Nutrition Society of Nigeria, 2017).

Dietetics

The entry-level education for dietitians is a BSc degree and diploma certification for dietetic technologists (sub-professional) cadres with supervised internship experience in a facility recognized by the federal government. The Dietitians Association of Nigeria is an offshoot of the Nigerian Dietetic Association that registered with the Corporate Affairs Commission and formally inaugurated on March 19, 2009. It is a national association for professional dietitians and dietetic technologists (sub-professional). The Dietitians Association of Nigeria is a member of the International Confederation of Dietetic Associations, incorporated in Canada.

The association in 2017 has only 250 registered members (Dietitians Association of Nigeria, 2017) and is striving to obtain approval from the federal government to establish the Dietitians Registration Council to regulate the professional training and practice. The Dietitians Association of Nigeria advocates for dietitians and provide a quality assurance program for accredited dietetics education programs, and dietetic internship (International Confederation of Dietetic Association, 2010).

Biomedical engineering

In 1969, a School of Biomedical Engineering was established in Zaria as an "on-the-job" training program to repair and maintain medical equipment within ABU Teaching Hospital and six northern states of Kano, Kaduna, Katsina, Kebbi, Sokoto, and Maiduguri. Biomedical engineering activities started in the 1970s when interprofessional collaborations evolved among engineers, physicians/dentists, pharmacists, and physicists. The establishment of the Nigerian Institute for Biomedical Engineering (NIBE) in 1999, which is the professional organization for biomedical engineers, further fostered the progress of biomedical engineering activities in Nigeria. The profession was also given a significant boost in 2007, when the Federal University of Technology, Owerri established the first undergraduate program and later offered MSc and PhD degree programs. Also, in 2016, the UNILORIN graduated its first cohort of BSc degree students in biomedical engineering. Six universities offer a degree program, while five other institutions provide certificate and diploma programs in biomedical engineering.

The College of Biomedical Engineering and Technology was established in 2009 by the General Assembly of the NIBE at its 10th annual general meeting to take over the scholarship functions. The five Faculties of the College are biological engineering and technology/bioengineering/biotechnology, medical engineering and technology, clinical engineering and technology, rehabilitation engineering and orthopedic technology, and biomedical physics and allied sciences. The College of Biomedical Engineering and Technology currently conducts professional and certification examinations. The professional examination includes a dissertation leading to the award of the prestigious fellowship of the College of Biomedical Engineering and Technology (FCBET) and other diploma and certificate credentials.

The over 5,000 members of the NIBE are mostly drawn from the related science and classical engineering disciplines of members employed at the universities and hospitals as well as from other institutions/organizations (NIBE, 2015). The profession is structured into five divisions: biological engineering, medical engineering, clinical engineering, rehabilitation engineering, and biomedical physics /allied sciences, to accommodate virtually every field in the sciences. In 2003, the NIBE was admitted as the 50th member of the International Federation for Medical and Biological Engineering, and the same year, the NIBE co-founded the African Union of Biomedical Engineering and Sciences while some of the members were on a Medical Equipment Training course in Ghana (Nkuma-Udah et al., 2005).

Prosthetic and orthotic

The Association of Prosthetic and Orthopedic Technologists was formed in 1967 by Nigerian prosthetics and orthopedic technologists who trained abroad. The association changed its name in 2011 to the Nigerian Prosthetic, Orthotic, and Orthopedic Technology Society (NPOOTS). At the inaugural meeting of the NPOOTS, the general assembly nominated the following national officers: Onwukamuche Chikwado Kingsley (President), Ohia Happiness Chidaka (Vice President), Emesurumonye Ugochukwu (Secretary), Cajetan Nwaiwu (Financial Secretary), Igbokwe Ifeabunike Sunday (Public Relations Officer), and Ezekaka Perpetua Oluoma (Treasurer). As of 2017, the number of registered members of NPOOTS has increased from nine people registered at the first meeting to about 100 and growing (NPOOTS, n.d.).

By 2010, there are less than ten qualified prosthetist and orthopedic technologists in the country. Given the shortage, the federal government proposed to establish training schools in the three National Orthopedic Hospital in Lagos, Kano, and Enugu, but only the one in Lagos was commissioned in 2008. It awards the ND and HND degrees in prosthetist and orthopedic technology (ISPO, 2020).

Clinical psychology

Clinical psychology as an academic discipline is a product of Western Europe. It became an independent occupation in 1879 when Wilhelm Wundt, the doyen of the profession, opened an experimental laboratory at the University of Leipzig, Germany, to investigate the nature of human consciousness. It took 85 years following the debut of the occupation in Western Europe before it was introduced in the higher education system in 1964 at the UNN by Professor Carl Frost. The first home-trained Nigerian psychologists graduated in 1967. By 1969, the CMUL established a full-fledged Department of Psychology to replace the unit that had been in existence since 1966 with the appointment of Professor Alastair Charles Mundy-Castle.

In 1976, Professor MH Zaidi, a London-trained Pakistani national, established another department at the University of Jos. By the end of the 1970s, new psychology departments were created at the UI by Professor DCE Ugwegbu in 1977, and at OAU by Professor AA Olowu in 1978. By 1990, there were ten departments of psychology in universities across the country (Ojiji, 2015).

In the early years, Western Europeans dominated the profession in Nigeria. The economic decline of the mid-1980s negatively impacted the development of the discipline as the country became an unattractive destination for foreigners and Western-trained Nigerian psychologists. Many of the expatriates employed in the country left as soon as their contracts expired, thereby creating a leadership vacuum that was taken up by Nigerian psychologists who mostly received their training in Western nations – Drs. Chris Onwuzurike, Amechi Nweze, Isidore S. Obot, EU Egwu, Frank Eyetsimitan, and James Gire in Jos; AF Uzoka, Isidore Eyo, ON Osuji, Emeka Okpara, BN Ezeilo, and JO Ozioko. By the end of 1990, psychologists educated in Nigeria have led all the departments of psychology in the universities and led the Nigerian Psychological Association (Ojiji, 2015).

The Nigerian Psychological Association (NPA), formed in 1984, represents the "first generation" of indigenous psychologists. The NPA, which is the highest body representing psychologists in the country, is currently registered with the Corporate Affairs Commission. The association operates as a nongovernmental organization without legal backing and unable to sanction its members nor regulate the education and practice of the profession in the country. Most psychology departments in the country do not have laboratories and even those that have one, lack the required equipment for instruction and research (Ojiji, 2015).

Ondo State University in Ado-Ekiti (now Ekiti State University) became the first state university to establish a psychology department in 1986. Subsequently, other states (Ekiti, Imo, Enugu, Benue, Ebonyi, Anambra, Ondo, Delta, and Nasarawa) followed. Also, five private universities (Madonna, Renaissance, Godfrey Okoye, Redeemer, and Covenant) have established a psychology department. The Nigeria Defense Academy, Kaduna, and the Police Academy, Kano, and the new Federal Universities in Yobe, have initiated a psychology program. Over 30 departments of psychology now exist in the country (Ojiji, 2015).

Public and environmental health

In Nigeria, the origin of environmental health dates back to the 18th century when the colonial government introduced the sanitary inspectors to the colony of Lagos to control the breeding of mosquitoes, which was a major killer of colonial settlers. In 1913, the senior municipal sanitary officer was appointed as a member of the legislative council on the amalgamation of both the southern and northern protectorates of Nigeria (Environmental Health Officers Registration Council of Nigeria, 2015). Environmental health services and training started in the 1920s, following the arrival of Dr. Isaac Ladipo Oluwole from Britain, where he trained as a public health physician. As the first African medical officer of health in the Lagos colony, he established the School Health Services for sanitary attendants. He also created the first Nigerian School of Hygiene at Yaba, Lagos, in 1920 (now School of Health Technology), where qualified persons from all over Nigeria were trained as sanitary inspectors awarded the Royal Society of Health Diploma. Sanitary inspectors' work was significantly recognized during the outbreak of bubonic plague in 1924 when Dr. Oluwole revitalized Port Health Services and sanitary inspection of ships and port premises. Their impact was much felt during the control of the yaws of 1930 and the smallpox of the 1970s. The development of environmental health has continued to increase regarding the number of practitioners trained and some schools educating the practitioners (Environmental Health Officers Registration Council of Nigeria, 2015).

In 1933, the Field Unit School located at Makurdi (in the Benue river in the north) was established to train sleeping sickness assistants. The school was later upgraded to train medical field unit assistants for the entire country. A six-month program was established at the Oji river settlement in the east to train leprosy inspectors and attendants. By 1954, four leprosy inspectors and 21 leprosy attendants were trained. The only institution for training dispensary attendants was in the north (Kano and Zaria). When the training of public health attendants (sanitary inspectors) and dispensary attendants was discontinued, in 1957, a similar training school was later established at the UCH, Ibadan. Although sleeping sickness is still a significant problem in many parts of the country, the training of sleeping sickness assistants has been eliminated. In the early 1950s, four Schools of Hygiene were established across the country to train public health attendants (known then as sanitary inspectors). The Lagos town council public health department operated one of the School of Hygiene and graduated only four sanitarians in 1954. The federal government-owned the other schools in Kano, Aba, and Ibadan, and they graduated 128 sanitarians (Scott-Emuakpor, 2010).

Environmental health remained unregulated until 2002 when the federal government recognized it with the enactment of the environmental health officers (Registration, etc.) Act 11 of 2002. The law established a Council charged with responsibility for regulating the standards of knowledge and skill of members and providing certificate or diploma education in environmental health. The professionalization of ecological health is retarded because of the dominant and superiority influence exerted by the medical profession, which annexed the occupation as part of clinical practice, even though the World Health Organization recognized environmental health as a distinct prevention–oriented discipline.

The duration of training as an environmental health officer is four years in the School of Health Technology or School of Hygiene or university, followed by a one–year compulsory practical internship. Following the training, the student is qualified to take the professional examination conducted previously by the Royal Society of Health, London, or the HND awarded by the West Africa Health Examination Board, a body approved by the National Board for Technical Education (Garba, 2004; Environmental Health Officers Registration Council of Nigeria, 2015). Recently, the Environmental Health Officers Registration Council of Nigeria (EHORECON), and the Federal Ministry of Environment in collaboration with UNICEF developed a degree program in environmental health (BSc/BTech). The degree program is presently offered at the Federal University of Technology Owerri and University of Ilorin (https://www. blogger.com/profile/11306623184660676106 Mohammed, 2011).

Chartered chemist

The Institute of Chartered Chemists of Nigeria (ICCON), a parastatal of the FMH, was created by Decree 91 of 1993 (now ICCON ACT CAP 1.12 LFN 2004) and charged with responsibility for regulating the teaching and practice of chemistry. The agitation of Nigerian chemists to get chartered dates back to the early 1980s, and finally bore fruit in 1993 when Decree 91 was signed into law by General Ibrahim Babangida. ICCON has over 2,400 members from different spheres of chemistry practice. The late President Umaru Musa Yar'Adua was inducted into the fellowship of the Institute on May 13, 2008 (Institute of Chartered Chemists of Nigeria, 2017).

Dental therapy

The roots of dental therapy in Nigeria dates back to the precolonial era. The poor oral hygiene and lack of proper nutrition in the early fifties caused the high incidence of periodontal diseases, which led to an increase in the awareness of the need for preventive measures. In 1958, a team of dentists from the United Kingdom led by Miss Vera Mary Creaton came to Lagos and started to train dental hygienists. The training school later morphed into the Federal School of Dental Technology and Therapy and relocated to Enugu. And in 1961, the Federal School of Dental Technology and Therapy was granted an initial 10-year full accreditation by a credentialing team from Britain led by Sir Williams Kesley Fry. Subsequently, the certification was renewed every ten years.

In 1986, the Nigerian Dental Therapists Association drew the attention of the FMH to establish a regulatory body for dental therapy and dental surgical assistants. The Dental Therapists Registration Board of Nigeria was promulgated on August 25, 1993, by Decree 81, and charged with responsibility for regulating and controlling the training and practice of dental therapy and dental surgical assistants. Successful completion of the dental therapy course and one-year internship program results in the award of the HND/BSc/(B. DTh) credential.

Public analysis

Determination of the composition of drugs, food, and chemicals are of vital public health concerns for government regulatory bodies, such as the National Agency for Food, Drug Administration and Control (NAFDAC), and Environmental Protection Agency (EPA). The Institute of Public Analysts of Nigeria (IPAN) is a parastatal under the FMH. It was established in 2004 by IPAN Act CAPI16 LFN (formerly Decree No 100 of 1992), as a professional regulatory body with mandates to train, examine, and regulate the practice of public analysts and analytical laboratories in Nigeria.

The entry-level qualification for registration as a student member is a BSc degree or HND in pharmacy, biochemistry, chemical engineering, food science and technology/engineering, microbiology, chemistry, industrial chemistry, and science laboratory technology. The applicant must have a minimum of five ordinary level credits in the GCE/WASC, including the English language and mathematics.

Social work

The Nigeria Association of Social Workers was established in 1975 and was recognized in 1976 by the International Federation of Social Workers. As of 2019, 4,000 practitioners are registered with the Nigeria Association of Social Workers. The organization operated as a professional body registered with the federal government as a nonprofit organization concerned with training, negotiation of salaries/conditions of service, and protection of its members.

The Institute of Social Work of Nigeria, based in Lagos, is the professional educational center established to certify social work professionals. The Institute is duly registered and approved by the office of the attorney general of the federation as a legal professional organization under CAP 59 of 1990. The Federal Ministry of Education also recognizes the Institute for training and certification in core social work practice disciplines. Besides, the Institute develops capacity, consults, and offers a broad range of social work services and care. It provides critical professional practices as well as an educational platform for addressing emerging social work issues in all ramifications.

The Institute also collaborates with educational organizations and research centers to foster efficient and productive social work practice. The Institute membership is conferred upon passing the social work proficiency certificate examination. The College of Social Work, the training arm of the Institute, offers a ND and HND and a postgraduate diploma in social work. It also provides professional Master's (MSW) and Doctor of Social Work degrees (ISOWN, 2019).

Health occupation (vocational) careers in Nigeria

Auxiliary health care workers (HCWs) are critically needed in the health care system because of the limited recourses and shortage of professionals that provide access to health care services. Auxiliary HCWs do not require a university degree or extensive education. Their duration of training is relatively short, leading to a certificate or diploma credentials. Within the health care system, they serve in supportive roles, usually under the supervision of the professionals regulating the discipline.

In Nigeria, there are several auxiliary HCWs within the health care system. Those recognized by the federal government are dental technologists/assistants, pharmacy technicians, medical laboratory technicians/assistants, occupational therapy assistants, physiotherapy aides and assistants, medical (health) records officers, and community health officers. Table 5.1 presents their entry-level education, year of training, and professional regulatory boards.

The training of the occupation (vocational) careers within the health care system in Nigeria is discussed below.

Training of nurses

The entry-level training of nurses and midwives occur at several institutions accredited by the Nursing and Midwifery Council of Nigeria. Nationwide, there are 90 certified Schools of Nursing, 47 School of Basic Midwifery, 37 School of Post Basic Midwifery, 52 School of Post Basic Nursing, 28 Department of Nursing (BSN), and eight Community Midwifery Programs distributed unevenly across the country. Admission to the Schools of Nursing and Midwifery is limited to 50 students per cohort, to maintain a high-quality standard (Nursing and Midwifery Council of Nigeria, 2019; Labiran et al., 2008).

Table 5.1 Auxiliary health workers, their entry-level education, year of training and professional regulatory boards

Serial #	Auxiliary workers	Entry-level credential	Years of training	Name of professional regulatory boards
1	Dental technologists/ assistants	HND/OD	3	The Dental Therapists Registration Board of Nigeria
2	Pharmacy technicians	Diploma/on-the-job training	3	Pharmacists Council of Nigeria
3	Medical laboratories technicians/ assistants	Diploma/on-the-job training	3	Medical Laboratory Science Council of Nigeria
4	Occupational therapy assistants	OD	3	Medical Rehabilitation Therapist Board
5	Physiotherapy aides and assistants	Certificate	2	None
6	Medical (health) records officers	OD, HND	3	Health Record Officers Registration Board of Nigeria,
7	Community health officers	OD, HND	3	The Community Health Practitioners Registration Board of Nigeria

Source: The Health Workforce Profile for Nigeria, 2008.

Training of pharmacy technician

There are 21 accredited schools/colleges of health technology, where the pharmacy technicians are trained and certified by the PCN (PCN, 2020).

Training of medical/health records

The Health Records Officers Registration Board certifies the educational program of the two categories (certificate and diploma) of medical/health records personnel trained. Nationwide, there are 19 accredited schools of health information management programs, and 87 schools of health technology (Health Records Officers Regulation Board of Nigeria, 2020).

Training of dental technologists and therapists

The dental technologists and therapists' training is regulated by the Dental Therapists Registration Board of Nigeria. There are three accredited dental technology and 21 dental therapy training institutions in the country (Dental Therapists Registration Board of Nigeria, 2020; Olabanji, 2020).

Training of community health care practitioners

Community health care practitioners (CHCP) were introduced in 1978 by the minister of health, Professor Ransome-Kuti, with the primary purpose of meeting the health care needs in rural areas. CHCP comprise of community health officers, community health supervisors (training stopped in 1990), community health assistants (renamed community health extension workers), and community health aides (renamed junior community health extension workers). CHCP remained the core occupation in the Nigerian primary health care system (Ibama et al., 2015). The Community Health Practitioners Registration Board of Nigeria was established on November 24, 1992, by President Ibrahim Babangida, and formally constituted in December 2000. The Board regulates the training and practice of CHCP as specified by the FMH parastatal decree 61 of 1992 (LFN CAP C19 DF 2004).

There are 14 institutions accredited for training community health officers and 43 for community health extension workers. Since the inception of the training program, over 200,000 CHCP have been produced. Health care delivery by CHCP is Nigeria's unique and impactful contribution to the global health care system (Ibama and Dennis, 2016; Uzondu et al., 2015).

Distribution of auxiliary health care workers

There is an uneven distribution of auxiliary HCWs within the health care system. The majority of the ancillary HCWs are employed in the southern region. For instance, over 30% of the environmental and public health workers, dental technologists and therapists, and pharmacy technicians are from the southwest region of the country (Table 5.2).

The number of nurses in Nigeria is five times more than physicians. All HCWs are concentrated mostly in the urban centers and the southern regions of the country. Many rural health centers, particularly in the northern states, are run by nurses (Scott-Emuakpor, 2010). In addressing the apparent disparities in the distribution of the auxiliary HCWs, President Olusegun Obasanjo's administration mandated nurses and midwives to spend one year in rural areas before they are registered with the Nursing and Midwifery Council of Nigeria. This requirement emanated from the recommendation of a committee constituted by his administration to investigate how to reduce the maternal mortality rate in the country. There is gender inequity within the auxiliary health care workforce (Table 5.3).

HCWs in dental technology, medical records, environmental health, chartered chemistry, and public analysis are predominately males. On the other hand, nursing, midwifery, and community health are female-dominated. Women make up 95% of nurses, 100% of midwives, and 59% of community health officers (Labiran et al., 2008).

Table 5.2 The distribution of auxiliary health care workforce by region

Serial #	Health profession	N	Northcentral %	Northeast %	Northwest %	Southeast %	South %	Southwest %
1	Nurses	128,918	16.4	11.7	13.5	15.3	27.8	15.4
2	Environmental and public health workers	4,280	9.4	11.3	18.9	12.4	15.7	32.1
3	Medical records officers	1,187	13.3	4.9	11.6	14.6	29.9	26.0
4	Dental technologists	505	14.1	5.9	5.9	13.0	16.6	44.5
5	Dental therapists	1,102	13.2	10.3	21.9	10.2	13.0	31.5
6	Pharmacy technician	5,483	6.2	9.1	18.0	8.6	11.8	46.0

Table 5.3 Gender distribution of the auxiliary health care workforce

Serial #	Occupation	N	% Female
1	Nurses	128,918	94.6
2	Midwives	90,489	100.0
3	Dental technologists/assistants	1,517	44.1
4	Pharmacists technicians	5,483	–
5	Medical laboratories technicians	2,936	–
6	Medical laboratories assistants	7,044	–
17	Chartered chemists	1,503	31.7
18	Environmental and public health workers	4,280	33.8
19	Public analysts	500	24.6
20	Medical records officers	1,187	47.3
21	Community health officers	19,268	59.4

Source: The Health Workforce Profile for Nigeria, 2008.

Discussion

This chapter explores the origin and developmental milestones of the major HCE programs in Nigeria. The information presented were acquired as a participant-observer in Nigeria at different time frames from 1955–1980, 1986–1991, and during several visits between 2015 and 2019 (Balogun, 2018). The literature review revealed only one previous investigation has systematically studied the developmental milestones of HCE in Nigeria (Balogun and Aka, 2018). The findings showed that the pace of professionalization for several occupations imported was timid. There was a considerable entrance gap, running into several centuries, between medicine introduced into the country by the Portuguese in 1472, and physiotherapy, whose date of entrance, 1945, occurred just 15 years shy of the country's independence in 1960. A similar gap, though nothing resembling the depth of the difference in the entry between medicine and physiotherapy, is also observable regarding legislative mandate to establish a regulatory board.

Medicine and dentistry were the first two occupations to be imported into the country in 1504 – 516 years ago. Pharmacy was the first health occupation to form a professional organization, followed by medicine, physiotherapy, veterinary medicine, dentistry, and optometry. The "first-generation" physiotherapy programs are all located in the southwest region of the country. The northern states did not have a physiotherapy program until 1990 when Bayero University was established. Much later in 2003, another physiotherapy program was initiated in the north at the University of Maiduguri. As of June 2020, entry-level professional BPT or BMR-PT degrees are offered in 13 (8%) out of the 170 existing universities in Nigeria. At seven (54%) of the 13 universities with a physiotherapy program, postgraduate (MS and PhD) programs are offered. It took physiotherapy the shortest duration of 14 years to form a professional association following their entrances into the country as compared to medicine and dentistry, which took an eternal 484 and 500 years, respectively (Balogun and Aka, 2018).

The duration for professional associations to achieve legislative permission for the regulatory board varied widely among the six different health disciplines studied. It took dentistry and medicine only 4 and 11 years, respectively, to receive legislative approval from the federal government. The timeline bears no comparison with pharmacy and physiotherapy, whose numbers are 65 and 33 years, respectively. Physiotherapy ranked fifth in the years it took to receive government approval to form a regulatory body following formation as a professional association. After importing the six health fields into the country, their developmental milestones progressed at varying paces. On a similar trajectory, a cross-national retrospective study in 2018 compared the developmental journeys of physiotherapy education in Nigeria with the landmarks of Australia, the United Kingdom, and the United States and found that the United States attained major educational milestones at a faster pace than Australia, the United Kingdom, and Nigeria, respectively (Balogun et al., 2018).

There are two types of medical curricula in Nigeria: the traditional curriculum with little emphasis on primary health care, exemplified by the UCH/UI, CMUL, and UNN, and the more primary health-care-oriented curriculum such as the OAU, ABU, and UNILORIN. An audacious and controversial transformation in medical education was initiated at OAU in 1972. As prime minister, the late Chief Obafemi Awolowo in the late 1960s saw the need for a medical school that will provide health care service to the citizen of the old western region. A planning committee was constituted to bring his vision to fruition at the newly established University of Ile-Ife (now OAU). Over three years, the committee scanned the environment for ideas and human and physical resources. The committee submitted its report to the university senate at the end of January 1971. They questioned many of the medical and dental education ideas at UCH/UI and CMUL and concluded that the two foundation universities had elitist curricula that are ineffective in responding to the crises within the Nigerian health care system at the time. And recommended the appointment of the late Professor Adesanya Ige Grillo as the founding dean of the proposed medical school.

The educational philosophy adopted by Professor Grillo and the pioneer faculty members went beyond the traditional domain of teaching, research, and institutionally based services. It aimed to emphasize primary health care and community service. From the start, OAU exerted its uniqueness by not adopting the "Faculty/College of Medicine" name but called itself the "Faculty of Health Sciences," a clear departure from the reigning nomenclature adopted at the time by UCH/UI, CMUL, and UNN. One of the primary missions of the faculty was to train various cadres of health professionals to work together as a functional unit capable of delivering quality health care in the community. OAU graduates were expected to be "general practitioners with a scientific approach to medicine" (Fatusi, 2012).

From the outset, the goal of Professor Grillo and the pioneer faculty was to develop a Bachelor of Science (BSc) degree in health sciences, as the entry-level education for admission into the medical (MBChB) and dental (BChD) degree programs. Professor Grillo also set a goal to develop the first BSc degree in nursing that admit students directly into the preliminary years, without the need for an RN credential. OAU also admitted students to BSc degree programs in environmental health, medical rehabilitation (BMR-PT), medical laboratory technology, nutrition, dietetics, and dental therapists/hygienists. The faculty deliberately set out to train physicians/dentists who are scientists prepared to pursue higher degrees in human biology, human pathology, and immunology.

The OAU foundation medical and dental students were admitted into the Faculty of Sciences (preliminary year) on September 15, 1971, and formally admitted into the Faculty of Health Sciences on May 8, 1972. Ten nursing students were admitted into the preliminary year in September 1973, and the first cohort of physiotherapy students was accepted into the BMR (PT) degree program in 1977. Thirty-six of the 48-pioneering medical and dental students graduated with a BSc (health sciences) degree in 1975 and progressed to the clinical year in October of 1975; 35 of the 36 students completed their medical and dental degree programs on April 26, 1978. The faculty taught their students to think holistically out of the black box and not be afraid to be different. The different curricula offered fostered team spirit as students in the various programs shared classes with other health care team members. They learned to respect every professional group in the health team.

Unfortunately, the environment into which OAU graduates began their medical careers was very hostile. For example, when the government of the Western region employed the foundation graduates, they were sent to the hospital to work before they had an opportunity to practice community-oriented medicine, their forte. The stakeholders (students and parents) vociferously complained about the extra one-year length of training. Both parents and students were anxious, restive, and eager to graduate as physicians/dentists within six years, like their peers at UCH/UI, CMUL, and UNN. Because of internal and external pressures, the OAU primary health care centered curriculum was changed.

Another reason for the change in the OAU curriculum mission was the inability of some students to continue their clinical education due to the MDCN's regulation, which stipulates that a student must earn a minimum cumulative score of 50%, rather than the 40% needed to graduate with a BSc (health sciences) degree. The students who scored below 50% and were not promoted into the clinical year were not qualified for the postgraduate program and were unable to get a job because prospective employers of that era were not familiar with the curriculum's general education focus. As a result of all the confusion and a new administration, the OAU faculty succumbed to the external pressure. They changed the innovative curriculum to conform to the status quo ante that the founding fathers criticized.

The innovative medical and dental curricula at OAU, initiated by Professor Ige Grillo in 1972, emphasized primary health care. This move was decades ahead of the other medical schools in Nigeria. It took the Nigerian government 15 years after Professor Ige Grillo initiated the OAU program to embrace primary health care; and several years for the global community to embrace primary health care as the cornerstone for health delivery (Marcos, 2004; Fatusi, 2012). Forty-five years after OAU introduced the BSc (Health Sciences) degree program as a prerequisite into its medical and dental programs, the curricula design that was once widely criticized at the time is no longer controversial. It became a mainstream benchmark that the NUC embraced in 2016 by mandating a BSc degree in the biological sciences as the admission requirement for medicine and dentistry.

One of the most significant challenges in the Nigerian academy today is the shortage of qualified faculty in the basic medical and laboratory sciences. If the training of physicians/dentists with a robust BSc scientific foundation had been pursued consistently at OAU, this unfortunate problem would not have arisen. The nation came to recognize the need for university-level education for medical laboratory scientists at the university level 30 years after OAU implemented it.

Implication

Africa had been marginalized effectively from the globalization process from the time of the slave trade. Ancient African science exploits include the construction of the pyramids, the first intensive agricultural schemes, mining and smelting of copper as far back as 4000 BC, including hieroglyphic writing system and the use of papyrus. These were notable accomplishments in terms of the mathematical and astronomical knowledge needed to build and concretize.

Sadly, the eminence of African academics on the global stage is fast dwindling. The contribution of African academics to the literature in science, technology, and engineering is the lowest in the world. The universities are at the bottom of global ranking, and the continent produces the least number of Nobel Prize winners in science. Scientists from the other parts of the world are solving a significant amount of African developmental challenges. Yet, Africa has several intellectually endowed academics contributing to knowledge in the northern nations where the novel breakthroughs drive global developments in health care, science, and technology. Chapter ten of this publication featured the elite Nigerian health care academics in different parts of the world engaged in transformative research.

Conclusion

This chapter chronicles the origin and developmental milestones of the major HCE programs in Nigeria. Before 1472, African traditional medicine, which includes herbalists, bonesetters, spiritualists, and surgeons, was the only health care delivery system in Nigeria. The birth of Western medicine occurred after

1914, and medicine and dentistry were the first health occupations to become entranced into Nigeria by the Portuguese allopathic physicians. Pharmacy, physical-and-occupational therapy, veterinary medicine, clinical psychology, public and environmental health, and dental therapy were also imported. The other health professions (speech therapy and audiology, radiography, medical laboratory science, optometry, nursing, and midwifery, medical records, nutrition, dietetics, biomedical engineering, prosthesis and orthotics, public and environmental health, chartered chemist, public analysis, and social work) were homebred. Following the importation of the different disciplines into the country, they progressed at varying paces in establishing educational programs and in their quest for true professional status and prestige.

References

Adeniyi, KO, Sambo, DU, Anjorin, FI, Aisien, AO and Rosenfeld, LM. (1998) An overview of medical education in Nigeria. *Journal of the Pennsylvania Academy of Science*, 71 (3):135–142. [online]. Available at: www.jstor.org/stable/44149234?readnow=1&seq=1#page_scan_tab_contents (Accessed: 10 February 2020)

Association of Science Laboratory Technologists of Nigeria. (2012) [online]. Available at: www.nislt.gov.ng/aboutus.php (Accessed: 10 February 2020)

Balogun, JA. (2016) Brief on the proposed National Postgraduate Physiotherapy College of Nigeria (NPPCN) [online]. Available at: www.researchgate.net/publication/310473802_Brief_on_the_proposed_National_Postgraduate_Physiotherapy_College_of_Nigeria_NPPCN (Accessed: 10 February 2020)

Balogun, JA. (2018) Echoes of my life as a physical therapist. [online]. Available at: www.amazon.com/Echoes-My-Life-Physical-Therapist/dp/099931470X (Accessed: 10 February 2020)

Balogun, JA and Aka, PC. (2018) Professionalization milestones of medicine and eleven other professional disciplines in Nigeria. *International Medical Journal*, 25(1): 2–8 [online]. Available at: www.researchgate.net/publication/322628378_Professionalization_Milestones_of_Medicine_and_Eleven_Other_Professional_Disciplines_in_Nigeria (Accessed: February 3, 2020)

Balogun, JA, Aka, PC, Balogun, AO, Mbada, C and Okafor, U. (2018) Evolution of physical therapy education in Australia, United Kingdom, United States of America, and Nigeria: A comparative analysis. *International Medical Journal*, 25 (2)103–107. [online]. Available at: www.researchgate.net/publication/323945677_Evolution_of_physical_therapy_education_in_Australia_United_Kingdom_United_States_of_America_and_Nigeria_A_comparative_analysis (Accessed: 02 May 2020)

Balogun, JA, Aka, PC, Balogun, AO and Obajuluwa, VA. (2017) A phenomenological investigation of the first two decades of university-based physiotherapy education in Nigeria. *Cogent Medicine*, 4(1) 10.1080/2331205X.2017.1301183. Available at: www.tandfonline.com/doi/pdf/10.1080/2331205X.2017.1301183 (Accessed: 10 February 2020)

Balogun, JA, Mbada CE, Balogun, AO and Okafor, UAC. (2016a) Profile of physiotherapist educators from Anglophone West African countries: A cross-sectional study. *International Journal of Medical and Health Sciences*, 3(9): 99–109.

Balogun, JA, Mbada, CE, Balogun, AO and Okafor, UAC. (2016b) The spectrum of student enrollment-related outcomes in physiotherapy education programs in West Africa. *International Journal of Physiotherapy*, 3(6), 603–612.

Bolaji, F. (2020) List of all universities in Nigeria approved by NUC – 2020 latest list. [online]. Available at: https://campusbiz.com.ng/list-of-universities-in-nigeria/ (Accessed: 10 February 2020)

Carr-Saunders, AM and Wilson, PA. (1944) *"Professions" Encyclopedia of the Social Sciences.* Chicago: University of Chicago Press.

Dental Therapists Registration Board of Nigeria. (2020) Dental therapists registration act. [online]. Available at: www.lawyard.ng/wp-content/uploads/2020/04/DENTAL-THERAPISTS-REGISTRATION-ETC.-ACT.pdf (Accessed: 10 February 2020)

Dietitians Association of Nigeria. (2017) [online]. Available at: http://dietitians.org.ng/?page_id=1358 (Accessed: 10 February 2020)

Ekundayo, HT and Ajayi, IA. (2009) Towards effective management of university education in Nigeria. *International NGO Journal,* 4(8):342–347. [online]. Available at: www.academicjournals.org/INGOJ https://academicjournals.org/article/article1381500283_Ekundayo%20and%20Ajayi.pdf (Accessed: 10 February 2020)

Eni, G. (2011) The genesis of university-based physiotherapy degree in Nigeria. The experience and challenges of the first graduate Godwin Eni [Ret.]. [online]. Available at: www.nigeriaphysio.net/media/archive1/docs/Genesis_of_UniversityBased_Physiotherapy_Education_in_Nigeria.pdf (Accessed: 10 February 2020)

Environmental Health Officers Registration Council of Nigeria. (2015) History of Environmental Health. [online]. Available at: www.ehorecon.gov.ng/welcome (Accessed: 10 February 2020)

Fatusi, AO. (2012) A short historical account of the College of Health Sciences. 40th anniversary commemorative publication. [online]. Available at: http://pdfdrug.com/c/chs.oauife.edu.ng1.html (Accessed: 10 February 2020)

Garba, A, Danbirni, S, Ahmed, A, Ambursa, AU, Suleiman, A, Mohammed, MN and Muhammed, ST. (2011) Veterinary laws and administration in Nigeria: Historical and current perspectives. Sarilla *Veterinarian,* 8(2):21–28. [online]. Available at: www.researchgate.net/publication/235726491_VETERINARY_LAWS_AND_ADMINISTRATION_IN_NIGERIA_HISTORICAL_AND_CURRENT_PERSPECTIVES (Accessed: 10 February 2020)

Garba, S. (2004) Environmental health in Nigeria, yesterday, today and tomorrow. *Environmental and Public Health Watch.* [online]. Available at: https://tsaftarmuhalli.blogspot.com/2011/04/environmental-health-in-nigeria.html (Accessed: 10 February 2020)

Health Records Officers Regulation Board of Nigeria. (2020). [online]. Available at: www.hrorbn.org.ng/list-of-approved-schools (Accessed: 10 February 2020)

Ibama, AS and Dennis, P. (2016) Role of community health practitioners in national development: The Nigeria situation. *International Journal of Clinical Medicine,* 7: 511–518. [online]. Available at: www.researchgate.net/publication/305642915_Role_of_Community_Health_Practitioners_in_National_Development_The_Nigeria_Situation (Accessed: 10 February 2020)

Ibama, AS, Dotimi, O, Atibinye, D and Obele, R. (2015) Community health practice in Nigeria – prospects and challenges. *International Journal of Current Research,* 01 (7):11989–11992

Institute of Chartered Chemists of Nigeria. (2017) History. [online]. Available at: http://icconng.com/index.php?option=com_content&task=view&id=1&Itemid=3 (Accessed: 10 February 2020)

International Confederation of Dietetic Association. (2020) Dietitians Association of Nigeria. [online]. Available at: www.internationaldietetics.org/Newsletter/Vol18Issue1/Dietitians-Association-of-Nigeria.aspx (Accessed: 12 October 2020)

International Society for Prosthetics and Orthotics (ISPO). (2020) [online]. Available at: www.ispoint.org/page/Nigeria (Accessed: 10 February 2020)

Irune, E. (2018) Migration and training: a British-Nigerian surgeon's perspective. *ENT and Audiology News*, 27 (1). [online]. Available at: www.entandaudiologynews.com/features/ent-features/post/migration-and-training-a-british-nigerian-surgeon-s-perspective (Accessed: 10 February 2020)

ISOWN. (2019) Doctor of social work (DSW). [online]. Available at: https://isownigeria.org.ng/doctor_of_social.html (Accessed: 10 February 2020)

Labiran, A, Mafe, M, Onajole, B and Lambo, E. (2008) Health workforce country profile for Nigeria. *Africa Health Workforce Observatory*, 8: 1–89.

LawNigeria.Com. (2017a) Community health practitioners (Registration, etc.) Act. [online]. Available at: www.lawonlinereport.com/community-health-practitioners-registration-etc-act/ (Accessed: 10 February 2020)

LawNigeria.Com. (2017b) Medical Laboratory Science Council of Nigeria Act. [online]. Available at: http://web.mlscn.gov.ng/ (Accessed: 10 February 2020)

Makinde, F. (2016) Establish postgraduate college for nurses, NANNM tells govt. *Punch*. [online]. Available at: https://punchng.com/establish-postgraduate-college-nurses-nannm-tells-govt/ (Accessed: 12 October 2020)

Marcos, C. (2004) The origins of primary healthcare and selective primary healthcare. *America Journal of Public Health*, 22 (94):1864–1874. doi:10.2105/ajph.94.11.1864. [online]. Available at: http://ajph.aphapublications.org/doi/10.2105/AJPH.94.11.1864 (Accessed: 10 February 2020)

Mohammed, SG. (2011) Environmental and public health watch. Training and functions of environmental health practitioners/environmental health officers. [online]. Available at:https://tsaftarmuhalli.blogspot.com/2011/07/training-and-functions-of-environmental_26.html (Accessed: 23 September 2020).

Nigerian Institute for Biomedical Engineering. (2020) Welcome to Nigerian Institute for Biomedical Engineering. [online] Available at: http://nigerianbme.org/ (Accessed: 12 October 2020)

Nigerian Prosthetic, Orthotic and Orthopaedic Technology Society (NPOOTS). (n.d.) Restoring Mobility through Orthopaedic and Rehabilitation Technology. [online]. Available at: www.nipots.yolasite.com/ (Accessed: 10 February 2020)

Nigerian Veterinary Medical Association (NVMA). (2018) [online]. Available at: www.nvma.org.ng/ (Accessed: 10 February 2020)

Nkuma-UdahE, KI, Agoha, KEC, Ejeta, K and Ndubuka, GI. (2005) Biomedical engineering in Nigeria: A developmental overview. World Congress on Medical Physics and Biomedical Engineering, June 7–12, 2015, Toronto, Canada pp 1643–1648.

Nurses Arena Forum. (2016) List of schools offering postgraduate-Masters and PhD nursing degree in Nigeria [online]. Available at: www.naijanursesforum.com/viewtopic.php?t=1504 (Accessed: 10 February 2020)

Nursing and Midwifery Council of Nigeria. (2019) Approved schools. [online]. Available at: www.nmcn.gov.ng/apschool.html (Accessed: 10 February 2020)

Nutrition Society of Nigeria. (2017) About us. [online]. Available at: https://nutritionnigeria.org/ (Accessed: 10 February 2020)

Obiorah, N. (2019) When was ADWA's degree-awarding status formally recognized by NUC? [online]. Available at: https://groups.google.com/forum/?utm_medium=email&utm_source=footer#!msg/usaafricadialogue/gvH5zYT4COY/4dE8kRW1BQAJ (Accessed: 10 February 2020)

Ogaji, JI and Ojabo, CE. (2014) Pharmacy education in Nigeria: The journey so far. *Archives of Pharmacy Practice*, [cited 2017 May 27]; 5:47–60. [online]. Available at: www. archivepp.com/text.asp?2014/5/2/47/132644 (Accessed: 10 February 2020)

Olabanji, I. (2020) What you need to know about dental therapy board of Nigeria. [online]. Available at: www.healthsoothe.com/what-you-need-to-know-about-dental-therapy-board-of-nigeria/ (Accessed: 10 February 2020)

Olaoye OA, Emechete AI, Onigbinde AT, Mbada CE. (2016) Awareness and knowledge of occupational therapy among Nigerian medical and health sciences undergraduates. *Hong Kong Journal of Occupational Therapy*. [online] Available at: https://journals. sagepub.com/doi/pdf/10.1016/j.hkjot.2016.02.001 (Accessed: 12 October 2020)

Oyiborhoro, MA. (1988) Audiology training in Nigeria—I: A training model. *Social Science & Medicine*, 26 (10):1035–1042 https://doi.org/10.1016/0277-9536(88)90221-3 (Accessed: 10 February 2020)

Ojiji, O. (2015) Fifty years of psychology in Nigeria: Are we still teaching science or folktales? *African Journal for the Psychological Study of Social Issues*, 18(2): 99. [online]. Available at: http://ajpssi.org/index.php/ajpssi/article/view/129/pdf_94 (Accessed: 10 February 2020)

Oshin, TA. (1999) Physiotherapy in Nigeria: Yesteryears, presently and in the next millennium [online]. Available at: www.nigeriaphysio.net/oshin-1999 (Accessed: 10 February 2020)

Pharmapproach. (2019) History of pharmacy, pharmacy education, career and ethics in Nigeria. [online]. Available at: www.pharmapproach.com/history-of-pharmacy-in-nigeria-2/ (Accessed: 10 February 2020)

PCN. (2020) Accredited Schools of Health Technology. [online]. Available at: www. pcn.gov.ng/webpages.php?cmd=N&pages=30&mt=Pharmacy%20Technician%20 Training&smt=Accredited%20Schools%20of%20Health%20Technology (Accessed: 10 February 2020)

Radiographers Registration Board of Nigeria. (2017) [online]. Available at: www.rrbn. gov.ng/about/ (Accessed: 10 February 2020)

Robinson, R. (2020) The evolution of education. [online]. Available at: www. mattchurch.com/talkingpoint/education-evolution (Accessed: 10 February 2020)

Scott-Emuakpor, A. (2010) The evolution of healthcare systems in Nigeria: Which way forward in the twenty-first century. *Niger Med J*, [cited 2017 Jun 30]; 51:53–65. [online]. Available at: www.nigeriamedj.com/text.asp?2010/51/2/53/70997 (Accessed: 10 February 2020)

Speech Pathologists and Audiologist Association in Nigeria, (2020) [online]. Available at: www.spaan.org.ng/ (Accessed: 10 February 2020)

Sule, J. (2017) Brief history of the Association of Radiographers of Nigeria (ARN). [online]. Available at: http://arn.org.ng/ (Accessed: 10 February 2020)

Uzondu, CA, Doctor, HV, Findley, SE, Afenyadu, GY and Ager, A. (2015) Female health workers at the doorstep: A pilot of community-based maternal, newborn, and child health service delivery in northern Nigeria. *Glob Health Sci Pract*, Mar; 3(1): 97–108. [online]. Available at: www.ncbi.nlm.nih.gov/pmc/articles/PMC4356278/ (Accessed: 10 February 2020)

Wikimedia Foundation, Inc. (2010) Audiology and hearing health professionals in Nigeria. [online]. Available at: https://en.wikipedia.org/wiki/Audiology_and_ hearing_health_professionals_in_Nigeria (Accessed: 10 February 2020)

6 Pioneer Nigerian health care academicians

Introduction

The first Portuguese voyage to West Africa in 1482 introduced Western medicine to Africans. However, the Western medical practice of that era was not too different from the traditional African medicine. The method of modern medicine occurred 400 years later, when all European settlements in Nigeria passed to the British in 1850. At the time, health care service focused on providing care for British soldiers, and the practice surged when an epidemic destroyed the entire British garrison in 1756. The health care services extended beyond military garrisons to include colonial civil servants, with the formal colonization of Lagos, Nigeria, in 1850. Health care was not extended to the local population. However, the missionaries leveraged health care services to propagate religion to the local communities and provide excellent health care to a select group of the local people working for the colonial government.

The establishment of medical training institutions early in the first half of the 20th century lured several qualified Nigerian health care academicians who studied abroad to return to the country. Unfortunately, the service and scholarship contributions of this patriotic Nigerians have primarily remained unrecognized. This chapter sets out to identify the pioneer Nigerian health care academicians and explores their service and scholarship contributions.

Methodology

An exhaustive search of the literature was conducted using the PubMed and Google search engines using the keyword "first Nigerian professor" in combination with the name of different health disciplines and medical specialties. The search also reviewed the Nigerian Academy of Science (NAS) website and other Nigerian affairs-leaning sites to identify pioneer health care academicians (Balogun, 2015; Straightnews.ng, 2018; Ranker, 2020; Akinpelu, 2019; Nwachukwu, 2016; Isaac, 2019). The search produced 19 eminent Nigerian academicians from different health fields. Fourteen physicians from various medical specialties (Oritsejolomi, Mabayoje, Nwokolo, Lambo, Ogunlesi, Odeku, Grillo, Udekwu, Ransome-Kuti, Lucas, Akinkugbe, Osuntokun,

Adeloye, and Osotimehin), and five other health professionals – nursing (Adebo), physiotherapy (Nwuga), pharmacy (Aguwa), optometry (Ogbueh) and psychology (Ugwuegbu). The biographic information and scholarship/ service accomplishments of the 19 eminent academicians were gleaned from different open access sources and summarized below.

Results

Oritsejolomi Thomas (1917–1979), Professor and Pioneer Maxillofacial Reconstructive and plastic surgeon

Oritsejolomi was born in 1917 at Sapele, a city in Delta state, Nigeria. He attended Methodist Boys' High School in Lagos and Birmingham University in the United Kingdom. Oritsejolomi, during his medical career, was a trail-blazer. He was the first Nigerian admitted as a member of the Royal College of Surgeons (RCSs) of England. In 1952, Oritsejolomi was appointed a senior lecturer and foundation maxillofacial reconstructive and plastic surgeon at the UCH. He operated on maxillofacial cases referred to the hospital from all parts of the country (NAOMS, 2016). In 1962, Oritsejolomi was appointed founder and first HOD of surgery at the College of Medicine, University of Lagos (CMUL). He also served as the foundation provost and the pioneer chief medical officer of the Lagos University Teaching Hospital (UTH). He also served as the editor of the *West African Medical Journal*.

During his career, Oritsejolomi served in various nonacademic capacities. In 1958, he served on the Federal Electoral Commission, and in 1969 served as the chairman of the advisory committee constituted to explore the establishment of the University of Benin (UNIBEN) Teaching Hospital. Oritsejolomi served as the VC of the UI from 1972 to 1975 and died in 1979. This skilled administrator and eminent maxillofacial surgeon was a great mentor to the first generation of surgeons at the CMUL (Nigerian Academic, n.d.).

John Oluyemi Mabayoje (1920–) first Nigerian professor of medicine at CMUL; first president of the West African College of Physicians

Oluyemi was born in Ilesa on March 31, 1920. He had his elementary education from 1926 to 1932 at St. John's School, Ilora, Ilesa, and secondary education at Government College, Ibadan from 1933 to 1938. He attended Higher College Ibadan from 1939 to 1940 and began his medical training at Yaba Higher College, from 1941–1946. He later attended the Royal College of Surgeon in Dublin from 1947 to 1948 and the postgraduate medical school in 1949. Oluyemi returned to Nigeria in 1952 and was appointed physician by the Federal Ministry of Health, Lagos, and served till 1969. He had further training at the Institute of Cardiology, London (1955), Institute of Neurology, London (1959), University of Toronto, Canada (1964–1965), and Johns Hopkins University (1965).

Oluyemi became professor and HOD of medicine at CMUL in 1969. His area of research interest was in sickle cell anemia, viral hepatitis, heart disease, and pregnancy. He was a member of the New York Academy of Science and a fellow of the Royal Society of Medicine, London. Oluyemi achieved many "first" status during his career – the first Nigerian elected as Fellow of the RCSs of Edinburgh (1938); first Nigerian member of the Royal College of Physicians (RCPs) of Edinburgh (1951); first Nigerian elected to the RCPs of Edinburgh (1960), and was elected to the fellowship in 1963. He served as a member of the University Provisional Council at the University of Ile-Ife (now Obafemi Awolowo University – OAU) from 1963 to 1966, president of the Association of Physicians of Nigeria (1965–1967), first registrar of the Nigeria Medical Council (1966–1975), the first Nigerian professor of medicine at CMUL (1969), first president of the West African College of Physicians (1976), and Member of World Health Organization (WHO) advisory panel on cardiovascular disease. He is married and blessed with five children (Njoh, 2000; Osso, 2017a).

Chukwuedu Nathaniel II Nwokolo (1921–2014), professor and second Nigerian to obtain the MRCP qualification; advisor to the WHO

Chukwuedu was born on April 19, 1921, at Amaimo, in Imo state by Nathaniel Ezuma Nwokolo and Matilda Nwokolo (nee Efobi). Both his parents worked for the Church Missionary Society (CMS) as an evangelist, and he was the first male child amongst seven children. Chukwuedu started primary school at Ezinihitte-Mbaise and attended Government College, Umuahia. In 1939, he was admitted to study medicine at Yaba Higher College and qualified as a physician in 1946. He had his internships at the General Hospital Lagos and Aba General Hospital, and later worked at General Hospital Enugu, and was one of the first set of assistant medical officers employed in the Department of Medicine at UCH in 1949 (Wikimedia Foundation Inc, 2019d).

In 1950, Chukwuedu proceeded to the United Kingdom and had his fellowship training at Queen Mary's Hospital and obtained the MRCP qualification in 1953. He was one of the few Africans and the second Nigerian to receive the MRCP – the first was Dr. Olu Mabayoje. He later returned to Nigeria and was employed in the civil service as a medical officer at General Hospital, Enugu. He received the fellowship of the RCPs in 1960 and subsequently worked at UI as a senior lecturer. In 1963, Chukwuedu trained at the University of Minnesota as a Rockefeller Foundation fellow in gastroenterology and returned to Nigeria in 1964 and was appointed associate professor of medicine at the UI.

Before the Nigerian civil war began in 1967, Chukwuedu left Ibadan for Enugu. The military governor, Chukwuemeka Odumegwu Ojukwu, established a UTH at Enugu General Hospital and a Faculty of Medicine (FOM) at UNN. He was appointed the first HOD of medicine and associate dean of medicine and was promoted professor in 1971 (Wikimedia Foundation,

2018; Nwakanma, 2006). During the civil war, he tailored his research to address the sequelae of starvation and malnutrition that were prevalent in Biafra. Chukwuedu specialized in tropical diseases and was recognized for mapping out the area of paragonimiasis lung disease in eastern Nigeria and investigated the disease in other African countries. He established the sickle cell research program to fight the disease in Nigeria and globally. Chukwuedu published nine articles and contributed to the book, *Principles of Medicine in Africa published by* Cambridge University.

Chukwuedu was a fellow of several academic organizations, including the RCPs, and the NAS. He garnered two honorary Doctor of Science (DSc) degrees (University of Maiduguri, and UI), and was appointed professor emeritus at the UNN. He also received the officer of the federal republic (OFR), and the Nigerian national order of merit awards. He served in various capacities at national and international levels, including advisor to the WHO and the National Science and Technology Development Fund, chairman of the Joint Council for the Nnamdi Azikiwe University, Enugu, chairman of the board of the UTH Calabar, chairman and vice president of the West African College of Physicians, pro-chancellor and chairman of the Council at ABU, chairman of the Medical Research Council of Nigeria, chairman of the governing board of the National Council for Medical Research, and president of the Association of Physicians of Nigeria. He was married to Miss Njideka Priscilla Okonkwo on July 4, 1953, and the union blessed with seven children.

Theophilus Oladipo Ogunlesi (1923–), first Nigerian professor of medicine

Oladipo was born on July 12, 1923, to a blacksmith father in Sagamu, Ogun state. He attended St. Paul's Primary School in Sagamu from 1931 to 1935 and the CMS school in Lagos from 1936 to 1940. He enrolled at Yaba Higher College in 1941 and graduated in 1942. Oladipo was admitted to the Yaba medical school in 1942 and completed the medical assistant education in 1947. He served as an assistant medical officer in the Nigerian medical department between 1947 and 1948. He won a scholarship to study medicine in the United Kingdom, which he completed in 1950 and was appointed house physician at Hammersmith Hospital in London. He attended the University of London postgraduate medical school in 1953 and the University of Minnesota, from 1957 to 1958. He became an FRCP in 1958 and returned to Nigeria (Osso, 2017b).

Oladipo was influenced by Chief Obafemi Awolowo, who wanted Nigerians to replace the British in charge of the Adeoyo Hospital, Ibadan. In 1958, he was appointed a specialist in the Department of Medicine at Adeoyo until 1961 (Adegbite, 2017). Oladipo joined the FOM at the UCH/UI in 1961 as a senior lecturer and was promoted as the first professor of medicine in 1965. He was the first Nigerian HOD of medicine at UCH and served in that capacity from 1969 to 1972. He voluntarily retired in 1983 at the age of 60 and was awarded the emeritus professor of medicine in 1985. He is a foundation fellow of the NAS and a past vice president of the Academy (NAS, 2019a).

The primary legacy of Oladipo is the generations of physicians he trained at UI, including Professor Isaac Adewole, the former VC of the UI, and former minister of health. Among those, he taught include the late Professor Kayode Oshuntokun, and the late Professor Yombo Awojobi, a distinguished surgeon who left UCH to establish the Awojobi clinic at Eruwa (Adegbite, 2017). In 1983, he was honored with the prestigious OFR award. He got married to Susan Peters in 1950, and the union is blessed with five sons and two daughters.

Thomas Adeoye Lambo (1923–2004), first Nigerian professor of psychiatry and former deputy director-general of the WHO

Adeoye was born on March 29, 1923, in Abeokuta, Ogun state, by parents who are not affluent. He attended Baptist Boys High School in Abeokuta from 1935 to 1940. After completing the West African School Certificate, Adeoye was admitted at the University of Birmingham medical school and graduated in 1948. Subsequently, he enrolled at London University for postgraduate studies in psychiatry and completed the program in 1952 and was appointed house surgeon at the General Hospital in Birmingham.

In 1954, Adeoye returned to Nigeria, where he was appointed the director of the newly built Aro psychiatric hospital in Abeokuta. He was a scholar, administrator, and psychiatrist credited for reintegrating individuals with mental illness into society and helped to shed the stigma associated with mental illness. Adeoye served as a medical officer and consultant and became famous for his work in ethno-psychiatry and psychiatric epidemiology. He later joined the faculty at the UI, where he was promoted professor and the dean of the FOM from 1966 to 1968.

Adeoye served as the VC of the UI from 1968 to 1971. At the end of his tenure, he was appointed assistant director-general of the WHO. Three years later, he was promoted deputy director-general and served in that position until 1988 when he retired. Adeoye was a recipient of several professional and national awards, including the Nigerian national merit award in 1979. In 1982, he established the Lambo Foundation to research mental illness and fund treatment for those who are indigent and cannot afford it. Adeoye, his three children, and British wife, Dinah, continued to work full-time at the Lambo Foundation until his death on March 13, 2004 (This DayOnline, 2004).

Emmanuel Olatunde Odeku (1927–1974), first professor of neurosurgery in West Africa

Olatunde was born on June 29, 1927, in Lagos, but his father was a native of Awe, and his mother was from Lagos. He attended Methodist Boys High School in Lagos. He passed the London matriculation examination in 1945, scoring higher than many of his teachers who took the examination that year.

Olatunde finished secondary school with the best grade in biology, chemistry, English, geography, and history. He enrolled in 1947 at Howard University on an academic scholarship, to study zoology, and graduated *summa cum laude* in 1950. He studied medicine at Howard and graduated in 1954. The following year he returned to Nigeria and was employed as a medical officer at the Lagos General Hospital (Wikimedia Foundation Inc, 2019b).

Olatunde returned to the University of Michigan (1956–1960) and joined the neurosurgery faculty at Howard in 1961. He trained in neurology at the Walter Reed Medical Center in Washington, DC, and in pediatric neurosurgery at the Children's Hospital of Philadelphia, where he worked under Dr. Eugene Spitz – the creator of the Spitz-Holter valve used for treating hydrocephalus. In 1961, he joined the College of Medicine at Howard as an instructor in neuro-anatomy and neurosurgery and became a fellow of the American College of Surgeons, in 1962. He was the second Black to be certified by the American Board of Neurological Surgery.

Although Olatunde received multiple job offers in the United States, including two distinguished academic neurosurgery faculty positions, but returned to his native land in 1962. He joined the UCH/UI as a senior lecturer and the first neurosurgeon in West Africa. In three short years, he became a professor of neurosurgery. He served from 1968 to 1971 as the HOD of surgery and the dean of the FOM. Olatunde was instrumental in founding the National and West African Postgraduate Medical Colleges and the initiation of the swearing-in and commencement ceremonies at the UI. The other medical programs in Nigeria later adopted this ritual. He contributed significantly to the neurosurgical literature by publishing 85 specialty articles and 13 other general articles in peer-reviewed journals within 12 years.

Olatunde was a genuine global neurosurgery pioneer. His selfless service in the United States and Nigeria opened the door for people from both countries to elevate the field of neurosurgery. He received the Howard University alumni award for distinguished service. His health began to fail in 1972, from complications of diabetes. Sadly, he died on August 20, 1974, at Hammersmith Hospital, London, at the tender age of 47, leaving many of his ideas unfulfilled. He was buried at St Peter's Church, Burnham, England, the home country of his wife, Katherine Jill. He married twice to physicians. The first marriage produced two children, and in 1971 he married Jill Katherine Adcock, a British, and the union produced two children (McClelland, Harris, 2007).

Thomas Adesanya Ige Grillo (1927–1998), first professor of anatomy in Nigeria

Adesanya was born on January 29, 1927, in Lagos, to Aina Osaoba and Adenike Omolara (Serrano) Grill. He attended primary school at the Baptist Academy, Lagos, and later the Hope Waddell Training Institution, Calabar. He continued his education at City College Norfolk, England, RCSs of Ireland, and St. Stephen Green, Dublin, Ireland. Subsequently, Adesanya earned a Master of Arts and PhD at St. John's College, Cambridge, England (1960), DSc at Trinity College in Dublin (1972), Doctor of Medicine at the University College in Dublin (1993). He was appointed supervisor St. John's College, Cambridge, United States (1955–1960), assistant lecturer at St. Mary's Hospital Medical School, University of London (1960), assistant professor at Stanford University (1960–1961).

Adesanya returned to Nigeria in 1961 and was appointed lecturer at UCH/UI and promoted to the rank of senior lecturer in 1962. In 1964, he was again promoted to the academic rank of associate professor and became professor and HOD of anatomy in1966-1972. Adesanya's early research work was on the embryogenesis of the pancreas, which he conducted at UCH/UI. He also investigated the role of infections in the pathogenesis of the calcification of the pancreas. Adesanya's colleagues in the West were astounded at the high quality of research he conducted in a developing country (Osso, 2017e)

Adesanya relocated to the OAU in 1972 as the founding dean of the Faculty of Health Sciences (FHS) and held the position until 1990. At OAU, he served as a consultant pathologist at the Ife UTH (1975–1984), professor of medicine (1972–1987), and on retirement was honored as professor emeritus. He established an innovative interdisciplinary HCE curriculum that required medical and dental students to complete a BS degree in basic medical science before enrolling in the clinical year for the MBChB/BDS degree. The curricula design also mandates medical and dental students to take their basic medical science courses in tandem with other members of the health care team and think holistically out of the box. Adesanya inculcated in his students that they should not be afraid to be different and always to respect every professional group in the health care team (Ogunsola, 2014).

Adesanya left OAU in 1988 for the University of Sierra Leone to establish a new medical school. He served as the principal of the College of Medicine and Allied Health Sciences, until 1992. During his illustrious career, he was a fellow of several academic societies and received the chieftain title as the Busegun of Ilesha (Nigeria). Adesanya served as a consultant for WHO and universities in Liberia, Sudan, and Malawi. He was president of the Association of African Medical Schools for many years. He also served as a visiting senior scientist at the International Institute for Cellular and Molecular Pathology, Brussels (1978–1979), visiting professor at the University of Khartoum, Sudan (1973–1986) (Lucas, 1998).

Adesanya was married to Baxter Dorothea, born in 1931 to a physician father in Kingston, Jamaica. Dorothea, professor of embryology with a specialization in pediatrics, was the first to obtain a PhD in anatomy in Nigeria. Dorothea has held faculty appointment in Jamaica and at the Universities of Ibadan, OAU, Maiduguri, and Benin. She has lived in Nigeria since the 1961 and continued teaching even after her husband's death in October 1998. She taught anatomy at the UNIBEN for over 30 years until 2019, when she ceremoniously retired at the age of 88 and died a year later on May 30, 2020. The Grillo's were reputed to have started Anatomy in Nigeria and taught close to three generations of physicians, dentists, and other health professionals (Eshemokha, 2020).

Olikoye Ransome-Kuti (1927–2003), first Nigerian professor of pediatrics and former WHO deputy director-general and minister of health

Olikoye was born in Ijebu Ode on December 30, 1927, by Reverend Israel Oludotun Ransome-Kuti, school principal, protestant minister and the first president of the Nigeria Union of Teachers and Funmilayo Ransome-Kuti, a prominent women rights activist. He attended Abeokuta Grammar School and was one of the pioneer students at the FOM at the UCH/UI, before enrolling at Trinity College Dublin, where he attended the medical school (1948–1954) (Wikimedia Foundation, 2020). He enrolled at Hammersmith Hospital for his postgraduate medical education between 1960 and 1962. Subsequently, he returned to Nigeria and worked as a house officer at the Lagos General Hospital, and senior registrar in pediatrics at the UCH (1962–1963), and later a senior lecturer at the CMUL (1967–1970). He served as acting director of the Institute of Child Health (1968–1970) and became a professor in 1970 and served as HOD of pediatrics from 1970 to 1976 and retired in 1988 (Hallmarks of Labor Foundation, 2002).

Olikoye was one of Nigeria's foremost pediatricians and health experts. He introduced universal primary care into the Nigerian health care system. He promoted immunization programs to curb the increasing rate of diarrhea among children and encouraged mothers to breastfeed their children for at least one year. He also supported the use of oral rehydration therapy by nursing mothers and gave a new lease of life to family planning programs that previous governments had ignored. He broke the stigma surrounding AIDS and raised awareness about it through public and media campaigns.

Olikoye was a recipient of several national and international awards that include UNICEF merit award (1990), Bureau of Public Health (1991), Chairman of the National Primary Health care Development Agency, and Leon Bernard Foundation Prize (1986), and the Maurice Pate Award (1990). In 1985, he served as the Health Minister in General Ibrahim Babangida military administration until 1992 when he joined the WHO as its deputy director-general. In 1983, Olikoye and two associates founded a health-focused NGO – Society for Family Health, Nigeria – to provide family planning and child health services.

Olikoye's career appointments are numerous. He served as a member of the WHO's expert advisory panel on maternal and child health, visiting consultant to the Department of Pediatrics at Makarere University Kampala Uganda (1969); consultant to the Zambia Ministry of Health (1973); member of the consultative group of the African Heads Training Institute at the University of North Carolina (1974–1978); and senior associate for the Department of International Health at Johns Hopkins University (1979–1983). He died in a London hotel on June 1, 2003, while attending a WHO conference and was survived by his two sons, a daughter and his wife of 50 years, Sonia Doherty Adefare (Hallmarks of Labor Foundation, 2002).

Adetokunbo Oluwole Lucas (1931–), Harvard professor and world renounced global health expert

Adetokunbo was born in Lagos in 1931, living two years of his infancy in the vicarage after his father in 1936 became the vicar of St. Paul's Breadfruit Church. His nephew, Ladipo Oluwole, a distinguished physician, inspired him to study medicine (Litcaf.com, 2019). He enrolled at Durham University medical school and graduated in 1956 with honors, followed by postgraduate degrees in internal medicine and public health. Adetokunbo returned to Nigeria in 1960 and joined the faculty at UCH/UI. He climbed the academic ladder and became a professor of internal medicine and public health in his early 1930s. At UCH/UI, he was interested in the issue of tropical diseases among Nigerians. (Wikimedia Foundation Inc, 2020a).. After 16 years at Ibadan, he retired and directed the newly established Tropical Diseases Research Program of the WHO in Geneva (1976–1986).

In 1990, Adetokunbo was named professor of international health at Harvard. In retirement, he is an adjunct professor in population health in the Department of Global Health and Population. He chairs the Global Forum for Health Research. He continues to serve on numerous expert and advisory committees on health issues for national and international organizations such as the Rockefeller Foundation, the Edna McConnell Clark Foundation, the Carter Center, and the Wellcome Trust Scientific Group on Tropical Medicine (Newcastle University, 2018).

Adetokunbo authored several articles in peer referenced journals and books in public health and received honorary doctoral degrees from several world primer universities – Emory, Tulane, Harvard, and the UI. He received several academic awards: fellow of the Royal College of Obstetricians and Gynecologists; London School of Hygiene and Tropical Medicine Honorary Fellowship; medal from the Foreign Associates of the Institute of Medicine at Harvard; Mary Kingsley medal of the Liverpool School of Tropical Medicine; Harvard School of Public Health alumni award of merit; Prince Mahidol award (1999), Centenary medal for Life-Time Achievements in Tropical Medicine (2007); Jimmy and Rosalynn Carter's humanitarian award (2013), and the National Foundation for Infectious Diseases award (2013) (Newcastle University, 2018).

Oladipo Olujimi Akinkugbe (1933–), professor and former principal and foundation VC of the University of Ilorin and VC of ABU

Oladipo was born on July 17, 1933, in Ondo City. His father was a chemist and druggist, who is related in some distant past to the wealthy marble family in Igbe, Oyo state. Oladipo was admitted to Ondo Boys High School in 1944 and later transferred to Government College, Ibadan, where he excelled in science subjects. He gained admission to the UI medical school in 1951. After passing his second MBBS examination in 1955, he was posted to the Royal Hospital of the University of London for his clinical clerkship and graduated in 1958. He worked briefly as a clinical assistant at the Royal Hospital from 1959 to 1960, during which he expanded his knowledge and expertise. He obtained a diploma in tropical medicine and hygiene from the University of Liverpool in 1960.

Oladipo returned to Nigeria in 1961 and joined Adeoyo Hospital, Ibadan. Later that year, he returned to Oxford for the D.Phil., and MD degrees, which he completed in 1964. And in January 1965 joined the Department of Medicine at the UCH/UI. He became a professor of medicine in 1968, HOD of medicine in 1972, and dean of the FOM from 1970 to 1974. He was a Rockefeller visiting fellow at Johns Hopkins, Yale, and Washington medical schools (1966), visiting professor of medicine at Harvard (1974–1975), and fellow at Oxford from 1981 to 1982 (Osso, 2016). Oladipo is a fellow of the RCPs (1968) and a foundation fellow of the NAS (1977b).

Oladipo served as principal and foundation VC of the University of Ilorin and VC of ABU. Furthermore, he served in different professional roles at national and international levels: committee member of the University Grants Commission to the Ugandan Government; foundation chairman of the Joint Admission and Matriculation Board; chairman National Implementation Communications on Review of Higher Education; chairman of the planning committee for Ondo State University, and the University of Abuja; scientific advisory panel for CIBA Foundation, and the Council of International Society of Hypertension; expert committees on WHO's cardiovascular diseases, smoking control; senior consultant on WHO technical advisory committee on health research; and secretary of WHO technical discussions on University and Health for All. He also served as pro-chancellor and chairman of council, University of Port Harcourt.

Oladipo is an outstanding professional and academic role model with a high degree of expertise, thoroughness, dedication, integrity, and transparency. He is widely published in peer-reviewed journals and authored three books (Prabook, n.d.). During his illustrious and productive career, he received several awards: National Honor of Cote De Voire, Order of the Niger, Boehringer Ingelheim award from the International Society of Hypertension. He is a recipient of two honorary DSc degrees – from the University Ilorin and the Federal University of Technology, Akure. He married Folasade Modupeore Dina on May 8, 1965, and the union is blessed with two sons (Hallmarks of Labor Foundation, 2004; Vesta Healthcare, n.d.)

Benjamin Oluwakayode Osuntokun (1935–1995), professor and pioneer neuroepidemiologist in Africa and the doyen of neurology in Nigeria

Kayode was born on January 6, 1935, at Okemesi, Ekiti. He had his primary school education at the Holy Trinity School, Ilawe Ekiti, and Emmanuel School at Ado Ekiti and secondary school education at Christ's School, Ado Ekiti. He enrolled as a medical student at UCH/UI, Ibadan, then a campus of the

University of London and graduated as a physician in 1961. In 1963, Kayode spent a year at Welsh National School of Medicine in Cardiff. Kayode returned to UCH in 1964, as a medical research fellow. He left again for further studies to work under the mentorship of both Henry Miller and John Walton – eminent neurologists. At Newcastle, he worked briefly at the National Hospital for Nervous Diseases, Queens Square, London, and returned to UCH in 1965.

In 1971, Kayode obtained the MD degree with a thesis on the neurological manifestations of diabetes mellitus in Nigerians from the University of London. Kayode was appointed consultant physician/ neurologist at the UCH and, in 1970, was promoted to the rank of professor of medicine. From 1972 to 1974, he served as the HOD of medicine, sub-dean of the postgraduate studies, and dean of the FOM from 1974 to 1978 and later the chief medical officer at the UCH. And in 1977, he received a DSc degree from the University of London (Wikimedia Foundation, 2020; Roman, 1997).

Kayode was a prolific writer, an erudite scholar, a great teacher-researcher, and an esteemed scientist who contributed significantly to the training of many burgeoning neurologists. He authored over 300 peer-reviewed publications in medical journals globally. Kayode served on several international bodies, including chairman of the WHO's Global Advisory Committee on health research (1987–1990), a founding member of the Pan African Association of Neurological Sciences (PAANS), secretary of the African Region of the World Federation of Neurology Research Group on Tropical Neurology (1972–1986).

Kayode received several awards, including fellow of the Nigerian and West African Medical Associations, honorary fellow of the Nigerian and West African Radiology Associations, Frederick Murgatroyd prize of the RCPs of London (1977), Commonwealth professorship in medicine at the University of London and Royal Postgraduate Medical School, Hammersmith Hospital, London (1978–1979), honorary DSc degree from the University of Maiduguri (1984), Dr. Charles R. Drew World medical prize award from Howard University (1989), Wellcome Trust Fellowship at the Cambridge University (1991), an OFR and the Nigerian national merit honor (1984), and two honorary chieftaincies titles as Chief Bobajiro of Ara-Moko and Asiwaju of Okemesi-Ekiti (Roman, 1997). Kayode died at the Evelyn Hospital, Cambridge, on September 22, 1995, at the age of 60 years after a brief illness and was buried in his native land at Okemesi. He is survived by his wife – professor of ophthalmology at UCH/UI – and five children, two of whom are physicians (Roman, 1997).

Adelola Adeloye (formerly Rufus Bandele Adelola Adeloye) (1935–), Professor and Nigerian foremost physician and surgeon

Adelola was born in Ilesa on July 18, 1935, to Ebenezer Ajayi and Elizabeth Ajisomo, who hails from Ikole-Ekiti. His father started as a schoolteacher but later opted to be an artisanal mechanic (invented Cassava grater, double grating the Cassava machine, and cotton wool spiner). Subsequently, he became a traditional medicine practitioner. Adelola is the first of five children in his family.

He attended St. Paul's CMS school, Ikole-Ekiti from 1941 to 1946, and Christ's School, Ado Ekiti from 1947 to 1952. He was a government scholar and graduated in 1952 with grade one in the Cambridge certificate examination.

After a brief stint working for the defunct western region in1953, Adelola received a government scholarship to study medicine at the UI. He obtained the University of London MBBS degree in 1960 and was the youngest in his graduating class. He was a college scholar and won the chemical pathology prize. In July 1965, Adelola passed the RCPs, Edinburgh examination in neurology, and the fellowship examination of the RCSs of England in 1966. Like the legendary late Sir Samuel Layinka Ayodeji Manuwa, he was the second Nigerian to obtain the specialist credential in surgery – FRCS from Edinburgh in 1938 and MRCP, FRCP, and FACS – he has double expertise as a physician and surgeon, and the second Nigerian (after Professor Odeku) to qualify as a neurological surgeon who trained in Nigeria, the United Kingdom, and the United States.

Adelola returned to UCH in 1967 as a postfellowship senior registrar (under late Professor Odeku). By July 1968, he was appointed consultant neurosurgeon and a temporary lecturer at UCH (1968–1969). He was promoted senior lecturer in 1969 and professor of neurological surgery in 1972. He served as the HOD of surgery from 1974 to 1977 (Idowu, 2019). Adelola spent his sabbatical leave at the University of Cincinnati as a Rockefeller research fellow in experimental teratology (1972–1973). He was the Ratanji Dalai scholar of the RCSs of England (1973–1974). In 1973, he completed a Master's degree in surgery from the University of London (Idowu, 2019).

Adelola took up appointments in the UAE and served in various capacities. In 1987, he had a brief stint as a locum consultant neurosurgeon at the King Faisal specialist hospital, Riyadh. A year later, he became the head of neurosurgery at Al-Adan government hospital. In 1991, he returned to the University of Malawi as the foundation professor and HOD of surgery. He also served as acting dean, acting principal of the College of Medicine, and a senator until 2001. Additionally, he served in various leadership roles at national and international levels, including honorary president for life by the World Federation of Neurosurgical Societies (2001) – the first Black African to be so honored; president of the neurosurgery section of the Nigerian Society of Neurological Sciences (1988); president of the Surgical Association of Malawi (1998–2000); foundation member (1972), vice president (1998–2000) and president (2000–2002) of the PAANS, and foundation president of the Neurosurgical Society of East and Central Africa (1999). He also served as a postgraduate examiner in surgery in several universities in Nigeria, Tanzania, Uganda, Scotland, Australia, and South Africa.

In addition to an equally rich array of scholarly publications on diverse subjects in neurosurgery and medical history, Adelola garnered a panoply of academic and clinical expertise in the course of his career. The highest point of his career was the description of the Adeloye-Odeku disease (congenital dermoid cyst of the anterior fontanelle). Second, he helped to institutionalize neurosurgical training in Nigeria and established the Department of Surgery at the University of Malawi. He is a prolific scholar who authored over a dozen books and received several academic and community awards – honorary DSc degree in neurological surgery by the International University Foundation (1987), emeritus professor of neurosurgery at the UI (2010), and a chieftaincy title as the *Atorise of Ikole-Ekiti* (2018). In October 1967, he married the late Dr. Kamala Codanda Kappala, a medical graduate of Madras University and a pediatrician. The union was blessed with three children as well as grandchildren.

Babatunde Osotimehin (1949–2017), professor and former minister of health, executive director of the United Nations Population Fund (UNPF), and under-secretary-general of the United Nations

Babatunde was born in Ijebu Igbo, Ogun state, on February 6, 1949, as the oldest of the eight children of Mr. Alaba Osotimehin, a teacher, and Mrs. Morenike (nee Olukoya), a businesswoman selling organic fruit. From 1966 to 1971, he attended Igbobi College and studied medicine at the UI. In 1979, Babatunde enrolled in a postdoctoral program at the University of Birmingham, and from 1979 to 1980, was a fellow in endocrinology at Cornell University. He returned to Nigeria in 1980 and joined the Department of Clinical Pathology at UCH/UI. Babatunde climbed the academic ladder quickly and became a professor and served as the provost from 1990–1994.

Babatunde served on the world stage in various positions as executive director of the UNPF (2010–2017), chairman of the National Action Committee on AIDS in Nigeria (2002–2007), project manager for the World-Bank assisted HIV/AIDS program development project (2002–2008), vice president of the 14th International Conference on AIDS and STIs in Africa (2005), chairman of the governing board for the Joint Regional HIV/AIDS Project in the Abidjan – Lagos Transport Corridor (2003–2008), and director-general, Nigerian National Agency for the Control of AIDS (2007–2008), African spokesperson for the Partnership for Maternal, Newborn and Child Health (2008–2010).

Babatunde also served as the health minister during President Goodluck Jonathan's administration (2008–2010). He spurred all the 36 states to implement the national health plan that focused on primary health care launched by Professor Ransome-Kuti (from 1975 to 1980). As the executive director of the UNPF, young people remained Babatunde's focus, and he ensured both genders have equal participation within society and in reproductive rights and health. In 2017, the director-general of WHO, Dr. Margaret Chan, in her eulogy, described Babatunde as "a champion of health for all, but especially for women and adolescent girls. His work to reduce preventable maternal deaths and family planning highlighted these issues on the global health agenda." He was survived by his wife, Olufunke Olukoya, their sons, four daughters, and four grandchildren (Wikimedia Foundation, 2020; Shutti, 2017).

Fabian Anene Ositadimma Udekwu (1928–2006), professor and pioneer cardiothoracic surgeon in Nigeria

Fabian was born in 1928 at Enugwu Agidi, Anambra state, and attended St. Charles Teachers Training College in Onitsha. After graduation in 1947, he was retained as a teacher and taught mathematics and geography. Fabian independently studied for the London matriculation exams, and after saving adequate money, proceeded to the United States in 1950 for further studies. He completed the prerequisite courses for medical school in Los Angeles and transferred to Chicago Loyola School of Medicine, where he graduated in 1957. He enrolled in the surgical training program at Cook County Hospital and specialized in general cardiac and thoracic surgery in 1964. Fabian was the first fully certified cardiothoracic surgeon in Nigeria.

Fabian returned to Nigeria in 1965 as a pediatric thoracic and cardiovascular surgeon and joined the faculty at UCH/UI. He fled from Ibadan at the beginning of the Nigeria-Biafra war in 1967. During the war, Fabian served as a surgeon and head of the Biafran Teaching Hospital in various locations, including Enugu and Emekukwu, and secretary of the Biafran Relief and Rehabilitation Association. After the war, he was appointed a distinguished professor and HOD of surgery at the UNN Teaching Hospital (UNTH), and the administrative head of the Enugu campus of the university.

Fabian established the Department of Surgery at UNTH despite unsuccessful attempts at obtaining funding from many organizations in the United States, the United Kingdom, Scandinavia. Through unparalleled determination and ingenuity, he was able to garner enough funds locally through the generosity of Nigerians to build the operating theater and buy the equipment needed for open-heart surgery in Enugu. On February 1, 1974, Fabian led the team that performed the first successful open-heart surgery in Black Africa. On February 2, 1974, the second open-heart operation was performed, and five other patients followed the landmark surgeries. Subsequently, General Buhari/Idiagbon military government designated UNTH as a Centre of Excellence for Cardiovascular Diseases (UNTH, 2010).

Fabian was one of the founding members of the NAS and a fellow of several professional and academic organizations, including the International College of Surgeons, American College of Surgeons, American Association for Thoracic Surgery, and the West African College of Surgeons. He was a prolific scholar who published several manuscripts in peer-reviewed journals. He married Miss Anna Brita Bystrom on April 28, 1956, and the union had ten children, Sadly, Fabian died on November 17, 2006 (Wikimedia Foundation Inc, 2019).

Elfrida O. Adebo (1928–), first Nigerian professor of nursing

Elfrida was born on March 3, 1928, at Abeokuta as one of the four children of Mr. and Madam Olaniyan. She trained as a staff nurse and midwife at St. Mercy's Hospital, Paddington, London (1957–1958), and at the University of

North Carolina, Chapel Hills (1976–1980). Elfrida returned to Nigeria and worked in Ibadan as a public health nurse from 1959 to 1962. She joined the Public Health Nursing School of Hygiene in Ibadan as an instructor in 1962 and migrated in 1967 to UI as a lecturer. She worked in that capacity till 1971 and climbed the academic ladder to become a professor and the HOD of nursing in 1984 – the first Nigerian professor of nursing.

During her career, she represented the Nursing and Midwifery Council of Nigeria at national and international levels. She also served as a consultant on the African health training project group on nursing, midwifery, and allied health professions, and on WHO experts' advisory panel on nursing (1973). She published nine monographs in nursing and 14 articles in peer-reviewed journals (Osso, 2017d).

Paul Ogbuehi (1936–2016), professor and father of optometry in Nigeria

Paul was born in September 1936 in Umuopara, Umuahia south local government area in Abia state to Chief and (Mrs.) Stephen and Lolo Ogbonna Ogbuehi. He attended Methodist College, Uzuakoli, for his secondary school education, and passed the Cambridge school certificate examination with grade one. He proceeded to Dennis Memorial Grammar School, Onitsha for his high school education and subsequently the UI, wherein 1959, earned a BSc (honors) second class upper division degree in physics. He obtained the Doctor of Optometry degree in 1974 from the New England College of Optometry, Boston.

Paul made giant strides and monumental contributions to the optometry programs in various universities worldwide – UI, UNN, UNIBEN, King Saud University, Saudi Arabia, and Abia state University, Nigeria. He was a professor of optometry for 26 years (1976–2002) and taught optometry at UNIBEN for 14 years (1974–1988). He established at UNIBEN the first university-based optometry program in Black Africa. Paul resigned his appointment at the UNIBEN in 1988 to establish the Department of Optometry in the College of Applied Sciences, King Saud University, where he was a professor of optometry for 12 years (1988–2000). He returned to Nigeria in 2000 to establish the Department of Optometry at Abia State University, where he taught from 2000 to 2002.

At the UNIBEN, Paul trained the first cohort of Nigerians to earn an optometry degree, and served as the secretary (1977–1986), and president (1986–1988) of the Nigerian Optometry Association. Between 2000 and 2001, he also served as chairman of the Optometry and Dispensing Opticians Registration Board of Nigeria and president of the Nigerian College of Optometrists from 2009 to 2016. During his illustrious career, Paul received a fellowship award from the Nigerian College of Optometrists, American Academy of Optometry, Nigerian Optometric Association, and the Nigerian Institute of Physics. In 2016, the Abia state government honored him with the prestigious title of the Enyi Abia in recognition of his efforts as one of the founding fathers of the state. Paul was the chairman of the Abia state advisory committee on disability and a member of Ridge Club in Umuahia. He was active in his community and received two chieftaincy titles, Mgborogwu of Umuokpara and Akachi of Ezeleke.

Paul was described by one of his mentees as "a pacesetter, role model, leader, and the patriarch of optometry in Nigeria." He is survived by his amiable wife, Chief Joanah Ogbuehi, a retired deputy director in the Federal Ministry of Labor and Productivity, a son, Kelechi Ogbuehi, professor of ophthalmology and daughter, Mrs. Ogonna Agbi, a chartered accountant. On January 21, 2017, he was laid to rest in his hometown, Umuokpara, Umuahia (Egboluche, 2017).

Vincent Chukumeka Babatunde Nwuga (1939–2015), first Nigerian professor of physiotherapy

Vincent was born on April 22, 1939, in Lagos to Mr. Christopher Aniemeka Nwuga and Mrs. Agnes Nwuga (nee Okolo). His father, born in Enugu, was a civil servant with the Federal Ministry of Finance, and his mother from Asaba was a primary school teacher. He attended Holy Cross Catholic Primary School from 1945 to 1952 and St. Gregory's College in Lagos from 1953 to 1958. He proceeded to the United Kingdom, in 1961, for his high school certificate education at the Polytechnic, Harrogate, in Yorkshire, where he studied physics, biology, and chemistry. Subsequently, he attended and graduated from the Royal Herbert Hospital School of Physiotherapy in Woolwich and became a registered member of the Chartered Society of Physiotherapy. Vincent worked at both Brook General Hospital and Lewisham Hospital in London from 1967 to 1969 and returned to Nigeria in 1969. He was employed as a physiotherapist at UCH from 1969 to 1972 and transferred his service in 1973 to the FHS at OAU as a graduate assistant.

In 1971, Vincent earned a Bachelor of Science (BSc) degree in physical therapy from the School of Medical Rehabilitation, University of Manitoba, Canada, and a Master's (MSc) degree in physical medicine from the University of Minnesota, Minneapolis (1974), and a PhD degree from OAU (in 1977). He was the first physiotherapist in Nigeria to earn postgraduate (MSc and PhD) degrees and the first appointed a consultant physiotherapist (Balogun, 2015). After the doctoral degree, he rose rapidly through the academic ladder from Lecturer I in 1978 and became a professor in 1983.

During his academic career, Vincent systematically repackaged the oscillatory manual therapy methods, popularized by osteopaths and chiropractors in North America. He termed them the "Nwugarian" technique, which he successfully used to manage patients with low back dysfunction. Vincent was a beacon of hope to many of his students who saw him as a "fatherly figure" whom they can confide, and many of the patients with low back pain whom he successfully relieved of many years of agony and despair. Vincent was a trailblazer and a visionary physiotherapist academic extraordinaire, a doyen clinician per excellence.

Vincent broke the glass ceiling of achievement within the physiotherapy profession. In 1985, he developed the first MSc physiotherapy degree program in Africa. He also conceived at OAU the first occupational therapy educational program in Nigeria. He served as acting HOD of the Department of Nursing and Rehabilitation from 1979 to 1980, vice-dean of the FHS (1980–1981), and HOD of medical rehabilitation (1983–1989). He also served as the dean of the Faculty of Basic Medical Sciences (1991–1994) and was honored with the emeritus professor of physiotherapy. He served two terms as president of the Nigerian Society of Physiotherapy (1978–1982) and brought stature and pizzazz to the physiotherapy profession during his tenure. He played a pivotal role in the federal government action that established the Medical Rehabilitation Therapist Board of Nigeria in 1988. He authored 5 books and 69 manuscripts published in peer-reviewed journals in his area of clinical expertise – musculoskeletal (orthopedic) physiotherapy. He was married twice and blessed with three sons and two daughters; the most recent union was to Gladys Olapeju Ajayi in 1964. He passed away to join his creator on June 30, 2015, after a protracted illness (Eni, 2015; Osso, 2017e).

Cletus Nzebunwa Aguwa (1942–), first professor of clinical pharmacy in Africa

Cletus was born on November 24, 1942, and started primary school at St. Joseph's School (now Central School), Eke Nguru in Aboh Mbaise LGA of Imo state. Through the Eastern Nigerian regional scholarship, he attended Holy Ghost College, Owerri, from 1960 to 1964. After that, he proceeded to Trinity High School, Oguta, for the high school certificate education (1965 to 1966). He obtained his BSc degree in pharmacy from Howard University, and registered to practice in the states of Maryland, Pennsylvania, and Washington DC. He had his postgraduate degree from the Philadelphia College of Pharmacy and Sciences and was employed as an assistant professor of clinical pharmacy at Howard from 1974 to 1978.

Cletus returned to Nigeria in 1978 and joined the Faculty of Pharmaceutical Sciences at UNN. He climbed the academic ladder and became the first professor of clinical pharmacy in Black Africa (1987). He is a fellow of the West African Postgraduate College of Pharmacists and the Pharmaceutical Society of Nigeria and made significant contributions by training several generations of pharmacists in Nigeria. He also authored some books in pharmacy (Folorunsho-Francis, 2016; Wikimedia Foundation Inc., 2018b).

Dennis Chima Ugwuegbu (1942–), first Nigerian professor of psychology

Dennis was born on November 2, 1942, in Orlu, Imo state, to Mr. Ugwuegbu Osuoha Uzoechi Nwaoha, a farmer, Mrs. Margaret Nwannediya (nee Nwaobire), a trader and farmer. Dennis attended Wayne State University for his undergraduate (BA, 1966) and postgraduate (MA, 1968) degrees in industrial/

organizational psychology. Subsequently, he enrolled for a PhD degree in psychology at Kent State University and graduated in 1973 (Osso, 2019). Dennis returned to Nigeria in 1973 and cofounded the Department of Psychology at UI. He rose rapidly through the academic rank as a senior lecturer in 1978 and, in 1982, became a professor and HOD and served for over 15 years. He was a visiting professor at the University of Waterloo, Canada (1982–1983), visiting professor at the University of Michigan (1999–2003).

Dennis is a prolific scholar who has published more than 150 articles in peer-refereed journals in psychology and coedited several books. He is a fellow of the Institute of Administrative Management of Nigeria and was named African father of management and administration (1998). He served as the board chair for the Owerri Digital Village (1980–1990), founder and president of the African Society for the Psychological Study of Social Issues, president of the Nigerian Psychological Society, and president of the Nigerian Association for the Gifted and Talented (1985), an executive member of the Igbo Community Development Association. For his civic contributions, he received two chieftaincy titles as the Owa N'di Igbo Ji Ahuzo, and Eze Ndi Igbo N'Ala Ibadan (2003). Dennis is founder and executive director of the Social Economic Research and Consultancy in Ypsilanti, Michigan (2006–present). He was married to Frances Cash on August 27, 1969 (divorced) and married Elizabeth Toyin Fayose (a social worker) on August 31, 1998. Between both marriages, he has five children (Encyclopedia.com, 2019)

Discussion

This chapter sets out to identify the pioneer Nigerian HCE academicians and to explore their service and scholarship contributions. After a rigorous search of the literature on the major databases using the keywords "bibliometrics, H-index, Faculty, health, and Nigeria," no relevant "hit" was obtained, suggesting no previous empirical study has been published on the research productivity of Nigerian health care academicians as a group. An analysis of the academic accomplishments of the 19 scholars, gleaned from open access sources revealed that Osuntokun and Lucas were the most prolific scholars. On the other hand, Mabayoje and Adebo's publications were few and far between. Lucas' innovative program designed for the WHO improved the control of malaria, schistosomiasis, filariasis, leishmaniasis, Chagas disease, African trypanosomiasis, and guinea worm cease-fire, and leprosy. These diseases till today affect millions of the most impoverished people in tropical Africa, Asia, and South America. Lucas later focused his research on maternal and child health to prevent maternal morbidity and mortality (Prince Mahidol Award Foundation, 2006; Wikimedia Foundation Inc., 2019).

Osuntokun was a great Nigerian who left his footprints in the sands of neuro-epidemiological time. He launched a productive career by investigating the ataxic neuropathy associated with the high consumption of ill-processed Cassava with little or no supplement Cassava in Epe. He posited that the disorders (peripheral neuropathy, myelopathy, sensorineural deafness, and optic atrophy) was due to the high level of cyanogenic glycosides in the Cassava – the syndrome called "tropical ataxic neuropathy." The neuropathy associated with the ingestion of ill-processed Cassava, due to cyanide intoxication, was named the "Osuntokun's sign" in the African medical literature. He and his colleagues saw over 10,000 neurological cases, and their astute clinical observation led them to describe congenital asymbolia and auditory imperception, which was referred to as "Osuntokun's disease." Unfortunately, outside the continent, the term is not widely known (Roman, 1997).

Additionally, Osuntokun and the late Bruce S. Schoenberg and his associates developed the WHO's protocol for community-based studies of neurological disorders called the "green forms." The procedure was used at Igbo-Ora and all over the world (Copiah County, Mississippi, United States, Quito in Ecuador, China, and India) to study neurological diseases. The modified version of the protocol is used for cultural comparisons and generation of hypotheses on disease etiology. Later in his career, Osuntokun studied dementia among Africans in the diaspora by using the transnational, cross-cultural method to identify the putative risk factors. He inspired research into possible environmental factors in Alzheimer's disease and posited that psychosocial stimulation contributes to cognitive decline among the elderly (Ogunniyi, 1995).

More than their scholarship productivity, as a group, the service performance of the pioneer Nigerian HCE academicians is perhaps the most poignant. At the international level, Lambo and Ransome-Kuti's appointment as deputy director-general and Osotimehin's role as the executive director of the UNPF elevated the image of Nigeria on the world stage. Lambo's tenure as the deputy director-general of WHO and his overall performance is golden moments of the world body. He strongly pursued the case to invest not only in Africa but in all low-income countries.

At the national level, Ransome-Kuti's tenure as health minister is the most enduring as he advocated universal primary health care (PHC) as the epicenter of the health care system based on the models recommended by the Alma Ata Declaration in 1978. In 1988, Ransome-Kuti launched Nigeria's first comprehensive national health policy by expanding PHC services to all of the 52 local government areas. The PHC strategy emphasized preventive health care services at the grass-root, promoted exclusive breastfeeding practice, introduced free vaccination to children. He also encouraged the use of oral rehydration therapy by nursing mothers, helped continuous nationwide vaccination, mandated the recording of maternal deaths, and pioneered effective HIV/AIDS campaign. His efforts provided universal child immunization for over 80% of the population. Sadly, the military government that took over in 1993 ended the giant strides recorded under Professor Ransome-Kuti's leadership.

Adesanya Ige Grillo deserves special commendation for his visionary insight for conceptualizing HCE programs at OAU that was out of step with the conventional medical and dental curricula at UCH/UI and CMUL. He was five decades ahead of his time because the NUC, in 2016, embraced the combined

BS/MBChB/BDS curricula philosophy that he launched in 1972 (National Universities Commission, 2016).

It is pertinent to mention that in addition to those featured in this chapter other academicians also contributed to the development of HCE in the early 20th century. Examples are Professor Jibril Muhammad Aminu, professor of medicine (1979–1995), and VC of the University of Maiduguri (1980–1985) and Nigerian Ambassador to the United States (1999–2003); Ambrose Folorunsho Alli (1929–1989) former executive governor of Bendel state and professor of morbid anatomy and HOD of pathology at UNIBEN (1974–1979); Professor Herbert C. Kodilinye, founding dean of the FOM at UNTH and UNN fourth VC; Professor Vincent E. Aimakhu, HOD of obstetrics and gynecology at UI. Others are Professor Joseph Chike Edozien, the first Nigerian professor of physiology; Professor Oladele Ajose (1907–1978), the first Nigerian professor of public health, VC of the OAU, and the first tenured African professor at the UI and in Nigeria; Professor Babatunde Oguntona, the first Nigerian professor of nutrition; Professor Paul Aibinuola Oluwande, the first Nigerian professor of public health engineering; Professor Adelani Tijani, the first Nigerian professor of nursing from northern Nigeria and the 13th professor of nursing appointed in the country; Professor Musa Kolawole Jinadu, the second Nigerian professor of nursing; and Professor Arinola Sanya, the first female Nigerian professor of physiotherapy and former commissioner for health in Oyo state.

Conclusion

All of the 19 pioneer HCE academicians featured in this chapter have one thing in common; they all received their professional education in the United Kingdom or the United States and returned to Nigeria. They contributed to the development of HCE programs in Nigeria and other countries around the world. These patriotic Nigerians deserve commendation because many of them turned down lucrative job opportunities in the West and returned to the country at a tremendous financial loss and personal sacrifice. As trailblazers, they crafted the research agenda in their disciplines, but their scientific impact remained unquantified to date. Bibliometric measures such as the number of publications, citations, co-authorships, and H-index scores of their research are needed to ascertain the gravitas of their contribution to knowledge in their specific discipline.

References

Adegbite, C. (2017) How I became Nigeria's first Professor of Medicine – Prof Oladipo Ogunlesi. *The Sun Newspaper*. [online]. Available at: www.sunnewsonline. com/how-i-became-nigerias-first-professor-of-medicine-prof-oladipo-ogunlesi/ (Accessed: 10 March 2020)

Adeloye, A. (1974) Some early Nigerian doctors and their contribution to modern medicine in West Africa. *Medical History*, 18:(3) 275–293. [online]. Available at: https:// doi.org/10.1017/S0025727300019621 (Accessed: 10 March 2020)

Adeniyi, KO, Sambo, DU, Anjorin, FI, Aisien, AO, Rosenfeld, LM. (1998) An overview of medical education in Nigeria. *Journal of the Pennsylvania Academy of Science*, 71 (3):135–142. [online]. Available at: www.jstor.org/stable/44149234?readnow=1&seq=1#page_scan_tab_contents (Accessed: 10 March 2020)

Akinpelu, O. (2019) 7 Nigerian scientists you have probably never heard of. [online]. Available at: www.legit.ng/1206274-7-nigerian-scientists-heard-of.html (Accessed: 10 March 2020)

Balogun, J. (2015) A special tribute in celebration of the life of physiotherapist icon, Professor Vincent C.B. Nwuga: A eulogy presented at the 7th Annual Convention of the Ife Physical Therapy Alumni Association held at Orlando, Florida on June 25–28, 2015. [online]. Available at: https://bit.ly/3jOXF8H (Accessed: 10 March 2020)

Balogun JA and Aka PC. (2018) Professionalization milestones of medicine and eleven other professional disciplines in Nigeria. *International Medical Journal*, 25(1): 2–8 [online]. Available at: www.researchgate.net/publication/322628378_Professionalization_Milestones_of_Medicine_and_Eleven_Other_Professional_Disciplines_in_Nigeria (Accessed: February 3, 2020)

Egboluche, O. (2017) Exit of an optometry legend: Tribute to the father of optometry in Nigeria. [online]. Available at: www.medicalworldnigeria.com/read.php?year=2017&month=01&slug=exit-of-an-optometry-legend-tribute-to-the-father-of-optometry-in-nigeria#.XmfnDKhKg2w (Accessed: 10 March 2020)

Encyclopedia.com. (2019) Ugwuegbu, Denis Chima E. 1942–. [online]. Available at: www.encyclopedia.com/arts/educational-magazines/ugwuegbu-denis-chima-e-1942 (Accessed: 10 March 2020)

Eni, G. (2015) In remembrance of my very dear friend and colleague Prof. Vincent Nwuga: The gentle human catalyst Prof. Godwin Eni [Ret] Vancouver, British Columbia, Canada. [online]. Available at: www.nigeriaphysio.net/media/archive1/docs/In_Remembrance_Of_My_Very_Dear_Friend_and_Colleague.pdf (Accessed: 10 February 2020)

Eshemokha, U. (2020) Emeritus Prof Baxter Grillo Dorothea, Uniben prominent professor dies at age 89. *Nigerian Health Blog*. [online]. Available at: https://nimedhealth.com.ng/2020/05/30/emeritus-prof-baxter-grillo-dorothy-uniben-prominent-professor-dies-at-age-89/ (Accessed: 10 March 2020)

Folorunsho-Francis, A. (2016) How pharmacy opened floodgate of success for me – Prof. Aguwa. [online]. Available at: www.pharmanewsonline.com/how-pharmacy-opened-floodgate-of-success-for-me-prof-aguwa/ (Accessed: 10 March 2020)

Hallmarks of Labor Foundation. (2004) Hallmarks of labor role model award: Prof. Oladipo Olujumi Akinkugbe, CON, MD, NNOM, HLR. [online]. Available at: https://hallmarksoflabour.org/citations/prof-oladipo-olujumi-akinkugbe-con-md-nnom-hlr/ (Accessed: 10 March 2020)

Idowu, BM. (2019) Adeloye A: Quintessential neurological surgeon, neurologist, distinguished academic, medical historian, and biographer. [online]. *Ann Ib Postgrad Med*. 17(1): 85–91. Available at: www.ncbi.nlm.nih.gov/pmc/articles/PMC6871196/ (Accessed: 10 March 2020)

Isaac, N. (2019) Nigeria: Geniuses – Nigeria's leading scientists and their inventions. [online]. Available at: https://allafrica.com/stories/201908230086. (Accessed: 10 March 2020)

John, EB. (2015) Memorial to Professor Vincent C.B. Nwuga, 1939–2015. [online]. Available at: https://vcbnwuga.muchloved.com/ (Accessed: 10 March 2020)

Litcaf.com. (2019) Lucas Adetokunbo. [online]. Available at: https://litcaf.com/lucas-adetokunbo/ (Accessed: 10 March 2020)

Lucas, A. (1998) Thomas Adesanya Ige Grillo. BMJ, 317(7172): 1596. [online]. Available at: www.ncbi.nlm.nih.gov/pmc/articles/PMC1114410/ (Accessed: 10 March 2020)

McClelland, S and Harris, KS. (2007) E.Latunde Odeku: the first African-American neurosurgeon trained in the United States. *Neurosurgery*, 60(4):769–72. [online]. Available at: https://pdfs.semanticscholar.org/dc2b/3bed9afbd14d2f5fc4fb0edcc2980e2ae2 57.pdf?_ga=2.256171336.2114099833.1583802950-8009808.1583802950;https://peoplepill.com/people/latunde-odeku/ (Accessed: 10 March 2020)

NAOMS. (2016) Nigerian Association of Oral and Maxillofacial Surgeons. [online]. Available at: https://naoms.com.ng/our-history/ (Accessed: 10 March 2020)

National Universities Commission. (2016) Medical students in Nigerian to spend 11 years in university for MBBS degree – NUC; March 2016. [online]. Available at: www.habanaija.com/medical-students-in-nigerian-to-spend-11-years-in-university-for-mbbs-degree-nuc/ (Accessed: 10 February 2020)

Newcastle University. (2018) Dr. Adetokunbo (Ade) Lucas O.F.R.: Global health leader for Africa. *Alumni Newsletter*. [online]. Available at: www.ncl.ac.uk/alumni/community/inspire/profiles/dradetokunboadelucasofr/ (Accessed: 10 March 2020)

Nigerian Academic. (n.d.) Orishejolomi Thomas. [online]. Available at: https://peoplepill.com/people/orishejolomi-thomas/ (Accessed: 10 March 2020)

NAS. (2019a) Fellows of the academy. [online]. Available at: https://nas.org.ng/all-fellows/ (Accessed: 10 March 2020)

NAS. (2019b) Visit to Nigeria's first professor of medicine. *Nigerian Academy of Science*. [online]. Available at: https://nas.org.ng/2019/06/11/visit-to-nigerias-first-professor-of-medicine/ (Accessed: 10 March 2020)

Njoh, J. (2000) Early Nigerian doctors, their Edinburgh connection and their contribution to medicine in West Africa. *Proceedings of the Royal College of Physicians Edinburgh*, 30:164–171. [online]. Available at: www.rcpe.ac.uk/sites/default/files/vol30_2.1_12.pdf (Accessed: 10 March 2020)

Nwachukwu, I. (2016) Top ten Nigerian scientists today. [online]. Available at: https://connectnigeria.com/articles/2016/07/top-ten-nigerian-scientists-today/ (Accessed: 10 March 2020)

Nwakanma, O. (2006) Nigeria: Nsukka and the death of an idea. [online]. Available at: https://allafrica.com/stories/200607030392.html (Accessed: 10 February 2020)

Ogunniyi, A. (1995) In Memoriam Benjamin O. Osuntokun (1935–1995): The Pioneer of Neuroepidemiology in Africa. [online]. Available at: www.karger.com/Article/PDF/109897 (Accessed: 10 March 2020)

Ogunsola, FT. (2014) Apocalypse Now: A call for a coordinated national response to antibiotic resistance. Memorial lecture at the 7th Professor T. Adesanya Ige Grillo at the College of Health Sciences Obafemi Awolowo University. [online]. Available at: https://chs.oauife.edu.ng/sites/default/files/7th%20Late%20Prof.%20T.A.I%20Grillo,%202014.pdf (Accessed: 10 March 2020)

Osso, N. (2016) Blerfs Who is Who in Nigeria. [online]. Available at: https://blerf.org/index.php/biography/akinkugbe-professor-oladipo-olujimi/ (Accessed: 10 March 2020)

Osso, N. (2017a) Blerfs Who is Who in Nigeria: John O. Mabayoje. [online]. Available at: https://blerf.org/index.php/biography/mabayoje-professor-john-oluyemi/ (Accessed: 10 March 2020)

Osso, N. (2017e) Blerfs Who is Who in Nigeria: Nwuga, Professor Vincent Chukumeka Babatunde. [online]. Available at: https://blerf.org/index.php/biography/nwuga-prof-vincent-chukuka-babatunde/ (Accessed: 10 March 2020)

Osso, N. (2017b) Blerfs Who is Who in Nigeria: Ogunlesi Theophilus Oladipo. [online]. Available at: https://blerf.org/index.php/biography/ogunlesi-prof-theophilus-oladipo/ (Accessed: 10 March 2020)

Osso, N. (2017d) Blerfs Adebo, Elfrida O. [online]. Available at: https://blerf.org/index.php/biography/adebo-professor-elfrida-o/ (Accessed: 10 March 2020)

Osso, N. (2017e) Blerfs Grillo, Prof. T. Adesanya Ige. [online]. Available at: https://blerf.org/index.php/biography/grillo-professor-t-adesanya-ige/ (Accessed: 10 March 2020)

Osso, N. (2018) Blerfs Dennis Chima Ugwuegbu. [online]. Available at: https://en.wikipedia.org/wiki/Dennis_Chima_Ugwuegbu (Accessed: 10 March 2020)

Prabook. (n.d.) Oladipo Olujimi Olujimi Akinkugbe: educator nephrologist cardiovascular scientist. [online]. Available at: https://prabook.com/web/oladipo_olujimi.akinkugbe/474318 (Accessed: 10 March 2020)

Prince Mahidol Award Foundation. (2006) Dr. Adetokunbo Oluwole. [online]. Available at: www.princemahidolaward.org/people/dr-adetokunbo-oluwole-lucas/ (Accessed: 10 March 2020)

Ranker. (2020) Famous professors from Nigeria. [online]. Available at www.ranker.com/list/famous-professors-from-nigeria/reference (Accessed: 10 March 2020)

Roman, GC. (1997) Obituary: Benjamin Oluwakayode Osuntokun. *Journal of Neurological Sciences,* 147: 1-3. [online]. Available at: www.jns-journal.com/article/S0022-510X(97)90012-5/pdf (Accessed: 10 March 2020)

Royal College of Physicians of Edinburgh Library & Archives. (1965) Collection of Professor Alexander Brown. [online]. Available at: https://archiveshub.jisc.ac.uk/search/archives/b690f729-6ab0-354a-8808-4298152f342d (Accessed: 10 March 2020)

Shutti, G. (2017) Babatunde Osotimehin obituary. The Guardian Newspaper. [online]. Available at: www.theguardian.com/world/2017/jul/04/babatunde-osotimehin-obituary (Accessed: 10 March 2020)

Straightnews.ng. (2018) First Nigerian professors in various disciplines. [online]. Available at: https://straightnews.ng/first-nigerian-professors-in-various-fields;www.nairaland.com/2273563/successful-nigerian-academics-worlds-top (Accessed: 10 March 2020)

This Day Online. (2004) Adeoye Lambo (1923–2004) *This Day Online.* [online]. Available at: https://web.archive.org/web/20070930165051/www.thisdayonline.com/archive/2004/03/24/20040324edi01.html (Accessed: 10 March 2020)

UNTH. (2010) Open Heart Surgery. [online]. Available at: www.unthenugu.com.ng/open_heartsurgery.html (Accessed: 10 March 2020)

Vesta Healthcare. (n.d.) Emeritus Professor Oladipo Akinkugbe. [online]. Available at: https://vesta-hcp.com/dt_team/emeritus-professor-oladipo-akinkugbe/ (Accessed: 10 March 2020)

WHO. (2017) Dr. Babatunde Osotimehin. [online]. Available at: www.who.int/news-room/detail/05-06-2017-dr-babatunde-osotimehin (Accessed: 10 March 2020)

Wikimedia Foundation Inc. (2018a) Herbert C. Kodilinye. [online]. Available at: https://en.wikipedia.org/wiki/Herbert_C._Kodilinye (Accessed: 10 February 2020)

Wikimedia Foundation Inc. (2018b). Cletus Nzebunwa Aguwa. [online]. Available at: https://en.wikipedia.org/wiki/Cletus_Nzebunwa_Aguwa (Accessed: 10 March 2020)

Wikimedia Foundation Inc. (2019a) Adetokunbo Lucas. [online]. Available at: https://en.m.wikipedia.org/wiki/Adetokunbo_Lucas (Accessed: 10 March 2020)

Wikimedia Foundation Inc. (2019b) Fabian Udekwu. [online]. Available at: https://en.wikipedia.org/wiki/Fabian_Udekwu (Accessed: 10 March 2020)

Wikimedia Foundation Inc. (2019c) Thomas Adesanya Ige Grillo. [online]. Available at: https://en.wikipedia.org/wiki/Thomas_Adesanya_Ige_Grillo (Accessed: 10 March 2020)

Wikimedia Foundation Inc. (2020a) Babatunde Osotimehin. [online]. Available at: https://en.wikipedia.org/wiki/Babatunde_Osotimehin (Accessed: 10 March 2020)

Wikimedia Foundation Inc. (2020b) Benjamin Oluwakayode Osuntokun. [online]. Available at: https://en.wikipedia.org/wiki/Benjamin_Oluwakayode_Osuntokun (Accessed: 10 March 2020)

Wikimedia Foundation Inc. (2020c) Richard Akinwande Savage. [online]. Available at: https://en.wikipedia.org/wiki/Richard_Akinwande_Savage (Accessed: 10 March 2020)

Wikimedia Foundation Inc. (2020d) Chukwuedu Nathaniel II Nwokolo. [online]. Available at: https://en.wikipedia.org/wiki/Chukwuedu_Nwokolo (Accessed: 10 March 2020)

Wikimedia Foundation Inc. (2020e) Isaac Ladipo Oluwole. [online]. Available at: https://en.wikipedia.org/wiki/Isaac_Ladipo_Oluwole (Accessed: 10 February 2020)

Wikimedia Foundation Inc. (2020f). James Churchill Vaughan. [online]. Available at: https://en.wikipedia.org/wiki/James_Churchill_Vaughan (Accessed: 10 February 2020)

Wikimedia Foundation Inc. (2020a) Agnes Yewande Savage [online]. Available at: https://en.wikipedia.org/wiki/Agnes_Yewande_Savage (Accessed: 10 February 2020)

7   Emerging paradigms in health care education in Nigeria

Introduction

Health care education (HCE) is a dynamic system that responds to global standards and regional needs to deliver high-quality and cost-effective academic programs. As a result of the national shifts in academic benchmarks and policies mandated by the National Universities Commission (NUC), the training of health care professionals (HCPs) in Nigeria, has also changed significantly. Regretfully, the changes remained unknown to the rest of the world.

HCE in Nigeria evolved from training in African traditional medicine to the modern western (European and American) system of health care. The need to train Africans in western medicine was conceived in 1861 by Reverend Henry Venn from the Church Missionary Society of Great Britain. Dr. O. Harrison started the first medical training institution in Abeokuta in 1862. The Yaba Higher College opened in 1930 and provided a medical officer's course that includes two years of premedical education and three years of clinical training. The first university-based medical training in Nigeria was launched in 1948 at the University College Hospital (UCH) of the University of Ibadan (UI), as a campus of the University of London.

Subsequently, between 1960 and 1972, the "first generation" medical schools started at the University of Lagos, Zaria, Enugu, Benin, and Ile-Ife. The establishment of these medical schools opened the floodgate for new federal, state, and private schools. The curriculum in the medical schools, except for Obafemi Awolowo University (OAU), was modeled after the UI, which includes preliminary education, preclinical, and clinical medical curricula. The Ministries of Education and Health, the NUC, and the Medical and Dental Council of Nigeria (MDCN, n.d.) provides oversight and ensure each program maintains minimum standards, but with varying degrees of compliance by the universities. The Joint Admission and Matriculation Board conducts the admission examination, and each university selects its students. The National Postgraduate Medical College of Nigeria provides advanced training in postgraduate fellowship in different specialties.

Besides medicine and dentistry, physiotherapy, nursing, pharmacy, and optometry programs were established in many universities across the country.

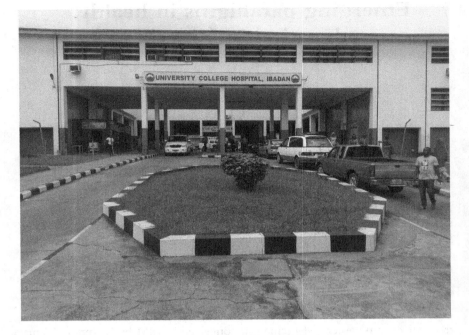

The main entrance to the University College Hospital, Ibadan.

The UI and OAU established physiotherapy, and nursing degree programs, University of Benin (UNIBEN) developed optometry and pharmacy degree programs. In contrast, Ahmadu Bello University (ABU), and the University of Nigeria, Nsukka (UNN) developed pharmacy degree programs. The history of HCE in Nigeria exists in the literature (Anonymous, 1991; Adeniyi et al., 1999; Ibrahim, 2007; Malu, 2010), but the developments in the last decade remain undocumented. There is an urgent need to bring the emerging events in HCE to the fore. This chapter analyzes the significant developments in Nigeria's HCE in the last ten years.

Overproduction of professors

One of the emerging paradigms in HCE in Nigeria is the perceived over-production of full professors. This widely held speculation is not empirically substantiated until now. The Google Scholar search engine was utilized to obtain related comparative information from universities in the United States, the United Kingdom, and Nigeria. The data were gleaned from open access sources and presented in Table 7.1. The findings revealed that the United States population in 2013 was 316.1 million, with over 4,000 higher learning institutions that enrolled over 20 million students. Forty percent of the institutions are private,

39% public, and 21% were for-profit institutions. By academic ranking, there were 181,530 full professors, 155,095 associate professors, 166,045 assistant professors, 99,304 instructors, 36,728 lecturers, and 152,689 other full-time faculty within the United States university system (Snyder, 2020; Multimedia Foundation, Inc., 2020).

As of June 2017, the United Kingdom had a population of 65.6 million (Office of National Statistics, 2017), and during the 2017/18 academic year, 164 higher education institutions enrolled 2.34 million students with 20,940 full professors (HESA, 2019). Of the 211,980 academic and nonacademic personnel employed in UK higher education, only 16% of the faculty were ethnic minorities, and 12% were nonacademic ethnic minority group. About 3,700 Blacks occupy professional positions, but only five managers, directors, and senior officials (HESA, 2019). In 2011, only 50 Blacks of African and Jamaican ancestry were full professors, and the number barely changed in eight years (Shepherd, 2011).

The population of Nigeria in 2016 was 186 million (World Population Review, 2020). As of July 2017, over 2,300 different academic programs exist in the 174 universities, employing 51,000 full professors. The student enrollment soared from approximately 2,000 in 1962 to over 1.9 million in 2017 (Rasheed, 2017).

The data in Table 7.1 revealed that for every full professor in the United States and United Kingdom universities, there were over 110 students, while in Nigeria universities, there were only 37 students. The number of full professors in Nigerian universities is three times higher than in the United Kingdom and the United States. A cursory review of the "*Directory of Full Professors in Nigerian Universities*" published by the NUC in 2017 revealed too many professors in several of the newly established universities with small enrollment (Rasheed, 2017).

Higher learning institutions often use a low student per faculty ratio (SFR) as a selling point for high-quality education because of the individual attention provided to students. Hence, a learning environment with fewer SFR will benefit low-performing students when the academic standard is more challenging (Henshaw, 2014). But this well-established educational paradigm does not hold in Nigerian universities, with more full professors and yet the quality of education is poor compared to United States and United Kingdom universities.

Table 7.1 Profile of United States, United Kingdom, and Nigerian universities

	Variable	United States in 2013	United Kingdom in 2017	Nigeria in 2017
1	Country population (millions)	316.1	65.6	186
2	Institutions of higher learning	4,000	164	174
3	Students enrolled (millions)	20	2.34	1.9
4	Number of full professors	181,530	20,940	51,000
5	Student-faculty (professor) ratio – (SFR)	110:1	112:1	37:1

Several highly respected academics have, over the years, lamented the low academic benchmark used in promoting lecturers to full professorship in the country. Social critics have questioned the credibility of the professorship conferred by Nigerian universities on the ground that several of the professors on *the Scopus* platform have H-index that is less than five. Many academics opined that the proposal by the NUC in 2019 to raise the academic bar and bring the promotion criteria for lecturers in Nigerian universities at par with global best practice as long overdue.

Collegiate system of university administration

The organizational structure and governance of the universities in Nigeria have been a source of debate for many decades (Olayinka, Adedeji, and Ojo, 2017). In the last ten years, the organization structure where the academic programs are located has changed from a "School" to a "Faculty" and the collegiate system. The later was introduced with the intention to fast track decision-making processes and ensure democratization of the operations of the Colleges of Medicine/Health Sciences. The collegiate system consists of many units offering different academic disciplines and varied from one university to another. Some of the Colleges (such as Medicine/Health Sciences, Agriculture, and Veterinary Medicine) operate independently as "mini university" and often located at a separate campus with separate administrative structures, infrastructures, and residential accommodation for students. The "mini university" are granted the authority to design and implement their academic programming (Babatola, 2017).

Although the collegiate system was introduced primarily to decentralize power and improve administrative efficiency, empirical data justifying its purpose and benefits in promoting democratic governance is mixed. In 2012, Itakpe evaluated the effectiveness of the collegiate system at the Universities of Ibadan, Benin, and Nsukka. The study sample consisted of 385 management, 748 academic, and 1,095 nonacademic staff from the three universities. The participants generally favored the collegiate system because it fosters decision making, centralization of powers, the delegation of authority, cross-fertilization of disciplines, and enhance the image of the institution, but the stakeholders have limited understanding of the rules guiding the collegiate system.

Conversely, the findings from a more recent study that evaluated the benefits of the collegiate system was unfavorable (Babatola, 2017). The case study concluded that the collegiate system "failed to justify its purpose and essence" in promoting effective university administration and democratic governance. The collegiate system has not been effective in enhancing HCE, in part, because the parent universities consistently grapple with limited resources and inadequate funding (Okonofua, 2019). The annual budget allocations to the universities by the NUC do not adequately fund the HCE programs. Previous recommendations by the MDCN and other medical academics (Okonofua, 2019) that the NUC should decentralize power for the Colleges of Medicine/Health Sciences by establishing independently administered specialized HCE universities are yet to be heeded. To date, perhaps only the College of Medicine at the UI has been able to garner adequate external funding to support its academic programs. UI, in 2016, was the first university in the country to crack the top 1,000 in the highly reputable Times Higher Education global ratings of universities and ranked 501-600 in 2020 (*Times Higher Education*, 2020).

One of the grotesque absurdities of the collegiate system is the position of the MDCN that the provost of the College of Medicine/Health Sciences and Vice-Chancellor (VC) of specialized University of Health Sciences must be a physician or dentist. As a result of this position, in many of the universities, there is constant friction between the provost and the deans of the basic medical sciences, who typically is a nonclinical scientist, and the deans of allied health, who usually belong to other clinical disciplines other than medical and dental professions. This long-held tradition is yet to be challenged legally. However, lecturers in the faculties of basic medical sciences and allied health sciences regard this view as an insult to their intellectual and administrative abilities. After all, they argue, the foundation of medicine is the basic medical sciences. This discriminatory policy is the root cause of tension and hatred between the MDCN and the other professional regulatory bodies in Nigeria. Critics argued that physicians and dentists do not have any specialized knowledge and skills in university administration, because the medical and dental curricula in Nigeria do not have contents in administration and management. Conversely, lecturers from the other health disciplines typically take administration or management courses during their postgraduate education. Hence, critics contends that any academically qualified professor in any health discipline should be eligible for the provostship of the College/Faculty of Medicine/Health Sciences and VC of the specialized University of Health Sciences.

Incoherent college nomenclatures

As of June 2020, there are 170 accredited universities by the NUC, 43 are owned by the federal government, 48 are state-funded, and 79 are private (Bolaji, 2020). Of the 170 universities, 44 of them offer HCE programs – 17 (39%) are funded by the federal government, 19 (43%) are state-funded, and the remaining 8 (18%) are private universities (Table 7.2).

The names of the academic setting where HCE programs are offered bore three distinct incoherent nomenclatures – College/Faculty of Medicine, College/Faculty of Health Sciences, and College of Medicine and Health Sciences (Table 7.3). The NUC approves all HCE programs, but the Colleges/Faculties are not independent entities, but an arm of the parent universities. Of the 44 universities offering HCE programs, 23 (52%) bore a name that is exclusive to medicine (College of Medicine). In contrast, the remaining 21 (48%) universities have names that are inclusive of all health professions (College of Health Sciences or College of Medicine and Health Sciences). The College

Table 7.2 Federal, private, and state universities offering medical and dental programs

Federal Universities
1. College of Medical Sciences, University of Maiduguri, Maiduguri, Borno State.
2. College of Medical Sciences, University of Calabar, Cross – Rivers State.
3. College of Medical Sciences, University of Benin, Benin City, Edo State.
4. College of Medicine, University of Nigeria Enugu Campus, Enugu, Enugu State.
5. Faculty of Medicine, Ahmadu Bello University, Zaria, Kaduna State.
6. Faculty of Medicine, Bayero University, Kano, Kano State.
7. College of Medicine, University of Ilorin, Ilorin, Kwara State.
8. College of Medicine, University of Lagos, Idi-Araba, Lagos State.
9. College of Health Sciences, Obafemi Awolowo University, Ile-Ife, Osun State.
10. College of Medicine, University of Ibadan, Ibadan, Oyo State.
11. Faculty of Medical Sciences, University of Jos, Jos, Plateau State.
12. College of Health Sciences, University of Port- Harcourt, Port Harcourt, Rivers State.
13. College of Health Sciences, University of Abuja, Abuja
14. Federal University of Health Sciences, Otukpo, Benue State
15. College of Health Sciences, Nnamdi Azikiwe University, Nnewi, Anambra State
16. College of Health Sciences, Usman Danfodio University, Sokoto, Sokoto State.
17. The Federal University of Medicine and Medical Sciences, Abeokuta, Ogun State

State Universities
1. College of Health Sciences, Abia State University, Uturu, Abia State.
2. College of Health Sciences, University of Uyo, Uyo, Akwa Ibom.
3. College of Health Sciences, Delta State University, Abraka, Delta State.
4. College of Health Sciences, Ebonyi State University Abakaliki, Ebonyi State.
5. College of Medicine, Ambrose Alli University, Ekpoma, Edo State.
6. College of Medicine, Enugu State Univ. of Science & Technology, Enugu, Enugu State.
7. College of Medicine, Imo State University, Owerri, Imo State.
8. College of Medicine, Lagos State University, Ikeja, Lagos State.
9. College of Health Sciences, Olabisi Onabanjo University, Ago Iwoye, Osun State
10. College of Health Sciences, Ladoke Akintola University of Technology, Ogbomoso, Osun State.
11. College of Health Sciences, Niger Delta University, Wilberforce Island, Bayelsa State.
12. College of Health Sciences, Benue State University, Makurdi, Benue State.
13. College of Medical Sciences, Chukwuemeka Odumegwu Ojukwu University, Uli, Anambra State.
14. College of Medicine, Ekiti State University, Ado-Ekiti, Ekiti State
15. College of Medical Sciences, Gombe State University, Gombe, Gombe State
16. Faculty of Medicine, Kaduna State University, Kaduna, Kaduna State
17. College of Medical Sciences, Yobe State University, Damaturu, Yobe State
18. University of Medical Sciences, Ondo City, Ondo State
19. Bayelsa State Medical University, Yenagoa, Bayelsa State

Table 7.2 Cont.

Private Universities
1. College of Health Sciences, Igbinedion University, Okada, Edo State.
2. College of Health Sciences, Madonna University, Elele, Rivers State
3. College of Health Sciences, Bingham University, Karu, Nasarawa State.
4. College of Health Sciences, Bowen University Iwo, Osun State
5. Babcock University, Ilishan-Remo, Ogun State
6. College of Health Sciences, Afe Babalola University, Ado-Ekiti, Ekiti State
7. PAMO Medical University, Port Harcourt , Rivers State
8. Eko University for Medicine and Health Sciences, Lagos, Lagos State

Total = 44

of Health Sciences or College of Medicine and Health Sciences terminology underscores the interprofessional education philosophy advocated in this book.

Some critics affirmed that the name "College of Medicine" literarily puts the other HCE disciplines on notice that they are persona non grata in their institutions. The terminology also conveys the wrong message to the general public and stakeholders, including prospective students interested in other health professions, that only medicine is offered at the institution, a factually inaccurate notion. The more politically correct and embracing nomenclature should be College of Health Sciences (CHS), or College of Health Professions. The term CHS will henceforth be used consistently in this book.

All the HCE programs, except for speech pathology and audiology, laboratory technology, optometry, nutrition, and dietetics, are organizationally "housed" within the CHS (Table 7.4). Speech language pathology (speech therapy) and audiology are within the Department of Special Education at the UI. At the Modibbo Adama University of Technology, laboratory technology is within the Faculty of Natural Science. Optometry is administratively within the Faculty of Natural Science at the UNIBEN, and nutrition is within the Faculty of Education at the UI. Nutrition and dietetics are administratively located within the Faculty of Agriculture in several universities – Imo State University, UNN, Bells University of Technology, University of Agriculture, Abeokuta, Nasarawa State University, Michael Okpara University of Agriculture, Wesley University of Science and Technology, and Bowen University. Biomedical engineering is within the Faculty of Engineering and Technology at the University of Ilorin (Balogun, 2017). These examples are an anomaly, and the issue must be addressed.

In some of the CHS, the process of assigning academic departments to Faculties or Colleges is based on political consideration rather than health disciplines with related curriculum core. For instance, at OAU, UNIMED, and Bowen University, several clinical disciplines such as physiotherapy, occupational therapy, nursing, and medical laboratory science are housed in the Faculty of Basic Medical Sciences instead of the Faculty of Clinical Sciences where they belong, as clinical disciplines. Health professions have unique ethos and

Table 7.3 Names adopted by universities offering medicine and dentistry in Nigeria

Medicine	Health sciences	Medicine and health Sciences
1 College of Medicine, University of Lagos, Idi-Araba, Lagos★	College of Health Sciences, Ebonyi State University, Abakaliki	College of Medicine and Health Sciences, Abia State University, Uturu, Abia State
2 College of Medicine, University of Ibadan, Oyo State★	College of Health Sciences, Obafemi Awolowo University, Ile-Ife, Osun State★	Eko University for Medicine and Health Sciences, Lagos, Lagos State
3 College of Medicine, University of Ilorin, Kwara State	College of Health Sciences, Ladoke Akintola University of Technology, Ogbomosho	
4 College of Medical Sciences, University of Calabar, Cross River State★	College of Health Sciences, University of Port Harcourt★	
5 College of Medicine, Lagos State University, Ikeja, Lagos State★	College of Health Sciences, Usman Dan Fodiyo University, Sokoto, Sokoto State	
6 College of Medicine, Ambrose Alli University, Ekpoma	College of Health Science, Madonna University, Okija	
7 Faculty of Medical Sciences, University of Jos★	Oba Okunade College of Health Sciences, Igbinedion University Okada, Benin City	
8 Faculty of Medicine, Bayero University, Kano State★	College of Health Sciences, Nnamdi Azikiwe University, Nnewi	
9 Obafemi Awolowo College of Health Sciences, Sagamu	College of Health Sciences, Delta State University, Abraka	
10 College of Medicine, Imo State University, Owerri	College of Health Sciences, University of Uyo	
11 College of Medical Sciences, University of Benin, Benin City, Edo State★	College of Health Sciences, Bigham University Karu, Nasarawa	
12 College of Medicine, University of Nigeria, Enugu Campus, Enugu★	College of Health Sciences, Niger Delta University, Wilberforce Island	
13 Faculty of Medicine, Ahmadu Bello University, Zaria	College of Health Sciences, Benue State University, Makurdi	

Table 7.3 Cont.

Medicine	Health sciences	Medicine and health Sciences
14 College of Medical Sciences, University of Maiduguri★	College of Health Sciences, Bowen University, Iwo	
15 College of Medicine, Enugu State University of Science and Technology	College of Health Sciences, Babcock University Ilishan-Remo, Ogun State	
16 University of Medical Sciences, Ondo City★	College of Health Sciences, University of Abuja	
17 College of Medicine, Ekiti State University, Ado-Ekiti	College of Health Sciences, Afe Babalola University Ado-Ekiti, Ekiti State	
18 College of Medical Sciences, Gombe State University		
19 Faculty of Medicine, Kaduna State University, Kaduna		
20 College of Medical Sciences, Yobe State University, Damaturu, Yobe State		
21 PAMO Medical University, Port Harcourt, Rivers State		
22 Bayelsa State Medical University, Yenagoa, Bayelsa State		
23 The Federal University of Medicine and Medical Sciences, Abeokuta, Ogun State		

Note: ★Offers a dentistry program (12)

language of communication that are distinctive and limited to the clinical/ hospital setting. Students assimilate the professional ethos and style of discussion during their education in the clinical/hospital milieu. Therefore, educating health professionals in contexts other than the CHS deprives the students' critical clinical experience that is antithetical to contemporary practice in HCE. This anomaly is a quality control issue that the NUC should address with the institutions concerned.

Ascertaining the quality of HCE programs in Nigeria is a subject of fierce controversy. This is because there are no objective and verifiable benchmarking criteria used to discern high-quality programs. That said, attempts are made by

Table 7.4 Universities offering other health care education programs

S/N	Program	University
1	Medical Rehabilitation/ Physiotherapy	University of Nigeria (UNN), Nnamdi Azikiwe University (UNIZIK), Obafemi Awolowo University (OAU), University of Lagos (UNILAG)/ University of Ibadan (UI), Bayero University Kano (BUK), University of Maiduguri (UNIMAID), University of Benin (UNIBEN), Bowen University (BOWENU), University of Ilorin (UNILORIN), Federal University, Dutse (FEDUD), Ondo State Univ. of Medical Sciences (UNIMED), Kaduna State University – (13)
2	Occupational Therapy	Obafemi Awolowo University (OAU) – (1)
3	Pharmacy	University of Lagos (UNILAG), University of Nigeria (UNN), University of Benin (UNIBEN), University of Ibadan (UI), University of Port Harcourt (UNIPORT), Ahmadu Bello University (ABU), Bayero University Kano (BUK)Delta State University (DELSU), Igbinedion University (IUO), Gombe State university (GOMSU), Nnamdi Azikiwe University (UNIZIK), Obafemi Awolowo University (OAU), Olabisi Onabanjo University (OOU), University of Jos (UNIJOS), University of Ilorin (UNILORIN), University of Maiduguri (UNIMAID), University of Uyo (UNIUYO), Usman Dan Fodio University (UDUSOK), Kaduna State University (KASU), Madonna University (MADONNA) – (21)
4	Optometry	University of Benin (UNIBEN), Federal University of Technology, Owerri (FUTO), Imo State University (IMSU), Abia State University (ABSU), Bayero University Kano (BUK), Madonna University (MADONNA) – (6)
5	Nursing/Nursing Science	Imo State University (IMSU), University of Lagos (UNILAG), University of Nigeria (UNN), Abia State University (ABSU), University of Benin (UNIBEN), University of Calabar (UNICAL), University of Ibadan (UI), University of Port Harcourt (UNIPORT), Ahmadu Bello University (ABU), Babcock University (BABCOCK), Bayero University Kano (BUK), Benson Idahosa University (BIU), Delta State University (DELSU), Ebonyi State University (EBSU), Igbinedion University (IUO), Nnamdi Azikiwe University (UNIZIK), Obafemi Awolowo University (OAU), Osun State University (UNIOSUN), University of Jos (UNIJOS), University of Ilorin (UNILORIN), University of Maiduguri (UNIMAID), Usman Dan Fodio University (UDUSOK), National Open University of Nigeria (NOUN), Madonna University (MADONNA), Niger Delta University (NDU), Ladoke Akintola University of Technology (LAUTECH), Afe Babalola University (ABUAD), Bowen University (BOWENU) and University of Medical Sciences (UNIMED) – (29)

Table 7.4 Cont.

S/N	Program	University
6	Medical Laboratory Science/ Laboratory Technology	University of Lagos (UNILAG), University of Nigeria (UNN), University of Calabar (UNICAL), Bayero University Kano (BUK), Nnamdi Azikiwe University (UNIZIK), University of Maiduguri (UNIMAID), Usman Dan Fodio University (UDUSOK)/ Modibbo Adama University of Technology (MAUTECH) – (8)
7	Medical Radiological Science/ Radiography	Bayero University Kano (BUK)/University of Lagos (UNILAG), University of Nigeria (UNN), University of Calabar (UNICAL), Bayero University Kano (BUK), Nnamdi Azikiwe University (UNIZIK), University of Maiduguri (UNIMAID), Usman Dan Fodio University (UDUSOK) (7)
8	Human Nutrition/ Dietetics	University of Calabar (UNICAL), University of Ibadan (UI) Afe Babalola University (ABUAD, Bowen University (BOWENU) – (4)
9	Prosthesis and Orthotic Technology	Federal University of Technology, Owerri (FUTO) (1)
10	Biomedical Technology/ Engineering	Federal University of Technology, Owerri (FUTO)/ University of (UNILORIN), Bell University of Technology, Achievers University, Owo, University of Lagos, University of Port Harcourt (6)
11	Public Community Health / Public Health/ Technology	Novena University (NOVENA – (1))/Bauchi State University (BASU)/Federal University of Technology, Owerri (FUTO), University of Calabar (UNICAL), Babcock University (BABCOCK), Osun State University (UNIOSUN), Madonna University (MADONNA), Bauchi State University (BASU) – (6)
12	Speech Pathology, Audiology	University of Ibadan

Source: https://myschool.com.ng/

individuals and franchise groups to rank academic programs. Example of the 2018 and 2020 ranking of the top medical schools in Nigeria from two different sources (Ezebuiro, 2018; Chinemerem, 2020) are presented in Table 7.5.

The College of Medicine at the UI is consistently considered the best medical program in Nigeria and one of the best in Africa. In 2020, UI was ranked the leading medical school in sub-Saharan Africa. It has ongoing research collaboration with several universities worldwide, including a student exchange program with the Feinberg School of Medicine at Northwestern University, Chicago, USA.

Upgrade in admission requirements

Medicine and dentistry are the two dominant (in power and prestige) health professions in Nigeria. The MDCN, established in 1963, serves as the regulatory

Table 7.5 Ranking of the ten best medical schools in Nigeria

Ranking	2018 Ranking	2020 Ranking
1	College of Medicine, University of Ibadan, Ibadan	College of Medicine, University of Ibadan, Ibadan
2	College of Health Sciences, Obafemi Awolowo University, Ile-Ife	College of Medicine, University of Lagos, Lagos
3	College of Medicine, University of Ilorin, Ilorin	College of Health Sciences, Obafemi Awolowo University, Ile-Ife
4	Faculty of Medicine, Ahmadu Bello University, Zaria	College of Medicine, University of Ilorin, Ilorin
5	College of Medicine, University of Lagos, Lagos	Faculty of Medicine, Ahmadu Bello University, Zaria
6	College of Medicine, University of Benin, Benin City	College of Medicine, University of Nigeria, Enugu
7	College of Medicine, Lagos State University, Ikeja	College of Medicine, Lagos State University, Ikeja
8	College of Health Sciences, Delta State University, Abraka	College of Medicine, Ambrose Alli University, Ekpoma
9	College of Medicine, University of Nigeria, Enugu	College of Health Sciences, Delta State University, Abraka
10	College of Medicine, Ambrose Alli University, Ekpoma	College of Medicine, University of Benin, Benin City

body for the two professions, including alternative medicine. The duration of the training and the regulatory board for all the health professions recognized by the NUC was discussed in Chapter 4 of this book (summarized in Table 4.1). The length varied widely from seven years for medicine and dentistry and four years for most of the other professions, except pharmacy, optometry, and physiotherapy.

Before March 2016, admission requirements for medical and dental programs are ordinary or advanced level General Certificate of Education or the West African School Certificate Examination qualification, and the duration of the training was six years. A significant change occurred in March 2016 when the NUC announced that medical and dental education would be seven years. And students must first spend four years to complete a bachelor's degree in anatomy, physiology, or biochemistry before proceeding to the three years clinical phase of the MBBS/MBChB/BDS degree programs. Final year nursing, pharmacology, physiotherapy, radiography, optometry, public health, and medical laboratory science students desirous of a career change were offered the opportunity to be admitted to the clinical year of the medical and dental programs (NUC, 2016a).

The admission policy proposed by the NUC is consistent with the practice in the United States where any degree, even in arts, social sciences, and humanities is the baseline qualification. In addition, applicants are required to pass the Medical

College Admission Test® (MCAT) – a standardized, multiple-choice, computer-based test. MCAT evaluates the knowledge in four primary areas 1) biological and biochemical foundations of living systems, 2) psychological, social, and biological foundations of behavior 3) chemical and physical foundations of biological systems, and 4) critical analysis and reasoning skills (Association of American Medical Colleges, 2019). An applicant must perform at a level higher than the 80th percentile to have a good chance of being admitted. The average cumulative grade point average and MCAT scores for applicants admitted in 2018 were 3.71 and between 510 to 511, respectively (Princeton Review, n.d.).

Transition of the entry-level education in some disciplines to doctoral level

Another major paradigm shift in the HCE landscape is the upgrade of the entry-level education in some disciplines to doctoral level. In the last decade, HCE has evolved significantly under the aegis of the NUC. In addition to medicine and dentistry, the entry-level education for pharmacy, optometry, and physiotherapy is now at the doctoral level. The remaining health disciplines (occupational therapy, medical laboratory technology, radiography, nutrition, dietetics, prosthesis and orthotics, biomedical technology/engineering, and public/community health) are still at bachelor's degree level. In 2014, both the NUC and the Pharmacists Council of Nigeria adopted a policy that upgraded the entry-level pharmacy education to the doctoral (PharmD) level in the 12 Schools of Pharmacy in the country. The PharmD curriculum first commenced in 2016 at the UNIBEN, and the other Schools of Pharmacy across the country are at different stages of implementation (Ogaji and Ojabo, 2014; Ozioko, 2018).

The implementation of the new entry-level doctoral education curriculum in pharmacy, optometry, and physiotherapy faces significant challenges due to the shortage of qualified lecturers in the universities, the mistrust, and rivalry between the pharmacy and medical boards (Erah, 2011). The Pharmacists Council of Nigeria contends that the transition of their entry-level education to the doctoral level would equip pharmacists with the skills to counsel patients on the management of minor illness and the adoption of healthy lifestyles.

The Nigerian Medical Association and the MDCN are against the idea of training other HCPs at the doctoral level. They averred that doctoral education would enable other health care providers to gain advanced clinical skills with the potential to blur the lines of clinical practice boundaries with the potential to confuse most patients, particularly those who are uninformed or illiterate. And other HCPs will be called "doctors," and "play physician" by practicing outside their ethical code (John, 2016). Critics contend that it is the quintessential mindset and ploy of many physicians and dentists to dominate and prevent other health occupations from attaining true professional status. They argued against the anachronistic and Neanderthal position of the MDCN as shortsighted and misinformed because entry-level training at the doctoral degree level for chiropractors, osteopaths, pharmacists, physiotherapists, and optometrists are now a common practice and requirement for licensure in the United States – a country with the educational and health care systems that are technologically the envy of the world.

Specialized health sciences universities

Several academics have advocated for the development of specialized Health Sciences Universities (SHSU). The typical model CHS affiliated with Universities Teaching Hospitals has not adequately addressed the needs in the HCE programs. Critics affirm that the existing CHS are unable to provide adequate resources needed to launch and operate world-class HCE programs. They posited that with sufficient funding, SHSU will have more flexibility in curriculum innovation and will be well-positioned to produce more graduates in many health disciplines (Okonofua, 2019).

For decades, SHSU have been in existence in the United States, the Caribbean Islands, Japan, South Africa, Sudan, Ghana, Tanzania, and Iran. However, the concept is nascent in the Nigerian educational landscape. The first SHSU was established in Nigeria on April 22, 2015, through the visionary leadership of the Governor of Ondo State, Dr. Olusegun Mimiko, a physician, and alumnus of OAU. Professor Friday Okonofua served as the founding VC. From inception, the University of Medical Sciences (UNIMED), sets itself apart from the existing CHS through innovative curricula and community development projects. UNIMED is the third SHSU in Africa (after South Africa and Ghana).

UNIMED commenced with seven faculties: Sciences, Nursing Sciences, and Allied Health, Basic Medical Sciences, Dental Sciences, Basic Clinical Sciences, Clinical Sciences, and in 2017 added a School of Postgraduate Studies. A Department of Herbal Medicine was created to train the first set of professional herbal medicine practitioners in West Africa. The School of Public Health is scheduled to start during the 2020/2021 academic year. The pioneer departments of the university (biochemistry, anatomy, and physiology) have submitted a proposal to NUC to offer several postgraduate degree programs – Master of Science (MSc), Master of Philosophy (MPhil), Doctor of Philosophy (PhD) and the Doctor of Medicine (MD).

In 2018, UNIMED became the first university in Nigeria to create a Faculty of Nursing Science as part of its academic division with four departments: Nursing Education and Administration, Community Health Nursing, Maternal, Neonatal and Child Health, and Adult Health (Okonofua, 2019).

UNIMED is also the first university in the country to establish a Faculty of Medical Rehabilitation in 2020. In addition to physiotherapy and occupational therapy currently offered, occupational therapy, audiology, speech therapy, and prosthesis/orthosis are in developmental phase. Since the inception of UNIMED in 2015, other SHSU have emerged. These include Peter and Mary Odili University of Medical Sciences in Port Harcourt and the Eko University for Medicine and Health Sciences, Lagos – both are private universities and have enrolled students. In 2017, the first Federal University of Health Sciences was established at Otukpo in Benue State. In 2018, the Bayelsa State

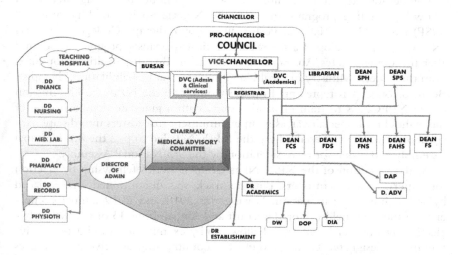

Figure 7.1 The organogram for a specialized university of health sciences.

Government established the Bayelsa Medical University (Godwin, 2017; Itodo, 2018; Punch Editorial, 2018). The Federal University of Medicine and Medical Sciences at Abeokuta was launched on March 3, 2020.

The organizational structure between the conventional universities (see Chapter 4, Figure 4.1) and SHSU universities is different. The SHSU Sciences does not have the position of provost in their organizational structure. The reporting channels in SHSU are fewer and less complex (Figure 7.1). Thus, communication is less bureaucratic and more efficient than in conventional universities.

The SHSU has a unified administrative structure. The executive officer of the University Teaching Hospital also serves as the deputy VC for administration and clinical services and the chairman of the Medical Advisory Committee. This powerful position is statutorily "zoned" to physicians and dentists. The conventional universities have a separate administrative structure. Their University Teaching Hospital is affiliated with the CHS and operates as a "mini university."

Fellowship programs

Physicians and dentists can specialize during the residency training in any of the 15 clinical specialties offered by the Faculty of the National Postgraduate Medical College of Nigeria (NPMCN) or that of the West African College of Physicians/Surgeons. Following successful completion of the required examination, they are inducted as fellows, and the qualification makes them eligible for appointment as a lecturer one and consultant in their specialties. Also, they become an automatic member of the Medical and Dental Consultants Association of Nigeria (MDCAN).

For decades, the other health professions, without success, agitated for a fellowship training program. In 2016, the Nigeria Society of Physiotherapy (NSP) launched the National Postgraduate Physiotherapy College of Nigeria (NPPCN) and developed a fellowship clinical specialists' program structured after the United States, Australian, and Canadian Board specialties. Nominees from the Federal Ministry of Health and the Medical Rehabilitation Therapists Board of Nigeria is represented on the Council of the NPPCN. The mission of the NPPCN is to train physiotherapists with a graduate degree in one of the eight clinical specialty areas in an environment that fosters interdisciplinary collaboration. The Bill establishing the NPPCN failed to pass the 8th National Assembly and is due for reconsideration by the 9th National Assembly.

At the inception of the NPPCN, its Council awards fellowship by election for experienced practitioners, but this track was discontinued and replaced by fellowship by examination. During the 2018 and 2019 annual conference of the NSP held in Port Harcourt and Abuja, about 43 of fellowship by-election awards were conferred. Fellowship by examination candidates receive training at designated centers around the country and take five core courses over 18 months period. After completion of the classes, they sit for the final exam. Out of the candidates qualified to sit for the fellowship through examination, 60% is the final stage of the program and will write the qualifying exam in 2021. The fellowship by examination is open to physiotherapists with a postprofessional graduate degree and a minimum of 11 years of practice experience and at least 3,000 hours of experience in the specialty. Candidates with fewer years of practice experience will qualify for the intermediate specialists' stage of the program. The fellowship by examination is temporary, and once the residency program starts, it will be phased out.

In addition to physiotherapy, a few other health professions now award fellowship following successful completion of examinations and dissertation at the end of an intensive residency program. They do not have a residency program, but award fellowship by examination or by experience to "distinguished members." The duration of the residency program offered is shorter and less intensive compared to the demand of the medical residency program that lasts four to six years, depending on the specialty. Only the physiotherapy profession has a Postgraduate College similar in design and operation as the NPMCN.

The Council of the NPPCN has approved the same University Teaching Hospitals and Federal Medical Centers recognized by the MDCN (2020) for its residency training. Candidates for the fellowship program take five courses and also write the final examination after satisfying the academic and clinical requirements. The eight specialties offered are in orthopedics and sports, cardiopulmonary, neurology and mental health, pediatrics, geriatrics, women's health, and community physiotherapy (Balogun, 2016). Fellowship by residency has three stages: prespecialist, intermediate, and final. There are more than 100 registered trainees who began their training in February 2020.

The School of Medical Laboratory Sciences at ABU Teaching Hospital (ABUTH), Zaria, now offers a 36 months or three years program leading to the award of the fellowship of the Medical Laboratory Science Council of Nigeria (MLSCN). Requirements for admission to the program include registration as an associate member of the MLSCN plus a minimum of one year postqualification experience, completion of the National Youth Service Corps or exemption certificate, and current license issued by the MLSCN (ABUTH, 2019, MLSCN, 2019).

The West African College of Nursing now offers a fellowship program by examination for qualified nurses. The duration of the residency program is three weeks long during each of the four years. Classes are held at the UI campus. Candidates for the fellowship are required to have earned the following qualifications:

1. BS degree in nursing and a minimum of five years post qualification experience
2. 15–20 years of postqualification experience for registered nurses/midwives
3. Honorary fellows of the College, and
4. Current license to practice nursing/midwifery in the country.

Nurses with a master's or PhD degree in nursing or any of the specialties approved by the Council are exempted from the Part I examination (West African College of Nursing, 2019).

The West African Postgraduate College of Pharmacists awards fellowship in four categories. Fellowship by examination (FPCPharm) is for registered pharmacists with at least three years' experience who passed the prescribed exams and satisfied all other academic requirements. Classroom instruction are held twice every year at Abuja, Benin, Enugu, Kano, Lagos, and Port Harcourt. Five years is the minimum duration required to complete the program; one year of the training is for primary phase, two years each for parts one and two. Candidates are required to attend at least two update classroom instruction to qualify for the primary examination of the fellowship program and attend at least four update classroom instruction to be eligible for the part one review. After passing the part two theory examinations (final), a candidate can defend the dissertation project that same year or the next year. Foundation fellows are awarded to pharmacists with a MSc or PhD degree in pharmacy with not less than ten years' postqualification experience. Elected fellows are members of the Council with more than 15 years' postqualification experience or pharmacists with a MSc or PhD degree in a pharmaceutical discipline with ten years' postgraduation experience. Pharmacists who have rendered extraordinary service to the College for not less than five years are eligible for fellowship. Honorary fellows (FPCPharm (Hon.) are nonpharmacists or pharmacists who have distinguished themselves and made a significant contribution to the growth of the College (West African Postgraduate College of Pharmacists, 2013).

The Association of Radiographers of Nigeria awards fellowship of the Nigerian Institute of Radiographers to qualified members with a MSc degree and a minimum of 12 years' experience (Association of Radiographers of Nigeria (n.d.). The College of Biomedical Engineering and Technology, the academic unit of the Nigerian Institute for Biomedical Engineering, awards two types of fellowship to distinguished and deserving members or professionals from cognate disciplines. The Nigerian Institute for Biomedical Engineering with over 5,000 members is a nongovernmental organization of biomedical engineers and technologists in hospitals, academia, industries, and research settings (Nigerian Institute for Biomedical Engineering, 2015). The fellowship of the College of Biomedical Engineering and Technology is awarded to members of the College with a minimum of seven years' experience who are in good standing and have earned a professional certificate, diploma, and advanced diploma or postgraduate diploma in biomedical engineering and technology. The fellowship of the College is also awarded to nonmembers with requisite educational qualification and 15 years' experience in biomedical engineering and technology or cognate disciplines in biological, medical, physical, engineering, environmental, or management/social sciences as it relates to health or human well-being. The honorary fellowship of the College is awarded to distinguished science professionals in the biological, medical, physical, engineering, environmental and management/social sciences (College of Biomedical Engineering and Technology, 2015).

Significance of inaugural lectures

Over the years, inaugural lectures have been an essential occasion of significance in Nigerian universities. Only professors who have delivered their inaugural lectures on many campuses can apply for the coveted VC position. Inaugural addresses allow newly promoted professors an opportunity to share their past, current, and future research work with the campus community and the general public at large. It also affords the newly promoted professors a unique opportunity to celebrate the significant academic milestone with families, friends, and colleagues, young and old. The occasion represents an essential public relations event for the university to recognize and showcase its faculty's academic achievements. It also helps the university to create a broader awareness of the latest developments in medicine, science, engineering, arts, humanities, law, and social sciences (Sunshine Bookseller, 2020).

During the inaugural lecture, the hosting professor, VC, and faculty echelons traditionally wear academic robes. This practice, borrowed from the British academy, does not feature in the US academy. In the British educational system, professors deliver their inaugural address within 12 months of their promotion (University of Bristol, 2020). In Nigeria, this timeline is often not adhered to, and in some cases, professors have refused to participate in the tradition. Inaugural lectures are typically marked by pomp and pageantry, and a carnival-like atmosphere on campus. The audience often sings the university anthem with gusto and the national anthem with sobriety. Regretfully, in some universities, instead of concentrating on the scholarship, over one-quarter of the presentation is devoted to the minutiae of thanking each member of the nuclear and extended families, friends, and colleagues present at the occasion.

Raising the academic bar for lecturers

In 2008, the former executive secretary of NUC, Professor Julius Okojie, declared in an address to the Association and Committee of Vice-Chancellors, that by 2009, all lecturers must possess a terminal (doctoral) degree. According to Professor Okojie, this declaration is in line with the benchmark minimum academic standard (BMAS) regulation on the essential qualification for appointment as a university lecturer (Fatunde, 2008). He told his audience that:

> *If you don't have a PhD, you cannot teach. It has been an old regulation in the university system. If you graduate with a first-class or second class upper, we take you as a Graduate Assistant. You are a Trainee Fellow. You are not a Lecturer. When you earn your masters, you become an Assistant Lecturer. You are still not a Lecturer.*

A decade later, the NUC's proposed PhD mandate is yet to be enforced, and a double standard inflicts the ivory tower.

All over the world, faculty evaluation for promotion is based on performance in three primary domains: scholarship of teaching and learning, scholarship of discovery, and scholarship of engagement or service. In Nigeria, the scholarship of discovery is highly weighted compared to the other two domains. Many of the universities do not have clear and measurable criteria for evaluating the scholarship of teaching and learning, and scholarship of engagement (service domain). Contemporary practice around the world is to give faculty options to declare their primary, secondary, and tertiary areas of evaluation for promotion and tenure. This common practice is still alien to the Nigerian academy.

The contemporary practice is the mystery and controversy surrounding the elevation of faculty to professorial rank – the pinnacle of achievement in the academy. Understandably, attainment of this status takes years of hard work in higher education. Presently, the evaluation process in Nigerian universities is flawed with inconsistencies, inequities, polemics, antics, occasionally animus, and long delays ranging from 2 to 5 years. At times, the dossier of candidates is sent to only connected or known assessors or intentionally sent to dead assessors. Some universities institute grading policy that encourages single-authored publication and penalizes multiple-authored work, a definite departure from the global practice that emphasizes interprofessional collaboration. Given that the world has become a global village, the pertinent question is, should the Nigerian professors be only local champions, or should they strive to be scholars with international repute?

In many of the universities, the criteria used for faculty evaluation are subjective and based on the number of publications (the proverbial counting of the beans) instead of considering the scientific impact of the research work. In some universities, lecturers receive a low score for publishing in international journals instead of local journals, which are preferred. In one university, lecturers receive low scores if the name of the editor of the journal in which their publications appear is not prefixed by the title "Professor"; the assumption is that the journal and publication must be sub-standard! This view is shortsighted because, in the United States academy, the title "Professor" is rarely used; instead, "Doctor" is preferred.

The 2018 NUC's "*Directory of Full Professors in the Nigerian University System*" publication prescribed a "minimum of 60 internationally-published works," of which 80% of the articles must be in high-impact international journals as the benchmark for professorship (Rasheed, 2018). But there was a situation of a lecturer lambasted by his provost for having "too many publications" and asked where he "had the time to do all that research"? And advised him to "cut the number of publications down to 50." His recommendation is arbitrary without a basis. In this uncomfortable situation, what will this lecturer do? Clearly, the provost has set him up for failure since he is the one who will defend the portfolio at the University Promotion Committee.

In furtherance of its regulatory mandate, the NUC in June 2019 released a report on the new guidelines for the promotion of lecturers in Nigerian universities, in line with global best practice. The NUC proposed the use of bibliometric parameters in addition to other less objective criteria for appointment and promotion of lecturers. The Google Scholar's H-index of 40 and i10 index of 30 was specified as the benchmark to appoint or promote lecturers in the science disciplines to full professorial rank. And an H-index of 10 and an i10 index of 18 for lecturers in the nonscience disciplines. Oddly, the i10 indexes proposed for both the science and nonscience disciplines are lower than the H-indexes. No evidence was provided by the NUC to justify the benchmarks and the selection of the Google Scholar database, instead of other more credible bibliometric platforms such as the *Scopus* or the *Web of Science*, which does not require scholars to set up an account. That said, an H-index of 40 is a utopian expectation for most Nigerian academics applying for promotion to professorial rank. (Balogun, 2019; Industrial Engineering and Operation Research, 2020).

Increased research productivity

Research output is the significant yardstick used in measuring the scientific and technological advancement of nations. Countries with low research productivity remain underdeveloped (Odeyemi et al. 2019). A 2017 study by Hassan et al. evaluated the scientific research productivity between 2008 to 2017 in six selected West African countries – Nigeria, Ghana, Senegal, Burkina Faso, Ivory Coast, and Niger. The findings revealed an increase in scientific publications, from 2,500 articles in 2008 to over 4,000 in 2017, comprising more than 50% of the total volume of the materials from West Africa. The increase was, in part, attributed to the fact that Nigeria is the most populous country in Africa and has the highest number of tertiary institutions in the sub-Saharan region.

A sectoral breakdown of the publications showed that the majority were from the public, environmental, and occupation health domain followed by tropical medicine and infectious diseases. The least prominent research outputs were from pharmacology, food science, and technology. During the ten years, Nigeria had the least research impact index and the fewest international collaborations compared to the other West African countries studied. Unexpectedly, the percentage of Nigeria's international co-authored publications surged from less than 25% in 2008 to around 55% in 2017.

The highest number of publications and international research collaborations was from the UI with 5,006 articles. In descending order, was the UNN (3,042), OAU (2,537), University of Lagos (2,311), ABU (1,731) and UNIBEN (1,408). The foremost nation that collaborated with Nigerian researchers was the United States, followed by the United Kingdom, South Africa, Malaysia, Germany, and China. The United States, globally reputed for its high-quality education and research output, issued over 10,000 student visas to Nigerians in 2017 and awarded scholarships and financial aids of up to $9 million to Nigerian students. The UNIBEN percentage publication co-authored internationally is around 20%, but only 54% of the articles were cited at least once. Conversely, the UI percentage publications co-authored internationally is approximately 40%, and about 60% were cited at least once. These findings underscore the influence of international collaboration in boosting research impact due to the increased number of publications cited.

Overall, this landmark study showed an increase in research publications from Nigeria, but the growth was not distributed evenly across disciplines. Most of the articles came from the life and health sciences compared to the social sciences and engineering. Despite the large volume of research output, the findings were not translated into any meaningful policy, patents, commercialized products, or tangible outcomes that created jobs, and prevent diseases. Hence, there is a need to strengthening national health research systems (capacity), develop good research practice (standards), and need to consolidate linkages between health research and action (translation) (Odeyemi et al., 2019).

Controversies surrounding the selection of vice-chancellors

The management of the Nigerian system typifies the decay and maladies in the larger society. The universities are mangled in corruption, tribalism, and mediocrity, as in every aspect of life in Nigeria. There was a time in the history of the country when the VCs were selected based on merit without ethnic consideration. For example, the UI appointed Professor Kenneth Onwuka Dike (1960–1967), Professor Thomas Adeoye Lambo (1967–1971), Professor Oritsejolomi Thomas (1972–1975), and Professor Tekena Tamuno (1975–1979) as the VC. Three of the four VCs who served between 1960 and 1979, were not from the western region (non-Yorubas). Today, the Nigerian academy has become tribal enclaves where only "natives" or individuals from the state of location of the universities are welcomed to apply for the VCs, even in federal government-owned universities. The traditional rulers in the jurisdiction of the institution are now the power brokers in the selection of VCs.

Under the Laws of the Federation of Nigeria (LFN, 2004) and Universities (Miscellaneous Provisions) (Amendment) Act, 2003, the University Council is empowered to advertise and screen qualified candidates with experience in university administration for the position of the VC. The VC must be less than 65 years of age with at least five years of experience as a full professor. The candidate must also be a distinguished academic and top-notch researcher with a proven track record of a significant number of impactful peer-reviewed articles or book publications. The other qualifications required include a terminal doctoral degree (PhD), mentorship of thesis and dissertation of graduate students, membership of learned societies and professional bodies, evidence of discoveries or inventions, administrative experience as dean or head of department, consulting services to local, national and international organizations. Shortlisted candidates' interview with the University Joint Council and Senate Selection Board, and the names of the top three candidates in ranking order forwarded to the "visitor," who makes the final decision.

In developed countries, experienced and discerning leaders administer the academy's different levels. Successful university administrators create a system that rewards meritocracy and not mediocrity. Such leaders are honest, flexible, confident, supportive, compassionate, caring, passionate with excellent persuasion abilities, and ability to leverage team strengths and serve by example. In the United States, the senior vice-president and provost is the chief academic officer of the university. The president is expected to have national and international visibility and fund-raising gravitas. The selection of the university provost and the president is based on merit, honor, and integrity. In the British system, the VC is the chief academic officer and a scholar par excellence who serves as a role model for the faculty. In Europe and North America, the process for selecting university leadership is settled and entrenched in the culture of the university.

Sadly, in Nigeria, the VC selection is fraught with an intense dispute and not a settled case. The criteria used have been a moving target for decades. For instance, in 2015, the Academic Staff Union of Universities (ASUU) and the MDCN sharply disagreed on the highest academic degree needed. Although the NUC, the statutory regulatory body for university, recognized the fellowship of the NPMCN to be equivalent to a PhD, but ASUU disagreed and insisted on a PhD degree. The MDCN argued that the duration of training for entry-level education to be a physician (Bachelor of Medicine and the Bachelor of Surgery degree) is 11 years against eight for other academic disciplines (NUC, 2016a). Besides, admission into the medical fellowship program is a highly competitive compared to the PhD program. The medical postgraduate fellowship program requires a minimum of six years to complete, while most PhD program requires only three years. Opponents argued that the PhD is an academic degree awarded by a university, the medical fellowship is a professional clinical degree awarded by a nonuniversity entity. They also opined that virtually all Faculties of Law in the country had mandated all lecturers who aspire to become a professor must earn a PhD (Fatunde, 2015). The controversy is still unresolved as both sides remain entrenched in their position.

The criteria used for the appointment of VCs are subjected to manipulation, unsavory schemes, and backdoor "fixes." By university statue, deans and provosts are voted into office by their colleagues, while the universities' Governing Councils elect VCs. However, the selection of VCs is now befuddled by nepotism and corruption. In 2015, there was a lecturer without a PhD degree and an H-index of two. Yet, this lecturer was appointed the VC of one of the "second generation" federal universities. The obvious question is, how did this happen when many highly qualified internal and external candidates also applied for the position? Critics affirm that the transparency needed for a successful selection outcome is often missing. This author advocates for an unbiased body such as the local chapter of the ASUU to coordinate all VC Search Committees.

Conclusion

This chapter chronicles the significant developments in Nigeria's HCE in the last ten years. The significant changes include overproduction of professors, collegiate system of university administration, incoherent college nomenclatures, upgrade in admission requirements into medical and dental programs, transition of the entry-level education in pharmacy, optometry, and physiotherapy to the doctoral level, the establishment of SHSU, and development of fellowship programs in several disciplines. Other evolutionary events include the significance of the inaugural lecture, raising the academic bar for faculty promotion, increased research productivity and controversies surrounding the selection of university leadership.

References

ABU Teaching Hospital – ABUTH (2019). School of Medical Laboratory Sciences, Fellowship Program. [online]. Available at: http://abuth.gov.ng/index.php (Accessed: 16 February 2020)

Adeniyi, KO, Sambo, DU, Anjorin, FI, Aisien, AO and Rosenfeld, LM. (1999) An overview of medical education in Nigeria. *Journal of the Pennsylvania Academy of Science,* 71 (3): 135-142. [online]. Available at: www.jstor.org/stable/44149234?seq=1 (Accessed: 16 February 2020)

Association of American Medical Colleges (2019) Association of American Medical Colleges. [online]. Available at: https://en.wikipedia.org/wiki/Association_of_American_Medical_Colleges (Accessed: 12 October 2020)

Anonymous. (1991) Nigeria: History of modern medical services. [online]. Available at: www.country-data.com/cgi-bin/query/r-9392.html (Accessed: 16 February 2020)

Association of Radiographers of Nigeria (n.d.). ARN Fellows. [online]. Available at: www.arn.org.ng/members/fellows/https://m.facebook.com/Radiography Nigeria/photos/rrbn-award-of-the-fellowship-of-the-nigerian-institute-of-radiographersapplicati/832642110204000/www.rrbn.gov.ng/ Accessed: 16 February 2020)

Babatola, JT. (2017) Collegiate system and university administration in Nigeria: A case study of Ekiti State University. [online]. Available at: www.researchgate.net/publication/315046480 (Accessed: 16 February 2020)

Balogun, JA. (2016) Brief on the proposed National Postgraduate Physiotherapy College of Nigeria (NPPCN). Available at: www.researchgate.net/ deref/ http %3A%2F%2Fdx.doi.org%2F10.13140%2FRG.2.2.34276.58245?_sg%5B0%5D= SO8741dBrKWMpdNnu35aoWKk3OdqZmf0GHrxAwNa_ZLU7KmHMuZOd 5HB2zjsyQRPVp_Yz8FgIfkctP8n5mIrfhgcLQ.vPp5cAgV6uNOA42G1NlzuVz1f r8flk57Uhsfm6up7_SeYKaiCM6KDJnhsRJzHM528b9dD1qTcSMHsCzG_SOgA (Accessed: 16 February 2020)

Balogun, JA. (2017) The case for a paradigm shift in the education of health professionals in Nigeria. Second Distinguished University Guest Lecture. Ondo, Nigeria: University of Medical Sciences. May 15, 2017. [online]. Available at: www.researchgate.net/ publication/317387397_The_case_for_a_paradigm_shift_in_the_education_of_ healthcare_professionals_in_Nigeria (Accessed: 16 February 2020)

Balogun, JA. (2019) Advocacy for research evidence in academic public policy development. *African Journal of Reproductive Health*, 23 (3), 2019. [online]. Available at: www. ajol.info/index.php/ajrh/article/view/191210/180384Accessed: 16 February 2020)

Bolaji, F. (2020) List of all universities in Nigeria approved by NUC – 2020 latest list. [online]. Available at: https://campusbiz.com.ng/list-of-universities-in-nigeria/ (Accessed: 10 February 2020)

Briggs, N. (2013) An overview of university education and administration in Nigeria. Guest lecture at the University of Port Harcourt [online]. Available at: www. nimibriggs.org/an-overview-of-university-education-and-administration-in-nigeria/ (Accessed: 4 February 2020)

College of Biomedical Engineering and Technology. (2015) Individual membership – Fellows of the college. [online]. Available at: www.nigerianbme.org/cbet/membership.html (Accessed: 16 February 2020)

Chinemerem, I. (2020) 17 best medical schools in Nigeria. [online]. *Worldscholarshipforum. com.* Available at: https://worldscholarshipforum.com/best-medical-schools-in-nigeria/ (Accessed: 16 February 2020)

Erah, PO. (2011) The PharmD Program: Prospects and challenges in Nigeria. *Nigerian Journal of Pharmaceutical Research*, 9 (1): pp. 30 – 48. [online]. Available at: www.ajol. info/index.php/njpr/article/view/74017 (Accessed: 16 February 2020)

Ezebuiro, P. (2018) About to study medicine? See the latest ranking of 10 best medical schools in Nigeria. *Buzz Nigeria*. [online]. Available at: https://buzznigeria. com/about-to-study-medicine-you-must-see-these-best-10-medical-schools/ (Accessed: 16 February 2020)

Fatunde, T. (2008) Nigeria: Lecturers without PhDs to lose their jobs. *University World News*. [online]. Available at: www.universityworldnews.com/post.php? story=20080327105613634 (Accessed: 16 February 2020)

Fatunde, T. (2009) Nigeria: Medical schools in crisis. University World News, Issue No:37. [online]. Available at: www.universityworldnews.com/post.php? story=2009091123250438 (Accessed: 16 February 2020)

Godwin, AC. (2017) Senate declares Federal University of Health Sciences, Otukpo 'a done deal.' [online]. Available at: http://dailypost.ng/2017/11/07/senate-declares-federal-university-health-sciences-otukpo-done-deal/ (Accessed: 16 February 2020)

Henshaw A. (2014) Student-to-faculty ratio: What does it mean? [online]. Available at: www.campusexplorer.com/college-advice-tips/0DC5BEE8/Student-to-Faculty-Ratio-What-Does-it-Mean/ (Accessed: 16 February 2020)

HESA. (2019) Higher education staff statistics: UK, 2017/18. [online]. Available at: www. hesa.ac.uk/news/24-01-2019/sb253-higher-education-staff-statistics (Accessed: 16 February 2020)

Princeton Review (n.d.) https://www.princetonreview.com/

Ibrahim, M. (2007) Medical education in Nigeria. *Medical Teacher*, 29(9):901–905. [online]. Available at: www.ncbi.nlm.nih.gov/pubmed/18158662 (Accessed: 4 February 2020)

Industrial Engineering and Operation Research. (2020) Scopus vs ISI WOS; Which one? [online]. Available at: https://ieconferences.com/scopus-vs-isi-wos-which-one/ (Accessed: 16 February 2020)

Itakpe, MA. (2012) Evaluation of the effectiveness of the collegiate system of adminis-tration in Colleges of Medicine in Nigerian federal universities [online]. Available at: http://80.240.30.238/handle/123456789/729 (Accessed: 4 February 2020)

Itodo, Y. (2018) Senate approves Federal University of Health Sciences, Otukpo. *Daily Post*. [online]. Available at: https://dailypost.ng/2018/07/06/senate-approves-federal-university-health sciences-otukpo/ (Accessed: 16 February 2020)

Malu, AO. (2010) Universities and medical education in Nigeria. *Niger Med J*, 51 (2): 84–88. [online]. Available at: www.nigeriamedj.com/article.asp?issn=0300-1652;year=2010;volume=51;issue=2;spage=84;epage=88;aulast=Malu (Accessed: 16 February 2020)

John, P. (2016). National postgraduate physiotherapy college of Nigeria: Before creating more problems in the health sector. [online]. Available at: www.medicalworldnigeria. com/2016/05/national-postgraduate-physiotherapy-college-of-nigeria-before-creating-more-problems-in-the-health-sector/#.V0piaDUrJdg (Accessed: 16 February 2020)

Medical and Dental Council of Nigeria (MDCN). (n.d.) [online]. Available at: https:// web.archive.org/web/20130603030344/www.mdcnigeria.org/ (Accessed: 16 February 2020)

Medical and Dental Council of Nigeria. (2020) Teaching hospitals approved for internship training with number of approved interns. [online]. Available at: www. mdcn.gov.ng/public/storage/documents/document_812954199.pdf Accessed: 16 February 2020)

MLSCN. (2019) Fellowship program. [online]. Available at: http://web.mlscn.gov.ng/index.php/register-as-fellow/ (Accessed: 16 February 2020)

Multimedia Foundation, Inc. (2020) Professors in the United States. [online]. Available at: https://en.m.wikipedia.org/wiki/Professors_in_the_United_States (Accessed: 16 February 2020)

Nigerian Institute for Biomedical Engineering. (2015) Welcome to Nigerian Institute for Biomedical Engineering. [online]. Available at: www.nigerianbme.org/ (Accessed: 16 February 2020)

Nigerian Institute for Biomedical Engineering. (2017) [online]. Available at: www. nigerianbme.org/Accessed: 16 February 2020)

National Universities Commission. (2016a) Medical students in Nigerian to spend 11 years in university for MBBS degree – NUC; March 2016. [online]. Available at: www.habanaija.com/medical-students-in-nigerian-to-spend-11-years-in-university-for-mbbs-degree-nuc/ (Accessed: 16 February 2020)

National Universities Commission. (2016b) Suspension of medical lab science. [online]. Available at: www.ngschoolz.net/nuc-has-suspended-laboratory-science-course-for-20152016-academic-session/ (Accessed: 16 February 2020)

Odeyemi, OA, Odeyemi, OA, Bamidele, FA and Adebisi, OA. (2019) Increased research productivity in Nigeria: More to be done. *Future Science OA* (Editorial). 5(2). Published Online. [online]. Available at: https://doi.org/10.4155/fsoa-2018-0083www.future-science.com/doi/full/10.4155/fsoa-2018-0083 (Accessed: 16 February 2020)

Office of National Statistics. (2017) UK population 2017. [online]. Available at: www.ons.gov.uk/aboutus/transparencyandgovernance/freedomofinformationfoi/ukpopulation2017 (Accessed: 16 February 2020)

Ogaji, JI and Ojabo, CE. (2014) Pharmacy education in Nigeria: The journey so far. *Archives of Pharmacy Practice*, 5:47–60. [online]. Available at: www.archivepp.com/text.asp?2014/5/2/47/132644 (Accessed: 16 February 2020)

Okonofua, F. (2019) The case for specialized medical universities – Part 4 *The Guardian Newspaper*. [online]. Available at: https://guardian.ng/opinion/the-case-for-specialised-medical-universities-part-4/ (Accessed: 16 February 2020)

Olayinka, I, Adedeji, SO and Ojo E. (2017) A brief review of governance reforms in higher education in Nigeria. (F Maringe and E Ojo, ed.). Chapter 6 (pp. 113–167) in *Sustainable Transformation in African Higher Education: Research, Governance, Gender, Funding, Teaching, and Learning in the African University*. The Netherlands: Sense Publishers.

Ossai, EN, Uwakwe, KA, Anyanwagu, UC, Ibiok, NC, Azuogu, BN and Ekeke N. (2016) Specialty preferences among final year medical students in medical schools of south-east Nigeria: Need for career guidance. *BMC Medical Education*, 16: 259. [online]. Available at: www.ncbi.nlm.nih.gov/pmc/articles/PMC5050581/ (Accessed: 16 February 2020)

Ozioko, C. (2018) History of pharmacy, pharmacy education, career and ethics in Nigeria. *Pharmapproach*. [online]. Available at: www.pharmapproach.com/history-of-pharmacy-in-nigeria-2/ (Accessed: 16 February 2020)

Premium Times. (2015) Nigeria needs 237,000 medical doctors but has only 35,000. [online]. Available at: www.premiumtimesng.com/news/top-news/192536-nigeria-needs-237000-medical-doctors-but-has-only-35000.html (Accessed: 16 February 2020)

Punch Editorial. (2018) Reforming Nigeria's university system. *Punch Newspaper* [online]. Available at: https://punchng.com/reforming-nigerias-university-system/ (Accessed: 16 February 2020)

Rasheed, AA. (2017) Directory of full professors in the Nigerian university system. National Universities Commission, 26, ISBN: 978-978-964-725-8. [online]. Available at: https://nuc.covenantuniversity.edu.ng/download/2017-Directory-of-Full-Professors.pdf (Accessed: 16 February 2020)

Shepherd, J. (2011) 14,000 British professors – but only 50 are black. *The Guardian (US Edition)*. [online]. Available at: www.theguardian.com/education/2011/may/27/only-50-black-british-professors (Accessed: 16 February 2020)

Snyder, JA. (2020) Higher education in the age of coronavirus. *Boston Review.* [online]. Available at: http://bostonreview.net/forum/jeffrey-aaron-snyder-higher-education-age-coronavirus (Accessed: 16 February 2020)

Sunshine Bookseller. (2020) Inaugural lectures and university lectures. [online]. Available at: www.sunshinenigeria.com/inaugural-lectures-and-university-lectures (Accessed: 16 February 2020)

Times Higher Education. (2020) World university rankings 2020. [online]. Available at: www.timeshighereducation.com/world-university-rankings/2020/world-ranking# !/page/0/length/-1/sort_by/rank/sort_order/asc/cols/stats (Accessed: 16 February 2020)

University of Bristol. (2020) Inaugural lectures. [online]. Available at: www.bristol. ac.uk/pace/public-events/inaugural/ (Accessed: 16 February 2020)

WES. (2017) Education in Nigeria. [online]. Available at: https://wenr.wes.org/2017/ 03/education-in-nigeria. (Accessed: 16 February 2020)

West African College of Nursing. (2019) Fellowship Program. [online]. Available at: www.nursingworldnigeria.com/2019/04/west-african-college-of-nursing-2019- fellowship-application-forms-on-sale and www.wacn-online.com (Accessed: 16 February 2020)

West African Postgraduate College of Pharmacists. (2013) Fellowship Program. [online]. Available at: www.wapharm.org/pm/webpages.php?id=37# (Accessed: 16 February 2020)

WHO. (2020) Achieving the health-related MDGs. It takes a workforce! [online]. Available at: www.who.int/hrh/workforce_mdgs/en/ (Accessed: 16 February 2020)

World Population Review. (2020) Nigeria Population 2020 (Live). [online]. Available at: https://worldpopulationreview.com/countries/nigeria-population/ (Accessed: 16 February 2020)

8 Contemporary challenges in Nigeria's health care education system

Introduction

Increasingly, the world is rapidly changing and more interdependent on one another. We now live in a world where knowledge and innovation are significant determinants of development. Good quality education and learning are becoming more important drivers of health and well-being, the progress of countries, and the quality of humanity's shared future (United Nations Educational, Scientific, and Cultural Organization – UNESCO – 2014). Regrettably, for over four decades, the Nigerian academy has witnessed the migration of its intellectuals seeking greener pastures. But the problem became more chronic in the last ten years with the rising wave of migration of faculty to the high-income countries and even African nations.

For decades, Nigerian public education, including the health care education (HCE) programs, was chronically underfunded. Undeterred by inadequate resources, the education sector hobbled along, but multiple challenges currently mar the system. The training of health care professionals changed significantly in the last decade (between 2010 and 2020), as described comprehensively in chapter 8 of this book. The developments have incurred several unintended events and challenges analyzed in this chapter.

Shortage of faculty in primary specialties

The migration of skilled HCE academics from Nigeria dates back to the civil war between 1967 and 1970. The exodus continues in the 1980s, with multiple coups d'état, the concomitant civil disruptions, and stunted economic growth from the structural adjustment program enacted by Ibrahim Babangida's military administration. By the early 1990s, the migration of lecturers from Nigeria was overwhelming economically, with many of the universities losing their most exceptional human resources to North America, Europe, and the United Arab Emirates. The "brain drain" significantly damaged a once-thriving Nigerian academy, with many physicians and dentists emigrated with their families, and left other loved ones behind (Irune, 2018).

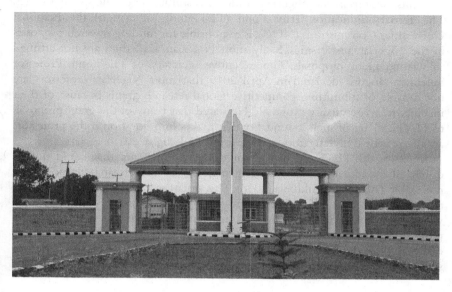

The main entrance to Bowen University, Iwo, Nigeria.

As of March 2020, there are 179 medical (consisting of 143 allopathic and 36 osteopathic curricula) and 66 dental schools in the United States. Comparatively, Nigeria has only 44 medical and 12 dental schools and experiencing an acute shortage of faculty and consultants in the primary specialties. As a result, some academics and technocrats have advocated for the establishment of additional College of Health Sciences (CHS) to meet the urgent national needs. This recommendation is ill-advised and not a panacea in solving the problem. The establishment of new Colleges will require a considerable amount of funding for personnel and physical infrastructures such as residential halls, libraries, classrooms, laboratories, and office spaces, as well as the purchase of instructional devices and research equipment. Such white elephant project is not a prudent option because of the suboptimal economic condition in the country, coupled with decades of neglect and dismal financial allocation for higher education by the federal government. Instead, increased funding to expand student enrollment, promote human capacity building, and physical resource development will be most beneficial.

Faculty limited capacity in grant writing

Grantsmanship is the process of acquiring funds from government, private community, and corporate foundations to support research, training of students, and capacity building projects that benefit the public. The concept of grantsmanship in the Nigerian academy is still in the developmental stages. The Tertiary Education Trust Fund (TETFund), an arm of the National Universities Commissions (NUC), is responsible for funding research proposals in the Nigerian universities. Sadly, most Nigerian academics are not attuned to writing grant proposals. The executive secretary of TETFund, Professor Suleiman Bogoro, declared in April 2019 that most Nigerian professors are not capable of submitting competitive global research grants because of their inability to write quality proposals. He stated that many of the grant proposals to TETFund are of such low quality that makes him question if the professors are the principal investigators of the project (Adedigba, 2019).

In 2018, the TETFund had about three billion Naira that could not be disbursed because the overwhelming majority of the research proposals are not viable (Alade and Aikulola, 2018). This situation is due, in part, to the fact that the skills set for writing successful grant proposals are very different from writing research articles for publication. Hence, many lecturers must require professional development training in grant writing to be successful in obtaining external funds (Walden and Bryan, 2010). Unfortunately, the opportunities for such critical training is not readily available in many Nigerian universities.

Underfunding of health care education

Nigeria has about 10.5 million out-of-school children, the world's highest. Sadly, since 1999 when the country returned to democratic governance, the annual budget allocation to education has been between four and ten percent, which is far below expectations. Other than Nigeria, none of the UNESCO's E9 (Bangladesh, Brazil, China, Egypt, India, Indonesia, Mexico, Nigeria, and Pakistan) or D8 countries (Bangladesh, Egypt, Nigeria, Indonesia, Iran, Malaysia, Pakistan, and Turkey), allocates less than 20% of its annual budget to education. Nigeria trailed far behind smaller and less financially endowed sub-Saharan Africa nations in terms of investment in education (Adedigba, 2017). In 2015, as a percentage of its gross domestic product (GDP), the United States spent less on education (6.1%) than its Organization for Economic Cooperation and Development (OECD) counterparts; Norway spent (6.4%), New Zealand (6.3%), and United Kingdom (6.2%). The average spending on postsecondary education as a percentage of GDP by OECD countries was 1.5%. The total government and private sector expenditures in the United States were 2.6%, Canada at 2.4%, Australia at 2%, and Chile at 2% (Investopedia, 2019).

The highest rate of education exclusion is in the sub-Saharan Africa region, including Nigeria. Over 20% of children between 6 and 11 years are not in school, followed by 33% of youth between 12 and 14 years. Approximately 60% of youth between 15 and 17 years of age are not enrolled in school. Urgent action is needed to ensure the situation does not get worse as there is a rising demand for HCE in the sub-Saharan Africa region due to a still-growing school-age population (UNESCO, 2020). In 2018, John Campbell asserted that the UNESCO recommends that developing countries seeking to develop rapidly, spend 25% of their national budget on education and that Ethiopia met this threshold. In 2018, Nigeria allocated 7.1% of its budget on education, which caused Bill Gates during a visit to Nigeria to criticize government officials for underinvestment in human capital (Campbell, 2018b). The education budget dipped to 6.7% in 2020. Critics assert averred that the decline in academic standard is due to decades of underfunding, and the "brain drain" of scholars to high-income countries and even other African nations such as Ghana and South Africa.

The source of the 26% education budget recommendation often ascribed to UNESCO is unknown and only exists in the Nigerian literature. The Minister of Education, Mr. Adamu Adamu, described "as a lie" this commonly referenced claim that the UNESCO, set a 26% benchmark funding for education. He stated that UNESCO officer "told him recently that it never established the controversial benchmark.... and they don't know where this lie originated from and why." Professor Peter Okebukola, the former executive secretary of NUC, in 2015, also denied the 26% allocation to education as "mythical." He speculated that the figure arose from an endorsement by a local UNESCO officer following a meeting held in Nigeria and does not bind the entire organization (Atueyi, 2015; Adedigba 2017).

The controversy is not without a basis. In two UNESCO reports titled "Education for all, EFA, 2000–2015: achievement and challenges" and "World education forum 2015" tagged – Dakar framework for action – established 15 to 20% as the international recommended benchmark for education (chapter 8, page 241 of the EFA report). The forward page of the EFA global monitoring report called for a significant increase in financial commitment to accelerate progress toward the EFA goals (Adedigba, 2017). Notwithstanding the controversy, Professor Okebukola advocated that 30% of the budget be earmarked to education because of the "deplorable state" of the education system. According to him, funds are desperately needed to "significantly" improve infrastructure for teaching and learning, teacher quality and welfare and curriculum delivery, and to provide access to over 10 million out-of-school children, improve school safety and to promote reading culture among youths and for overall improvement in the quality of delivery of "education" (Atueyi, 2015).

Given the exponential increase in students' enrollment, and the cost aggravated by inflation, the budget allocation to HCE programs has been grossly inadequate. Nigeria allocated $1.86 billion (6.7% of the federal budget share) of its 2020 budget to primary, secondary, tertiary education, including universities (Amoo, 2020). Comparatively, the United States government budget budgets nearly $79 billion (2.7%) annually for primary and secondary education programs (New America, 2015; Resilent Educator, 2020). Public education is funded by the state governments, as there are no federal universities in the United States, but private universities are dominant. Education spending in the United Kingdom, in 2010, peaked at £104 billion (5.7% of the GDP) at the 2018/19 exchange rate (Table 8.1). The allocation has declined to £91 billion (4.2%) in 2018/9 (Bolton, 2019). Almost 80% of education expenses in the United Kingdom is earmarked to primary and secondary schools. The relatively low share of higher education allocation is because the data excluded the subsidy component of student loans, which make up the majority of higher education spending (Britton, Farquharson and Sibieta, 2019).

The United Kingdom spends more on university education per capita than the United States and Nigeria. The estimated expenses on education (per person) in the United States is $246.3, $1,701.4 in the United Kingdom and a paltry $8.8 in Nigeria (Table 8.1).

The differences in the method of funding education in the three countries must be realized. Unlike Nigeria, the federal government in the United States and the United Kingdom have a minimal role in the funding of university education. The comparable information available from open sources for the three countries were used. However, the inferences drawn from the data presented should be taken with a dose of caution because the three countries' education budget and expense data were not for the same year. Nevertheless, the general education budget can serve as a proxy for HCE allocation.

The neglect of the University Teaching Hospitals (UTHs), which is at the apex of the nation's health care delivery system, is influenced politically because the ruling class does not receive their health care in Nigeria. The COVID-19 pandemic exposes the weakness and decay of the health care system to the elites who have no other option but to receive health care at home. Before the COVID-19 crisis, the Nigerian aristocrats engage in "medical tourism" in India, South Africa, and European countries for their medical treatment. For instance, President Muhammadu Buhari and his family receive their medical

Table 8.1 Education budget and expenses in the United States, the United Kingdom and Nigeria

	Variable	United States	United Kingdom	Nigeria
1	Country population (millions) ★	320.7 (in 2015)	66.3 in 2018/9	205.3 in 2020
2	Institutions of higher learning	4,000	164	174
3	Students enrolled (millions)	20	2.34	1.9
4	Annual education budget★★	$79 billion (in 2015)	£91 billion ($112.8 billion) in 2018/9	N 691.07 billion ($1.8 billion) in 2020
5	Education allocation as a % of budget	2.7%	4.2%	6.7%
6	Expenses on education per person	$246.3	$1,701.4	$8.8

Notes: ★World Population Review. (2020).
★★The exchange rate as of May 7, 2020 = £ = 1.24 $; N = 0.0026$.

treatment and annual check-ups abroad. Nigerians spend over $1billion annually on medical treatment abroad, and this massive foreign exchange waste can be better utilized to upgrade the dilapidated infrastructure at the UTHs. This move will adequately address the deficiencies that this book chronicles and end the disgraceful practice of medical tourism while promoting high-quality HCE in Nigeria.

For several decades, patients admitted to the UTHs pay for their services. But in the last decade, the federal government eliminated the fees with the promise to increase funding. This pledge was never kept and led to a significant decrease in the number of patients. As government subsidies to UTHs dwindled, patients were again requested to pay for their services, and admission further plummeted. In many hospitals, only the elites who can afford to pay, but with uncomplicated diseases (for which they traveled abroad) often show up. This development has negatively affected the depth of clinical education experience that students receive (Fatunde, 2009).

Annually, Nigeria produces over 2,000 physicians/dentists. Unfortunately, many of the graduates' struggle to find placements for the one-year internship experience in the facilities approved by the Medical and Dental Council of Nigeria (MDCN, n.d.). The shortage can be prevented by having each state government hire additional consultants and seek accreditation for the internship program in at least two General Hospitals in their state. A significant constraint to the training of consultant is the acute shortage of fellowship positions in the UTHs (MDCN, 2020). The journey to becoming a consultant begins with the completion of the entry-level professional (MBBS/MBChB/BDS) degree. The next barriers are the internship experience and residency training program – an institutional-based structured training for physician and dentist graduates.

The National Postgraduate Medical College of Nigeria (NPMCN) and the West African Postgraduate Medical College offer residency training at 48 approved hospitals across the country. The duration of the residency program range from four to six years, depending on the specialty. The 15 specialties currently offered by the NPMCN include anesthesia, dental surgery, family medicine, family dentistry, internal medicine, pediatrics, obstetrics and gynecology, ophthalmology, orthopedics, otorhinolaryngology, pathology, psychiatry, public health, radiology, and surgery (National Postgraduate Medical College of Nigeria, n.d.). Upon successful completion of the competency exams in the residency program, the graduates are awarded the fellowship of the College. This qualification makes them eligible for an appointment as a lecturer one and consultant at the UTHs.

The postgraduate training in medicine and dentistry is acutely underfunded because the law that created TETFund (the federal agency that provides funding for tertiary education in the country) did not include HCE disciplines in its resource allocation. Under the current dispensation, the Federal Ministry of Health and the State Ministries of Health are responsible for funding the UTHs and Specialist Hospital Centers, where postgraduate training occurs. Regrettably, these institutions do not receive funding allocation from the federal government for postgraduate HCE. As a result, they are without the financial support needed to deliver world-class postgraduate training. In June 2018, President Muhammadu Buhari signed into law the Medical Residency Training Act, to address the many challenges facing postgraduate medical training. The long-overdue law, when implemented, will hopefully ensure high-quality medical training, and build further confidence in the country's health care system.

As discussed in Chapter 7 of this book, the fellowship and clinical residency program in physiotherapy, pharmacy, and nursing are nascent and not currently funded by the federal government. Fundamentally, the underfunding of HCE is compounded by the NUC's financial policies, which is subjected continuously to constant review. This situation makes any long term planning difficult. The economic crisis makes the development of HCE to be stagnant. Additional funding will be needed to maintain the existing infrastructure, develop the operational system, execute capital projects, promote research, and pay staff and faculty salaries. Despite the inadequacy of funds to the universities, allocations made available are often mismanaged through the corrupt practices of those entrusted with the implementation of university projects.

Antiquated resources and egregiously high faculty-student ratio

Other confounding problems in many of the country's HCE programs are the aging of the facilities and instrumentation, and the lack of funds to purchase state-of-the-art research and instructional equipment. Another graphic illustration of the decay in HCE is inadequate infrastructures. Many of the academic programs are today housed in the same facilities and space used five decades ago. Meanwhile, the number of students enrolled has more than quadrupled. Many of the courses offered in the preliminary and preclinical years have over 800 students packed in hot and overcrowded classrooms. In many universities, scheduled laboratory sessions in basic medical science courses such as chemistry, biochemistry, and microbiology are often canceled due to insufficient chemicals and reagents.

Highly disconcerting is the small number of cadavers available in the Department of Anatomy in many of the universities. It is now common to have 40 students assigned to one corpse instead of eight students as the global standard mandates. The situation in the clinical courses is equally chaotic and appalling. The faculty-student ratio (a measure of class size and proxy for the quality of education offered) in many of the HCE programs is as high as 1:66 instead of 1:10 recommended by the NUC (Balogun et al., 2016). In the United States, the faculty-student ratio at many of the elite medical schools, including Harvard University, is 1:13. Having a low faculty-student ratio is beneficial in many ways. With a low faculty-student ratio, students can receive individual attention from instructors, and their different learning styles are better accommodated. In such a learning environment, students are less likely to get "lost in the system" because they readily get attention from their faculty. The close interaction between the faculty and student promotes lasting relationships, which can be beneficial when students need references for postgraduate school or job prospects.

Unethical academic misconduct

All over the world, unethical academic misconduct cases such as data falsification, coercive citation by reviewers, and plagiarism are on the rise. About 34% of researchers worldwide to unethical research practices, which include embellishing data to improve study outcome and dubious exposition of data. Other dishonorable activities include withholding details of methodology or data analysis, exclude data points from statistical analyses because of "gut feeling" that they were inaccurate and false reporting of the experimental research design and results (Fanelli, 2009).

There is now a disturbing pattern of plagiarism at different levels of the academy in Nigeria (Maina, Maina and Jauro, 2014). A recent study revealed that piracy is prevalent in articles published in African journals (Rohwer et al., 2018). Only 26% of the 100 online African journals published in 2016 had a plagiarism policy, and only 16% of them use plagiarism software to screen manuscripts submitted. Of the 495 articles reviewed in the study, 63% showed evidence of plagiarism, ranging from one to greater than six copied sentences (Rohwer et al., 2018). This unethical and unprofessional practice begs for reforms and vigilance by African journal editors and book publishers. Consistent with best practice, increasing numbers of journals around the world now employ text-matching software to screen manuscripts submitted. Unfortunately, the cost of the software license is prohibitive, and many journal publishers in developing countries cannot afford.

An exposé in a national newspaper revealed how university students now outsource their thesis and dissertation project to "mercenaries" who operate unchecked, as business center operators on campuses, and online merchants. Professor Okebukola confirmed that about 60% of undergraduate independent study projects were not their original work and 15% of Master's theses and 8% of PhD dissertation projects were plagiarized (Punch, 2020).

There were many other cases of academic dishonesty brought to the public domain in recent years. For instance, in 2013, former President Goodluck Jonathan appointed a "fake" professor as the director-general for the National Space Research and Development Agency. Also, in 2013, fifteen lecturers from Ebonyi State College of Education were demoted for certificate forgery and false declaration of doctoral and master's degrees from foreign universities. Nine of the 15 lecturers were downgraded to lecturer III, two of them to assistant lecturers, and the remaining two to clerical staff position. None of the lecturers was charged for a criminal act.

Many lecturers in Nigerian public and private universities forge their way to the top. In 2018, the Independent Corrupt Practices and Other Related Offences Commission arrested and detained the rector of a Polytechnic in Osun state and indicted him for a fraudulent PhD degree in economics allegedly obtained from the University of Ibadan. In March 2019, the University of Calabar, set up an Academic Fraud Committee to investigate two lecturers in the Faculty of Law accused of obtaining promotion to the rank of full professor without a PhD degree (Lawal et al., 2019). The NUC, on December 20, 2019, announced that they uncover and jailed over 100 "fake'" professors in tertiary institutions for fraud and academic dishonesty. By not publishing the names of the "fake" professors and their institutions, critics indicted the NUC for demonizing the entire educational system (Lawal et al., 2019).

The upsurge in academic misconduct, many experts, posited, is due to the lack of formal training on proper methods of citing published work, absence of misconduct policies in many universities, and operationally vague policies on plagiarism. Other experts asserted that the increase is due to philosophical arguments among faculty about what constitutes originality, intellectual property, and authority (McCuen, 2018). A concerted effort in each university is needed to address the unethical academic misconduct in the educational system if Nigeria is to maintain its global credibility in education.

Incessant closure of universities

In Nigeria, student unrests, union strikes, and economic turmoil often lead to the closure of institutions of higher learning and disruption of the academic calendar. The continuous industrial action is due to deplorable conditions of service and the failure of the government to implement contractual employment agreements (Oleribe et al., 2016, 2018). At times, the salaries of the Academic Staff Union of Universities (ASUU) members and nonacademic staff are for months not paid in some universities. The aftermath of all major strikes often leads to the shut-down of campuses, and suspension of lectures, examinations, and enrollment of newly admitted students. These actions often extend HCE programs beyond the regularly scheduled period. For example, undergraduate medical training is seven years in duration, but often extends to eight or more years (Irune, 2018). This situation must be addressed as it is disconcerting to the students and their parents.

Gender inequity

A retrospective review of the records of dental and medical practitioners in Nigeria from 1981 to 2000 revealed that the percentage of female dentists was consistently higher than the female medical practitioners. In 1981, only 15.3% of dental practitioners were female, but by 2000, the statistics increased steadily to 35.1%. Comparatively, the rate of female medical practitioners in 1981 was 15.0% but increased to only 19.0% by the end of 2000 (Ogunbodede, 2004). Another retrospective review of the records of 1,490 physiotherapist graduates from the Nigerian universities from the inception of the first program at the University of Ibadan in 1966 until 2003 revealed that only 38% of the graduates were women, and 62% males (Odebiyi and Adegoke, 2005).

In recent years, women are beginning to take the lead in HCE in Nigeria. Of the 1,996 students enrolled at the University of Medical Sciences (UNIMED), Ondo City during the 2018/2019 academic year, 57% were women and 43% men. At the first convocation ceremony of the university held in December 2019, women won all the seven prize awards, and a woman bagged the only first-class degree in biochemistry. These achievements are a sign of good omen for Nigerian women. UNIMED is leading a silent that will see Nigerian women take their rightful place by positively changing the trajectory of HCE in the country.

Although global progress had occurred regarding gender equity, the educational gap remains in many developing countries where women are considered "second class" citizens. In many African countries, gender inequality in education exists from primary school to tertiary institutions in favor of males. The percentage of male enrollment at different levels of education is usually higher than the females in many countries in Africa. Some experts argued that gender inequity is due to the preference of parents for male children because of the traditional belief that they will sustain the name of the family. In some countries, female children are not equally enrolled in school because of the cultural mindset that western education will interfere with marital life. Many Nigerian women view motherhood as their primary purpose of existence. It that role, they are expected to give birth to children, cook, washcloths, and take care of their husbands and be subordinate to them. Because of the patriarchal system, a Nigerian male child has a preference in access to education which confers rights of inheritance on them (Omoregie and Abraham, 2009).

Poorly conceived academic policies

Nigeria has the most extensive higher education system in Africa but lags behind other emerging global economies like Thailand, Turkey, South Africa, Egypt, and Brazil. Emulating the educational model of the European countries, the NUC in 2011, proposed establishing the National Research and Innovation Foundation to accelerate the growth of innovation-based entrepreneurship and to create the commercialization of research findings in the universities and research institutes (Mba and Ekechukwu, 2019). But the NUC is notorious for proposing academic policies that are poorly conceived and often take years to implement. A few examples will be provided to bolster this contention. The National Research, and Innovation Council (NRIC) was relaunched on February 18, 2014, after years of several revisions of the National Science Technology and Innovation Policy, which was first constitutionally recognized in 1986. Two years after its inauguration, the NRIC Bill was formally passed into law to cement its constitutional provisions and pave the way for its implementation. The NRIC had to be relaunched yet again on March 25, 2019, with new Council members. The absence of young experts and recognizable technocrats within the ranks of the members did not go unnoticed. It raised concerns about whether the country is genuinely ready for the digital economy since the older generation rarely critical matters of research and innovation (Ndiomewese,

2019). Almost a decade after the National Research and Innovation Foundation was first proposed, it is yet to be fully implemented.

Again, in March 2016, the NUC former executive secretary, Professor Julius Okojie announced at a public lecture delivered at UNIMED that applicants to the medical and dental programs in Nigeria must first obtain a bachelor's degree. The degree must be in any of the medical sciences, such as anatomy, physiology, or biochemistry. This new requirement extends the duration of training of medical and dental students to seven years; four years to obtain a bachelor's degree, and three years in the clinical year phase of the program. He also announced that qualified graduating nursing, pharmacology, physiotherapy, radiography, optometry, public health, and medical laboratory science students be admitted directly to the clinical year of the medical and dental programs. And complete the degree program in four years. Likewise, in 2017, the NUC announced that "all medical and dental schools must have an approved and appropriately utilized, clinical skills/simulation center" (NUC, 2017). As of June 2020, none of these two critical NUC's policy pronouncements have been implemented in any of the universities.

Adversarial relationship between the College of Health Sciences and the teaching hospitals

In Nigeria, the relationship between the CHS and its affiliate UTHs is often contentious and adversarial. In conventional universities, the two institutions are administered in a parallel fashion that tends to delimit the training mission of the UTHs. This schism is because the UTHs are presently run as commercial outlets with little consideration for their traditional primary purpose in research and clinical training of undergraduate and postgraduate students. The hospitals affiliated to the conventional universities often fail to budget for teaching and research activities, with the view that the parent universities should provide the resources needed.

The rivalry between conventional universities and the UTHs tend to reduce collaboration and morale severely. Having a unified administrative structure as in specialized University of Health Sciences instead of the separate organizational structure in conventional universities significantly reduces the cost of running the HCE program. The failure of the collegiate system to deliver world-class HCE led many to advocate that the traditional medical schools in the country should be converted to specialized University of Health Sciences (Okonofua, 2019).

Campus brigandage and cultism/insecurity

In the last two decades, cultism is one of the contemporary issues that have impacted many aspects of life. It remains a real social menace and a serious obstacle to peace and tranquility in many universities in southern Nigeria (Arijesuyo, 2011). Their activities trigger many of the university problems, and efforts by the government to eradicate campus confraternities have not yielded any positive results, despite decree 47 of 1989, which prescribed a five-year jail term for students belonging to campus cults. Through administrative panels of inquiries, some universities have suspended or rusticated students for fueling cult-related activities and violence, but they proved challenging to eradicate.

It is common knowledge that highly placed university staff, elite and prominent Nigerians belong to secret cults, and many serve as "godfathers" to the student cult members. This support makes finding solutions to campus cult violence difficult to overcome. The campus confraternities' actions constitute a significant obstacle to quality assurance of universities as their activities threaten the very essence of university education (Okoli, Ogbondah and Ewor, 2016).

Sexual harassment

Sexual harassment is now a common plague in Nigerian universities and is dubbed "sex-for-grade" act. A survey study explored the sexual harassment experiences of female graduates in Nigeria. The findings revealed that male classmates and lecturers had sexually harassed 70% of the study respondents. About 48% of them reported physical and sexual harassment, and 66% experienced nonphysical contact sexual harassment. About 58% reported unwanted sexual comments, and 32% experienced demand for sex in exchange for a favorable grade. Physical, sexual harassment included unwanted touching (29.4%) and intentional body contact in a sexual way (28.9%). Following the incident, the victims experienced depression and perceived insecurity on campus (Owoaje and Olusola-Taiwo, 2008).

In 2019, several high profile nationally debated cases of sexual harassment were reported against male lecturers in different universities in the country. The female students and graduates openly accused their lecturers of sexual harassment on Facebook, and Twitter. An undercover journalist reported the most shocking allegations. One of the students tweeted that "lecturers don't just ask to sleep with you, they also demand "threesome," and you must pay for the hotel room, and they still end up giving you E." The tweet went viral and generated nationwide outrage. The most infamous of the five was a case of the sexual assault allegation against a lecturer taped demanding sex-for-grade. The audio conversation leaked to a third party who posted it on the internet. Barely one month after, another student from a different university accused another lecturer of sexually harassing her in his office, and to bolster her allegation, she released the nude pictures of the lecturer (Ifijeh, 2019).

Corruption in the educational system

Nigeria has invested trillions of dollars toward university education for many years during the military rule and at the dawn of democratic government in 1999, but without corresponding positive outcomes. Allegations of corrupt

Table 8.2 Ranking of the top corrupt parastatals in Nigeria, 2003–2007

Rank	Organization	Corruption index Year: 2003–2005	Corruption index Year: 2005–2007
1	The police	96	99
2	Ministry of education – universities and tertiary institutions	63	74
3	Federal road safety corps	42	51
4	Custom and excise duty	65	61
5	Power holding company of Nigeria	83	87
6	Immigration/passport office	56	48
7	Local government authority	47	56
8	Independence national electoral commission	–	38
9	Federal inland revenue service	36	36
10	Ministry of health	27	31
11	Presidency	24	29
12	Nigeria national petroleum commission	27	28
13	Federal housing authority	26	28
14	Nigeria port authority	33	24

practices among faculty and senior administrative officers in the universities are well known. Specifically, there were often allegations of abuse of due process, mismanagement of funds, immorality, and fraud. These allegations led in 2016 to the commissioning of an ad-hoc committee to investigate petitions brought against ten tertiary institutions (Todowede, 2016).

The drivers of corruption in the Nigerian educational sector is well documented in the existing literature (Egbefo, 2012; Ifedayo, 2015; Todowede, 2016; Nwaokugha and Ezeugwu, 2017; Campbell, 2018a; Samuel, 2018; Noko, 2019; AZ Research Consult, n.d.; Chukwuma, n.d.). Ifedayo (2015) reported the findings from a survey study conducted by the Independent Advocate Project and Anti-Corruption group from 2003 – 2007 that revealed that the education sector is the second most corrupt organization in Nigeria after the police (Table 8.2).

On an optimistic note, as of 2016, the education sector was no longer on the list of the top corrupt parastatals. The Nigeria's statistics agency interviewed a nationally representative sample of 33,067 households and found that 32.3% of the adults reported paying at least six bribes in the previous period, totaling about N5,300 (about US$17), estimated at nearly one-third of the average monthly salary of a Nigerian worker. The survey concluded that 82.3 million bribes occurred and cost N400 billion (US$1.31 billion), or nearly 40% of the combined federal and state education budget in 2016. The exchange rate at the time of the study was N305/US$, and the value of the bribes estimated at US$4.6 billion when the cost of living is factored in (Ajikobi, 2017). Ninety percent of the bribes were paid in cash, and the remaining ten percent exchanged

Table 8.3 Parastatals who received the most brides in 2016

Rank	Parastatals	% of bribes paid	Average bribe paid (USD)
1	Police officers	46.4	14
2	Prosecutors	33.0	33
3	Judges/magistrates	31.5	61
4	Immigration service officers	30.7	10
5	Car registration/driving license agency	28.5	14
6	Tax/revenue officers	27.3	5
7	Customs officers	26.5	290
8	Traffic officers	25.5	9
9	Public utility officers	22.5	11
10	Land registry officers	20.9	29
11	Members of the armed forces	19.3	10

for food and drinks, another service or favor. The adults in the survey who interacted with a public official, 67% of them indicated that they were not asked for bribes. But 27% of them stated they paid bribes "regularly," 4% did so "periodically," while 1.3% "refused" to pay. In the survey, the police still topped the list taking the most bribes, followed by prosecutors, judges, and immigration officials (Table 8.3).

The custom officers solicited the most bribes, followed by immigration and elected state and local representatives. The top reasons for paying bribes is to speed up procedures, evade fines, or to avoid losing an essential utility such as power or water (Ajikobi, 2017).

Another depravity practice is the concurrent employment of lecturers at multiple universities in addition to their primary institution. Although the NUC approved only one adjunct/visiting appointment, there are many instances of abuse of this academic freedom work protection. It is now standard practice for lecturers to be employed in two or more universities concurrently. The teaching workload of the lecturers engaged in this "multi-dipping" practice is impractical for them to be effective in their faculty roles. In the Nigerian academy, this well-known festering dirty little secret, despite the immorality associated with it, is not discussed but condoned. The NUC recently issued a directive that universities should closely monitor the background of all newly appointed lecturers to curtail this practice. Without an up-to-date register of all lecturers in Nigerian universities, the implementation of the directive will be ineffective.

Corruption in the university system threatens equal access, as well as the quantity and quality of education, and it affects more people than corruption in other government sectors, by breeding ill-prepared citizens and leaders. For example, several projects sponsored by foreign donors to reform and upgrade university education standards often collide with the brick wall of an entrenched corrupt system, and they are unable to produce the desired outcomes.

Conclusion

This chapter analyzed the significant unforeseen circumstances in Nigeria's HCE, including the shortage of faculty in primary specialties due to mass migration to high-income countries in search of greener pastures, limited capacity in grant writing, underfunding of institutions/programs, and failure to enforce existing academic policies. Other untoward challenges are unethical misconduct in research, plagiarism, and falsification of credentials, incessant closure of universities due to student unrest and union strikes, gender inequity, poorly conceived academic policies, adversarial relationship between the CHS and the UTHs, campus brigandage, sexual harassment. It will be an arduous task to effectively solve the ongoing challenges in HCE because of the endemic corruption, tribalism, and nepotism practices that have permeated the fabric of the Nigerian society.

References

Adedigba, A. (2017) Fact check: Did UNESCO ever recommend 26 percent budgetary allocation to education? *Premium Times*. [online]. Available at: www.premiumtimesng.com/news/headlines/251927-fact-check-unesco-ever-recommend-26-per-cent-budgetary-allocation-education.html (Accessed: 16 February 2020)

Adedigba, A. (2019) Why Nigerian professors aren't getting research grants – TETFund boss. *Premium Times*. [online]. Available at: www.premiumtimesng.com/news/top-news/326893-why-nigerian-professors-arent-getting-research-grants-tetfund-boss.html (Accessed: 16 February 2020)

Ajikobi, D. (2017) Everyday corruption in Nigeria – who is on the take? [online]. Available at: https://africacheck.org/factsheets/factsheet-everyday-corruption-in-nigeria-who-is-on-the-take/ (Accessed: 16 February 2020)

Alade, B and Aikulola, S. (2018) TETFund's N3 billion research funds yet to be accessed, says NUC. *The Guardian Newspaper*. [online]. Available at: https://guardian.ng/news/tetfunds-n3billion-research-funds-yet-to-be-accessed-says-nuc/ (Accessed: 16 February 2020)

Amoo, A. (2020) Nigeria allocates 6.7% of 2020 budget to education ministry. Nigeria education budget. [online]. Available at: https://educeleb.com/nigerian-2020-budget-education-ministry/ (Accessed: 16 February 2020)

Ani, NA. (2018) Decades of corruption have held Nigeria back — it's time for change. [online]. Available at: https://apolitical.co/solution_article/decades-of-corruption-have-held-nigeria-back-its-time-for-change/ (Accessed: 16 February 2020)

Arijesuyo, AE. (2011) Theoretical perspectives on campus cultism and violence in Nigeria universities: A review and conceptual approach. *International Journal of Psychological Studies* (3)1: 106–126. [online]. Available at: http://citeseerx.ist.psu.edu/viewdoc/download?doi=10.1.1.679.3723&rep=rep1&type=pdf (Accessed: 16 February 2020)

Atueyi, U. (2015) Nigeria should strive for a minimum of 30 percent budget on education. *The Guardian*. [online]. Available at: https://guardian.ng/features/education/nigeria-should-strive-for-a-minimum-of-30-per-cent-budget-on-education/ (Accessed: 16 February 2020)

AZ Research Consult. (n.d.) The effect of corruption on Nigerian education system (2005–2015). [online]. Available at: www.azresearchconsult.com/2018/04/19/ effectcorruptionnigerianeducationsystem2005-2015/ (Accessed: 16 February 2020)

Babatola, JT. (2017) Collegiate system and university administration in Nigeria: A case study of Ekiti State University. . [online]. Available at: www.researchgate.net/publication/315046480 (Accessed: 4 February 2020)

Balogun, JA. (2016) Brief on the proposed National Postgraduate Physiotherapy College of Nigeria (NPPCN) [online]. Available at: www.researchgate.net/publication/310473802_Brief_on_the_proposed_National_Postgraduate_Physiotherapy_College_of_Nigeria_NPPCN (Accessed: 16 February 2020)

Balogun, JA. (2017) The case for a paradigm shift in the education of health professionals in Nigeria. Second distinguished university guest lecture at UNIMED, Ondo City, Nigeria. May 15, 2017. [online]. Available at: www.researchgate.net/publication/317387397_The_case_for_a_paradigm_shift_in_the_education_of_healthcare_professionals_in_Nigeria (Accessed: 4 February 2020)

Balogun, JA. (2019) Advocacy for research evidence in academic public policy development. *African Journal of Reproductive Health,* 23 (3), 2019. [online]. Available at: www.ajol.info/index.php/ajrh/article/view/191210/180384 (Accessed: 16 February 2020)

Balogun, JA, Mbada, CE, Balogun, AO and Okafor, UAC. (2016) The spectrum of student enrollment related outcomes in physiotherapy education programs in West Africa. *International Journal of Physiotherapy*, 3(6): 603–612. [online]. Available at: www.researchgate.net/publication/311477857_The_Spectrum_of_Student_Enrollment-Related_Outcomesin_Physiotherapy_Education_Programs_in_Westafrica (Accessed: 4 February 2020)

Basiru, A. (2019) Pervasive intra-party conflicts in a democratising Nigeria: Terrains, implications, drivers and options for resolution. *African Journal on Conflict Resolution*, (19)1: 109–131. [online]. Available at: www.accord.org.za/ajcr-issues/pervasive-intra-party-conflicts-in-a-democratising-nigeria/ (Accessed: 16 February 2020)

Bolton, P. (2019) Education spending in the UK. [online]. Available at: https:// commonslibrary.parliament.uk/research-briefings/sn01078/ (Accessed: 16 February 2020)

Briggs, N. (2013) An overview of university education and administration in Nigeria. Guest lecture at the University of Port Harcourt [online]. Available at: www.nimibriggs.org/an-overview-of-university-education-and-administration-in-nigeria/ (Accessed: 4 February 2020)

Britton, J, Farquharson C and Sibieta L. (2019) Annual report on education spending in England. Institute for Fiscal Studies. [online]. Available at: www.ifs.org.uk/publications/14369 (Accessed: 16 February 2020)

Campbell, J. (2018a) Corruption denies millions access to quality education in Nigeria. [online]. Available at: www.cfr.org/blog/corruption-denies-millions-access-quality-education-nigeria (Accessed: 16 February 2020)

Campbell, J. (2018b) Uproar over parliamentary salaries in Nigeria, again. Africa in Transition. [online]. Available at: www.cfr.org/blog/uproar-over-parliamentary-salaries-nigeria-again (Accessed: 16 February 2020)

Chukwuma, C. (n.d.) Corruption and challenges of educational delivery in Nigeria with special emphasis on leadership and management of education. [online]. Available at: www.academia.edu/30531141/CORRUPTION_AND_CHALLENGES_OF_EDUCATIONAL_DELIVERY_IN_NIGERIA_WITH_SPECIAL_EMPHASIS_ON_LEADERSHIP_AND_MANAGEMENT_OF_EDUCATION (Accessed: 16 February 2020)

Egbefo, D. (2012) Corruption in the Nigerian educational system: It's implication in manpower and national development in the age of globalization. Journal of Arts and Education, Vol.6, No.2, ISSN: 2006-280X. *Journal of the Faculty of Education and Arts, IBB University Lapai, Niger State,* 149–266[online]. Available at: www.researchgate. net/publication/323390666_Corruption_in_the_Nigerian_Educational_System_ It's_Implication_in_Manpower_and_National_Development_in_the_Age_of_ Globalization (Accessed: 16 February 2020)

Fanelli, D. (2009) How many scientists fabricate and falsify research? A systematic review and meta-analysis of survey data. *PLoS ONE,* 4:e5738. [online]. Available at: https:// journals.plos.org/plosone/article?id=10.1371/journal.pone.0005738 (Accessed: 16 February 2020)

Fatunde, T. (2009) Nigeria: Medical schools in crisis. *University World News.* [online]. Available at: www.universityworldnews.com/article.php?story=2009091123250438 (Accessed: 16 February 2020)

Hassan, W, Akil, A, Amine, T and Owango, J. (2018) Scientific research in West Africa: key trends and observations, 1–16. © 2018 *Clarivate Analytics.* [online]. Available at: https://bit.ly/2H1r0y8 (Accessed: 16 February 2020)

Ifedayo, O. (2015) Socioeconomic implication of corruption and corrupt practice on Nigerian educational system. *Developing Country Studies,* 5(16). [online]. Available at: https://pdfs.semanticscholar.org/6c67/eaec4496a2c6302642253febcf80223 08c55.pdf (Accessed: 16 February 2020)

IIfijeh, F. (2019) Harvest of sexual misconduct in ivory towers. [online]. Available at: https://www.pressreader.com/nigeria/thisday/20191012/281754156081272 (Accessed: 16 February 2020)

Irune, E. (2018) Migration and training: a British-Nigerian surgeon's perspective. *ENT and Audiology News,* 27(1). [online]. Available at: www.entandaudiologynews.com/ features/ent-features/post/migration-and-training-a-british-nigerian-surgeon-s-perspective (Accessed: 16 February 2020)

Itakpe, MA. (2012) Evaluation of the effectiveness of the collegiate system of adminis-tration in Colleges of Medicine in Nigerian federal universities [online]. Available at: http://80.240.30.238/handle/123456789/729 (Accessed: 4 February 2020)

Investopedia. (2020) Universal healthcare coverage. [online]. Available at: www. investopedia.com/terms/u/universal-coverage.asp (Accessed: 24 October 2020)

John, EB, Pfalzer, LA, Fry, D, Glickman L, Masaaki, S, Sabus, C, Okafor, UAC and Al-Jarrah, MD. (2012) Establishing and upgrading physical therapist education in developing countries: Four case examples of service by Japan and United States physical therapist programs to Nigeria, Suriname, Mongolia, and Jordan-39. *Journal of Physical Therapy Education,* 26(1): 29. [online]. Available at: https:// pdfs.semanticscholar.org/6520/aebb7b1b952616be65632ffacdc76e64e208.pdf (Accessed: 16 February 2020)

Lawal, I, Atueyi, U, Njoku, L, Akhaine, S, Umeh, K, Adewale, M and Agboluaje, R. (2019) Inside Nigeria's ivory tower where fake professors' nurture' tomorrow's leaders. *The Guardian Newspaper,* December 20. [online]. Available at: https://guardian.ng/ features/inside-nigerias-ivory-tower-where-fake-professors-nurture-tomorrows-leaders/?utm_medium=Social&utm_source=Facebook&Echobox=1576827981 (Accessed: 16 February 2020)

Maina, AB, Maina, MB and Jauro, SS. (2014) Plagiarism: A perspective from a case of a northern Nigerian university. *International Journal of Information Research and Review,* 1(12): 225–230. [online]. Available at: www.researchgate.net/publication/ 271704467_PLAGIARISM_A_PERSPECTIVE_FROM_A_CASE_OF_A_ NORTHERN_NIGERIAN_UNIVERSITY (Accessed: 16 February 2020)

Mba, D and Ekechukwu, V. (2019) Nigeria's universities are performing poorly. What can be done about it? [online]. Available at: https://theconversation.com/nigerias-universities-are-performing-poorly-what-can-be-done-about-it-112717 (Accessed: 16 February 2020)

McCuen, RH. (2018) Advancing scientific knowledge: Ethical issues in the journal publication process. *Journal Publication Process*, 6(1): 1 [online]. Available at: www.mdpi.com/2304–6775/6/1/1 (Accessed: 16 February 2020)

Medical and Dental Council of Nigeria (MDCN). (n.d.) [online]. Available at: https://web.archive.org/web/20130603030344/www.mdcnigeria.org/ (Accessed: 16 February 2020)

Medical and Dental Council of Nigeria. (2020) Teaching hospitals approved for internship training with number of approved interns. [online]. Available at: www.mdcn.gov.ng/public/storage/documents/document_812954199.pdf Accessed: 16 February 2020)

National Postgraduate Medical College. (2017) [online]. Available at: http://npmcn.edu.ng/Nigeria (Accessed: 16 February 2020)

National Postgraduate Medical College of Nigeria (NPMCN) (n.d.) [online]. Available at: https://npmcn.edu.ng/faculties/ (Accessed: 16 February 2020)

National Postgraduate Medical College of Nigeria. (n.d.) [online]. Available at: https://npmcn.edu.ng/faculties/ (Accessed: 16 February 2020)

National Universities Commission. (2017) Stakeholders review endorse OER national policy. *Monday Bulletin*, 12:38, page 14. ISSN 0195 September 18, 2018. [online]. Available at: http://nuc.edu.ng/wp-content/uploads/2017/10/MB-18th-September-2018-ilovepdf-compressed.pdf (Accessed: 16 February 2020)

National Universities Commission. (2019) Draft of the Benchmark Guidelines for Appointment and Promotion of Academic Staffing Nigerian Universities

New America. (2015) Federal Funding. [online]. Available at: www.newamerica.org/education-policy/topics/school-funding-and-resources/school-funding/federal-funding/ (Accessed: 16 February 2020)

Ndiomewese, I. (2019) Nigeria has a National Research and Innovation Council that oversees matters of innovation in the country. *Techpoint Africa*. [online]. Available at: https://techpoint.africa/2019/04/05/national-research-and-innovation-council/ (Accessed: 16 February 2020)

Noko, JE. (2019) Corruption in the Nigeria education sector. *Mensch Mind*. [online]. Available at: https://educacinfo.com/corruption-nigeria-education-sector (Accessed: 16 February 2020)

Nwaokugha, DO and Ezeugwu, MC. (2017) Corruption in the education industry in Nigeria: Implication for national development. *European Journal of Training and Development Studies*, 4 (1): 1–17 [online]. Available at: www.eajournals.org/wp-content/uploads/Corruption-in-the-Education-Industry-in-Nigeria-Implications-for-National-Development.pdf (Accessed: 16 February 2020)

Odebiyi, D and Adegoke, BOA. (2005) Gender distribution of physiotherapy graduates from Nigerian universities. *Journal of Nigeria Society of Physiotherapy*, 15(2).

Ogunbodede, EO. (2004) Gender distribution of dentists in Nigeria; 1981 to 2000. *Journal of Dental Education*, 68(7) suppl 15–18. [online]. Available at: www.jdentaled.org/content/68/7_suppl/15.full (Accessed: 16 February 2020)

Okoli, NJ, Ogbondah, L and Ewor, RN. (2016) The history and development of public universities in Nigeria. *International Journal of Education and Evaluation*, 2 (1): 60–73. [online]. Available at: www.iiardpub.org (Accessed: 16 February 2020)

Okonofua, F. (2019) The case for specialized medical universities – Part 4 *The Guardian Newspaper* [online]. Available at: https://guardian.ng/opinion/the-case-for-specialised-medical-universities-part-4/ (Accessed: 4 February 2020)

Olayinka, I, Adedeji, SO and Ojo E. (2017) A brief review of governance reforms in higher education in Nigeria. (Maringe, F and Ojo. E, ed.). Chapter 6 in *Sustainable Transformation in African Higher Education: Research*, Governance, Gender, Funding, Teaching, and Learning in the African University. The Netherlands: Sense Publishers.

Oleribe, OO, Ezieme, PI, Oladipo, O, Akinola, EP, Udofia, D and Taylor-Robinson, D. (2016) Industrial action by healthcare workers in Nigeria in 2013–2015: An inquiry into causes, consequences, and control – A cross-sectional descriptive study. *Human Resources Health*, 27;14(1):46. [online]. Available at: https://pubmed.ncsi.nlm.nih.gov/27465121 (Accessed: 16 October 2020)

Oleribe, OO, Udofia, D, Oladipo, O, Ishola, TA and Taylor-Robinson SD. (2018) Healthcare workers' industrial action in Nigeria: a cross-sectional survey of Nigerian physicians. *Hum Resour Health*, 16: 54. [online]. Available at: www.ncsi.nlm.nih.gov/pmc/articles/PMC6192190 (Accessed: 16 October 2020)

Omoregie, N and Abraham, IO. (2009) *Persistent Gender Inequality in Nigerian Education*. Nigeria: Benson Idahosa University, Benin-City. [online]. Available at: https://in.nau.edu/wp-content/uploads/sites/135/2018/08/Persistent-Gender-Inequality-in-Nigerian-Education-ek.pdf (Accessed: 16 February 2020)

Owoaje, E and Olusola-Taiwo, O. (2008) Sexual harassment experiences of female graduates of Nigerian tertiary institutions. *International Quarterly of Community Health Education*, 30(4):337–348. [online]. Available at: www.researchgate.net/publication/49790933_Sexual_Harassment_Experiences_of_Female_Graduates_of_Nigerian_Tertiary_Institutions (Accessed: 16 February 2020)

Princeton Review. (n.d.) What is a good MCAT score? [online]. Available at: www.princetonreview.com/med-school-advice/what-is-a-good-mcat-score (Accessed: 16 February 2020)

Punch. (2020) Racketeers partner lecturers turn varsity final-year projects to money-making machines. [online]. Available at: https://punchng.com/racketeers-partner-lecturers-turn-varsity-final-year-projects-to-money-making-machines/ Accessed: 16 February 2020)

Rasheed, AA. (2017) Directory of full professors in the Nigerian university system. *National Universities Commission*, 26, ISBN: 978-978-964-725-8. [online]. Available at: https://nuc.covenantuniversity.edu.ng/download/2017-Directory-of-Full-Professors.pdf (Accessed: 16 February 2020)

Resilent Educator. (2020) 10-Year Spending Trends in US Education. March 2020. [online]. Available at: https://resilienteducator.com/news/10-year-spending-trends-in-u-s-education/ (Accessed: 16 February 2020)

Rezzonico, A and Parthemore, C. (2019) Briefer: Nuclear, climate, and security issues in Nigeria. [online]. Available at: https://climateandsecurity.org/2019/08/28/briefer-nuclear-climate-and-security-issues-in-nigeria/ (Accessed: 16 February 2020)

Rohwer, A, Wager, E, Young, T and Garner, P. (2018) Plagiarism in research: a survey of African medical journals. *British Medical Journal Open* 8. [online]. Available at: https://bmjopen.bmj.com/content/bmjopen/8/11/e024777.full.pdf   (Accessed: 16 February 2020)

Samuel, GO. (2018) How corruption is affecting basic education in Nigeria. *International Anti-Corruption Conference*. [online]. Available at: https://iaccseries.org/blog/how-corruption-is-affecting-basic-education-in-nigeria/ (Accessed: 16 February 2020)

Todowede, BJ. (2016) Corruption and the future of Nigeria's educational system. *International Journal of Arts and Sciences*, 09(02): 325–334.

UNESCO. (2014) UNESCO education strategy 2014–2021. [online]. Available at: https://unesdoc.unesco.org/ark:/48223/pf0000231288 (Accessed: 16 February 2020)

UNESCO. (2020) Education in Africa.[online]. Available at: http://uis.unesco.org/en/topic/education-africa (Accessed: 16 February 2020)

Wahab, B. (2018) 5 times lecturers have been accused of sexual harassment in 2018. . [online]. Available at: www.pulse.ng/communities/student/sex-for-mark-5-times-lecturers-have-been-accused-of-sexual-harassment-in-2018/6pffvzq (Accessed: 16 February 2020)

Walden, PR and Bryan,VC. (2010) Tenured and non-tenured College of Education faculty motivators and barriers in grant writing: A public university in the south. *Journal of Research Administration*, XLI, 3: 85–98. [online]. Available at: www.missouristate.edu/assets/longrangeplan/Faculty_Motivators_and_Barriers_in_Grant_Writing.pdf (Accessed: 16 February 2020)

World Population Review. (2020) Nigeria Population 2020 (Live) https://worldpopulationreview.com/countries/nigeria-population/

9 Reforming Nigerian's health care education system

Introduction

The first step to reforming Nigeria's health care education (HCE) system is to address all the challenges enumerated in Chapter 8 of this book. The issues discussed in this chapter will be a value-added approach towards enhancing the country's quality of HCE. The students are the most crucial person in a university. Without them, there would be no need for lecturers and staff. The students are not cold enrollment statistics but a human being with feelings and emotions and not someone to be tolerated – the personnel dependent on them to make a living. Therefore, the primary goal of every institution of higher learning is to provide all its students the opportunities they need to excel and become academically productive, be able to develop economically sustainable livelihoods and be able to meaningfully contribute to peaceful and democratic societies. To achieve these lofty goals, a university is as good as the sum of its parts in terms of the quality of its personnel, curriculum, and resources.

Universities that provide high-quality education have certain characteristics in common; effective leaders at all levels, reputable faculty with research credentials, competent faculty with an institutional reputation for teaching scholarship, robust faculty development program, and low student-faculty ratio. They also have rigorous curricula with critical thinking as the instructional framework, interprofessional education (IPE) philosophy, entrepreneur contents, and a comprehensive assessment program that uses findings to drive programmatic change. Institutions with high-quality education also provide adequate resources inform of state-of-the-art instructional technology (simulation/computer), including research labs, start-up funds for newly hired faculty to launch their research agenda. They also have program development budget for training and retooling, sponsor faculty to attend conferences to network and present their research findings and a positive learning environment that promotes research productivity and innovation. Any attempt at reforming the Nigerian educational system must utilize the stated recipe as the framework for change.

Improving the quality of HCE in Nigerian universities has been a subject of national interest for decades. There are numerous peculiar challenges and barriers to delivering quality education in the country. These hurdles underscore the need to find innovative solutions that address the unique circumstances of the Nigerian academy. A formative and summative evaluation of the HCE system was conducted between 2015 and 2019 to uncover the peculiar challenges. The assessment includes a written survey and unstructured interviews. The findings from the system assessment form the basis for the recommendations proffered in this chapter.

Methodology

The experience of the author as a faculty member and administrator at Obafemi Awolowo University (OAU), Ile-Ife, from 1986 to 1991 and half a dozen visits to several Nigerian universities between 2017 and 2019 provided the background and context for the information presented in this chapter. Formative and summative system evaluation was conducted over four years, from 2015 to 2019. It included visits to different parts of the country and presentation of two keynote speeches at professional conferences and three workshops to a diverse health professional audience. The experience created unique opportunities to network and engage in academic discussions and unstructured interviews with lecturers and administrators at the University of Medical Sciences (UNIMED), Ondo City, Bowen University, OAU, University of Ibadan, Lagos, Benin, and Maiduguri.

Phase one formative evaluation, conducted in 2017, was designed to assess curriculum and program assessment practices in HCE programs in Nigeria. An

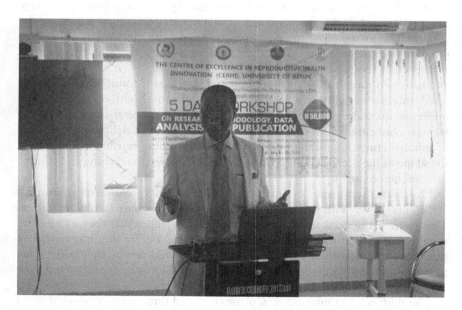

Professor Balogun delivering a lecture at a workshop at the University of Benin on July 8, 2019.

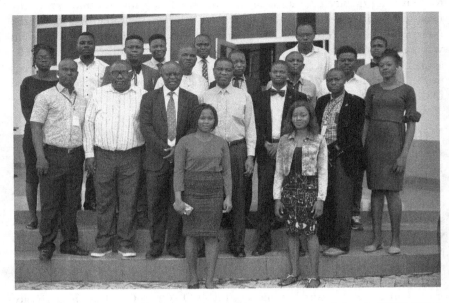

Group picture with a cross section of physiotherapists at a workshop in UNIMED in June 2019.

open-ended questionnaire was sent to four faculty members (with an average of over 30 years' teaching experience) from different geopolitical regions of the country. The survey asked three primary questions: the mechanism utilized for program assessment and the procedure used for assessing teaching effectiveness, and whether the process is published.

Phase two formative evaluation, conducted in 2018, consisted of unstructured interviews with five lecturers from different health disciplines. The interview questions sought information on department operations and effectiveness: core curriculum contents and perceived areas of deficiency, adequacy of infrastructures, continuing education opportunities, instructional methods, the scope of the accreditation process, formal education in teaching and administration before hiring.

Phase three summative evaluation, conducted in 2019, consisted of unstructured interviews with 11 (eight men and three women) faculty members. They were asked to share their views on the challenges that they experience in performing their role as faculty or administrator. Before the interview, they were reassured that their names and identities would not be divulged in any publications that may emerge from the discussion. The opinions expressed were compiled and analyzed for major themes.

The unstructured interviews in phases two and three were conducted like a natural conversation, and the questions were modified to suit the respondent's specific experiences (Cohen and Crabtree, 2006). The respondents were informed that their names and identities would not be mentioned in any publications that may emerge from the interview.

Results

Curriculum and program assessment practices

When the lecturers were asked whether their university has a mechanism for program assessment, they expressed similar but nonfactual perspectives. The quotes below represent typical points of view expressed by participants interviewed. A physician faculty has this to say:

> We have the mechanism for program assessment by the NUC, the NMDC, the Nursing and Midwifery Council of Nigeria (NMCN), and other professional associations. Each of them has scheduled for carrying out these assessments. For example, the NUC has what they call a resource verification visit before a program starts followed after that by the accreditation of the program. The NMDC undertake four visits before any institution can graduate a medical doctor or dentist. Thus far, the NUC has done its resource verification in our university and will be visiting for the accreditation of the basic medical sciences program next month. The NMDC has also done its advisory visit and is waiting to do their second visit very soon. And we are ready for them.
>
> (Respondent #1)

The other three faculty members responded to the question as follows:

> Program assessment is done by NUC. Program faculty are also expected to assess their program periodically; every five years.
>
> (Respondent #2)

> Yes. Every five years by the NUC. The Medical Rehabilitation Therapists Board of Nigeria (MRTBN) has also commenced accreditation of physiotherapy training programs using a template that differs slightly from that of NUC. Programs that obtain interim rather than full accreditation are revisited by the NUC after two years.
>
> (Respondent #3)

> Yes, by the NUC. Once in 5 years.
>
> (Respondent # 4)

The four faculty members erroneously equated program assessment with the accreditation process undertaken by the NUC and the professional regulatory boards (MRTBN, MDCN, National Association of Nurses and Midwifery of Nigeria [NANMN], and Pharmacists Council of Nigeria – PCN). While the NUC and professional regulatory boards are expected to evaluate compliance with accreditation standards, program assessment is an ongoing evaluation that occurs at the university department level, and it involves monitoring of students learning faculty teaching effectiveness and department operational effectiveness. This issue was discussed comprehensively in Chapter 4 of this book.

Quite often, too many decisions are made in the ivory tower, without empirical evidence. This situation is concerning, particularly in this globally acclaimed era of evidence-based practice. It is clear that program assessment, based on the criteria discussed in Chapter 4, is not practiced in HCE programs in the country. When the four faculty members were asked of the procedure used in their university for assessing teaching effectiveness and whether the process is published, they expressed varying perspectives. A physician faculty has this to say:

> *Yes, we have a mechanism for staff evaluation by students. And we also have a mechanism for the overall assessment of the University and students. The NUC provided this mechanism, and we have done and published this first assessment.*

(Respondent #1)

The three-HCE faculty declared that:

> *Yes, but in its initial stage. Lecturers are to be assessed by students at the end of each course using a questionnaire. The instrument is still undergoing revision and hence not yet published. The College initiated the idea.*

(Respondent #3)

> *The University has not adopted any mechanism for teacher's assessment, and no publication on this are in place as of now. The university accepts it in principle, but this has not been put into effect.*

(Respondent #2)

> *Faculty assessment plan is in progress.*

(Respondent #4)

The faculty members' responses suggest that their universities were at varying stages of developing a formal process for evaluating teaching effectiveness. The overall findings from the interview revealed that program assessment is presently not widely practiced in Nigerian universities. This situation must be rectified, and program assessment institutionalized in all the universities. And both the NUC and the professional regulatory boards should make program assessment an integral component of the accreditation process. The relevant information on program assessment is presented in Chapter 4 of this book.

Department effectiveness

The lecturers expressed several concerns on the operations of their academic department and on the effectiveness of their curriculum in meeting the

21st-century practice needs. The lecturers indicated graduate unemployment as an area of concern in addition to a lack of formal education or training in andragogy before hiring. Furthermore, the academic department chairs or heads of departments indicated they accepted the position without any formal managerial education or administrative training on their roles and responsibilities. The medical and dental lecturers indicated their curricula have no contents in teaching process, management and health economics. Interdisciplinary team concepts are currently not taught in any of the health disciplines.

Challenges in performing faculty or administrative roles

In response to the challenges they face in performing their roles and responsibilities, the sentiments expressed by the lecturers and administrators were divergent and illuminating, but two major themes emerged – resources and academic issues. Highlighted phrases or sentences were selected to capture as fully as possible the underlying questions asked. The academic matters identified were deficiencies in curriculum evaluation, and program assessment practices discussed previously. The human and physical resources related issues identified include underfunding, corruption, cronyism and nepotism, inadequate infrastructure, plagiarism, sexual harassment, gender inequity, campus cultism, dilapidated facilities, insufficient number of qualified lecturers, poor conditions of service, low remuneration, and the continuous brain drain of faculty to other countries.

Follow-up questions were posed to probe further any perceived limited response to the primary issue. The interview findings revealed that corruption in the education sector takes different forms, such as bribes paid by parents to university administrators and faculty to ensure admission into HCE programs, and grafts paid to obtain good grades in the promotion exams. When the participants were asked to comment on their experiences with corruption, the responses presented below captures their shared experience:

> *undue influence and "envelopes" are exchanged to obtain the license required to start new universities and to bypass the stringent criteria for the establishment of academic programs.*
>
> (An administrator)

A senior faculty member opined that:

> *the members of visiting accreditation teams also receive "kola" to cover up glaring deficits in accreditation standards.*

A female faculty member responded that:

> *it is well-known turpitude for new universities to borrow instructional and research laboratory equipment from the more established neighboring universities and display them in their labs for the visiting accreditation teams to inspect. Under the disguise of*

carrying out oversight functions, legislators during their visit often demand "egunje" from university administrators.

A Head of Department administrator has this to say:

> *... corrupt practices include the admission of unqualified students through the back door, mismanagement of educational budget, the appointment of corrupt politicians to serve on University Boards who often politicize the system. Other wrongdoings include sexual harassment, illegal pursuit of entitlements.*

Other related perversion addressed by the sample of convenience includes lack of autonomy, cronyism, and nepotism in the award of construction contracts, the procurement of equipment, the selling of examination questions and piracy. The following responses shield light on the scope of the problem.

When the participants were asked about their opinion on university autonomy, one faculty member stated:

> *ASUU is threatening to embark on an industrial strike to resist the decision of the federal government to convert the university payroll system to the civil service computer system that is fatally flawed. It will not work for lecturers because we receive monthly salary from more than one source. We'll continue to resist this total takeover of our academic freedom.*

In response to the question regarding their perception about cronyism and nepotism, one female faculty member shared this view:

> *The total collapse of power (energy) and road networks in the country due to the corrupt attitudes of both the past and present leaders who have eroded the ethical base of the society. Moreover, due diligence, excellence, honesty, merit, and integrity are no longer cherished. We have nonacademic administrators collecting "envelopes" to admit students.*

Another administrator confided on the issue of cronyism and nepotism:

> *We are forced by the "power from above" to admit some students who did not make the cut for certain discipline.*

The quote below provided by a dean was a recurring theme when participants in the study were asked about plagiarism and cover up:

> *I know of a lecturer in my department who submitted a PhD dissertation without collecting any data and none of the examiners said a thing before the degree was awarded. The university is still investigating this scandal.*

When the opinion of the participants was sought on the issue of sexual harassment and gender inequity, one female lecturer responded that:

Sex for a good grade and cultism are now rampant in our universities. Discrimination based on gender is a fact of life and a daily struggle for Nigerian women in the academy.

Recommendations to address the various issues raised during the unstructured interview will next be discussed.

Discussion and recommendations

Previous national attempts at revising the medical and dental curricula

Medical education in Nigeria started in 1934 at Yaba Higher College and moved to the University College Ibadan in 1948 (Rasheed, 2017). From its inception, the Faculty of Medicine at the University of Ibadan (UI) adopted the traditional British medical and dental curricula and transplanted them to the other newly established institutions. The newer medical schools embraced the curriculum of the first-generation universities with little modification. They failed to respond to the global trend of using assessment as a tool in curriculum revision. Many of the lecturers in the universities have no formal training in andragogy/heutagogy and no program assessment experience. Regional and national efforts made in the past to revise the medical and dental curricula and improve the quality of education have not yielded the desired results (Ibrahim, 2007). Given the myriad of intractable challenges in the educational system as described in Chapter 8 of this book, it is astonishing that the 1948 British medical and dental curricula imported to the country have not undergone any significant content revision despite appeals for reforms from different scholars (Ojo and Akinwumi, 2015; Oleribe et al. 2016; 2018; Alubo and Hunduh 2017; Balogun, 2017b).

In recognition of this untenable situation, a Technical Working Groups of the National Advisory Committee for the undergraduate medical and dental curricula was constituted by the federal government in January 2007 to design medical and dental curricula for the nation. The collaborative project was sponsored by the Federal Ministry of Health (FMH), Medical and Dental Council of Nigeria (MDCN), the NUC, and the Diaspora Unit of the FMH. The United States Agency for International Development (USAID) provided funding through its Health Systems 20/20 Project. The Technical Working Groups were formed by tapping into the national and global experience of Nigerians in the academy, clinical practice, and administrative communities. They were charged, inter-alias, to produce new medical and dental curricula that will be "the gold standard" for quality and relevant medical training and to "produce competent, compassionate, and confident graduates who will engage in ethical practice and who will be socially responsive and accountable and globally relevant" (FMH, 2012).

The White Paper of the Health Systems 20/20 report project, proposed several changes in the undergraduate medical and dental curricula offered in Nigerian universities. The report retained the general framework of the traditional British curricula, but contemporary "clinical" and "nonclinical" contents were recommended. The "nonclinical" items proposed focused on the education's socialization, humanistic, and administrative/management elements. They also put forward contents in health economics, health administration/management, professionalism, communication and interpersonal skills, medical ethics and jurisprudence, clinical decision-making, evidence-based practice, human nutrition, complementary and alternative health care practices, social responsibility, and social accountability. In addition to the specific curriculum-related content proposed, the Committee recommended the adoption of the "multidisciplinary" teaching method. This recommendation is a step in the right direction toward improving communication among health professionals. However, the multidisciplinary instructional strategy is short of the IPE teaching method – the contemporary (cutting-edge) best practice in HCE. The differences between multidisciplinary and IPE teaching methods were discussed in Chapter 1 of this book.

Interprofessional instructional model framework, implementation, challenges and barriers

The unstructured interview findings in phase two of the investigation revealed that interdisciplinary team concepts are currently not in the curriculum of any health disciplines. The barriers impeding high-quality education are due, in part, to lack of cooperation among the disciplines. The solutions to address this challenge, implementation strategies, challenges, and barriers will next be discussed. The White Paper of the Health Systems 20/20 project was published in 2012 and was embraced by the NUC for adoption by all the College of Medicine/Health Sciences in the country. Sadly, this recommendation is yet to be implemented.

As of June 2020, only three of the 44 universities in Nigeria offering HCE programs have embraced the multidisciplinary education model. The origin of a multidisciplinary instructional method started at the UI in the early 1970s, later at the University of Ife (now OAU) in the 1980s and more recently in 2015 at the UNIMED, Ondo City. Three of the university's mandates medical, dental, physiotherapy, and nursing students to take anatomy, physiology, and biochemistry courses together (Balogun et al., 2017a). Unfortunately, the multidisciplinary instructional method adopted in the preclinical year never extended to the clinical courses. Consequently, the full potential of IPE was never realized. Little wonder the level of interprofessional conflict is still high in the health sector that is besieged with disharmony and court cases (John, 2016). The multiple challenges highlighted in Chapter 8 of this book underscores the need to adopt the IPE instructional model and to revise the curricula in line with global best practice.

The five core competencies proposed by the Institute of Medicine in the United States provides the curriculum framework for the development of the IPE instructional model *(Figure 9.1)*. The recommendation calls for revision

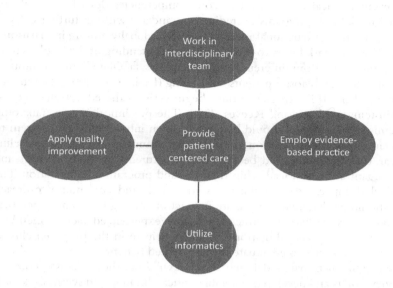

Figure 9.1 Five core skills that clinicians must utilize in the 21st century.

of the curriculum of all HCE programs to ensure all entry-level graduates can work in an interdisciplinary team, provide patient-centered care, employ evidence-based practice, apply quality improvement strategies to mitigate medical errors and utilize informatics to communicate effectively (Institute of Medicine of the National Academies, 2001; 2003).

In providing patient-centered care, the clinician must always respect and value patients' expressed needs, differences, and preferences. They must listen to, communicate with, and educate patients, relieve their pain and suffering, and share decision-making and management with the other health care team members. Also, the clinician must continuously advocate disease prevention and promote wellness, healthy lifestyles, including a focus on community health. And must work in interdisciplinary teams by cooperating, collaborating, communicating, integrating, and coordinating care continuously and reliably. At all times, the clinician must utilize evidence-based practice by combining the best research with clinical expertise and considering the patient values for optimum care and engaging in ongoing research activities.

The clinician must apply quality improvement skills to identify medical errors and hazards in the clinical environment and implement safety design principles by standardizing and simplifying operations. Understanding and assessing the quality of care in terms of structure, process, and outcomes reflect patient and community needs is also critical. To improve quality, the clinician must test interventions that change processes and systems of care. Finally, the clinician must utilize information technology skills to communicate, manage knowledge, and prevent medical error. The five core competencies described should be included in all HCE programs' accreditation standards without further delay.

Today, the IPE instructional method is shared globally among international organizations and task forces to promote the understanding of the faculty's roles and responsibilities from different health disciplines, facilitate better communication, and ultimately foster patients' well-being (Lavin et al., 2001). The implementation of the IPE experience must begin early in the educational process (Zwarenstein, Goldman and Reeves, 2009). The preclinical courses (anatomy, biochemistry, physiology) should be broken down into a credit unit system to engender genuine collaboration among students and faculty. In the first clinical year, the students should be provided structured case study reviews and taught organization and leadership theories, and program administration. The clinical clerkship experience during ward rounds and community outreach events should be designed to facilitate interaction among the faculty members and students from different professions. Only experienced faculty members who model effective collaboration should participate in the proposed clinical instructional activities to effectuate the anticipated benefits.

The IPE instructional model's actualization will force the students to consider other viewpoints and develop transferable critical thinking and synthesis skills. It will also enable students to consolidate their learning by synthesizing ideas from diverse perspectives, exploring alternative ways of knowledge acquisition, and motivating them to pursue new knowledge outside their disciplines. The institutional change will allow the students to cover topics in more depth because they will approach the problem utilizing their diverse training and life experiences. The experience will develop the students' research skills with the potential for greater creativity. The evolution will create a positive learning environment and foster mutual respect between the faculty from different health care fields (Gill, 2015; OpenLearn, 2015). The anticipated instructional and learning benefits, in its totality, will produce the competent faculty that is desperately needed to teach and manage the nation's education and health care systems.

The proposed seismic change can improve the quality of communication among faculty and modulate the disharmony and conflicts among the health care professionals. The move will go a long way in sanitizing the education and health care sectors by decreasing the stereotyping among the different health professions. There are six daunting logistical challenges to overcome in the implementation of IPE. First, due to time constraints, adding new information to any curriculum is always a contentious issue among faculty. Second, internal politics and turf protection among the faculty are plausible reasons for inaction. Third, for self-preservation purposes, faculty members who want to maintain the status quo will sabotage any curriculum reform. Fourth, the paradigm shift may generate unfair competition for discipline identities, values, and cultures. Fifth, the introduction of IPE initially might further promote the stereotyping of other professions, with the potential for conflicts. Finally, given that a few health disciplines have no collaboration experience bringing these professions along to embrace the new way of doing things will be a challenge to overcome.

Workforce capacity development

The lack of formal training in andragogy is among the lecturers' concerns during phase two of this investigation. Critics affirmed that this deficiency is partly responsible for the poor quality of instruction in HCE across the country. The underlying issues about this issue was discussed in more significant detail in Chapter 2 of this book. As a policy recommendation, each university should host workshops on curriculum/course design and instructional methods at the beginning of every semester for newly employed lecturers. And the workshop should cover the following topics:

1. Learning domains and Bloom's taxonomy
2. Program students learning objectives
3. Course goals and course objectives, curriculum mapping
4. The knots and bolts of creating a syllabus
5. Evidence-based practice applied to instruction
6. Effective teaching strategies
7. Learning theories and principles of learning
8. Adult and youth learning characteristics: Implications for teaching
9. Effective teaching strategies for large and small class sizes
10. Philosophy, principles, and characteristics of good assessment
11. Test construction: Essays, and multiple-choice questions
12. Communication skills in clinical practice
13. Methods of testing practical/clinical knowledge
14. Plagiarism in higher education
15. Use of technology in the classroom

Many of the above topics are presented in Chapter 2 of this book.

Another area faculty expressed the need for professional development is in grant writing. Many of the country's academics do not have the grant writing skills needed to compete for international agencies and foundations grants focusing on innovative programs and centers of excellence in health. Innovative research and development should be by the Vice-Chancellors and made the central focus of scholarship in public universities. The NUC should annually organize grant writing in universities located across the six geopolitical zones in the country.

Nigeria can learn from research universities in the United States, where external funding from grantsmanship is a significant percentage of the institutional budget. In these universities, track record in grant-funding is a requirement for faculty promotion and tenure. Requiring similar academic standards in Nigeria may spur more lecturers to engage in grant writing with great potential to increase institutional revenue. In the United States, there are 26 federal grant-awarding agencies funding over 900 grant programs in 20 categories. The foremost private philanthropic organization by a Nigerian is the Theophilus Y. Danjuma Foundation established in 2009 to improve the quality of life of the economically-disadvantaged. The foundation supports primary health and education intervention programs for youth and women groups (TY Danjuma Foundation, n.d.). The top international foundation funding sources in Nigeria are Bill and Melinda Gates Foundation, Open Society Foundations by philanthropist George Soros, Ford Foundation, William and Flora Hewlett Foundation, Children's Investment Fund Foundation (the only United Kingdom-based foundation), United Nations Foundation, John and Catherine MacArthur Foundation, Conrad Hilton Foundation, Rockefeller Foundation, and Gordon and Betty Moore Foundation (FundsforNGOs, 2019).

There is a need to ensure that ongoing research in the universities address local developmental challenges, promote economic growth, and improve citizens' quality of life. Thus, the funding allocation to HCE should be increased to foster research productivity and garner state of the art laboratory infrastructures. Furthermore, the establishment of a national publications database and a functional National Research Council to formulate research priorities and oversee collaboration at national and international levels, will go a long way in improving HCE and health care system in the country.

Entrepreneurship education

The lecturers interviewed in phase two of the investigation shared their concern on the ongoing graduate unemployment despite the need for their services. The panacea to this issue is entrepreneurship education to free the program graduates from the shackles of dependency on government jobs. Entrepreneurship courses should be designed to the students about innovations in technology, the development of therapeutic tools, and the conversion of creative ideas into commercial products. The courses should also emphasize the business aspects of health care, including the nuts and bolts of operating a private practice.

The UNIMED at Ondo city is the first and so far, the only university in Nigeria that has incorporated entrepreneurship contents into all the undergraduate HCE programs. This feat is commendable because, even in developed countries, the inclusion of entrepreneurship in HCE is relatively new. In the United States, the Accreditation Council for Graduate Medical Education has approved the training of residents in quality improvement. Still, entrepreneurship education is yet to be incorporated fully into the undergraduate and residency curricula (Ju and Nguyen, 2018). As of 2016, only 13 (7.4%) of the 175 (141 MD and 34 DO degree-granting) medical schools in the United States have integrated entrepreneurship content in their curriculum. Among the universities that have included entrepreneurship in their curriculum is the School of Medicine at Case Western Reserve, which, in 2018, developed an innovative entrepreneurship course. The course is offered in the preclinical year, and it includes biweekly seminars and a mentoring project.

The Feinberg School of Medicine at Northwestern University also offers a six-month IPE course that introduces the students to the development of medical technologies. Similarly, the School of Medicine at the University of

Michigan initiated an entrepreneurship course to teach surgical innovation. In the United Kingdom, about 100 newly qualified medical graduates in 2017 completed a "clinical entrepreneur training program" offered by the National Health System in collaboration with Health Education, England. Many of the physicians have transformed their creative ideas into innovative commercial products, apps, and services to improve health care and promote learning (Limb, 2017). When the entrepreneurship education proposal is implemented, it will curb unemployment and encourage the self-actualization and financial independence of newly qualified health care graduates.

Accreditation process

Two separate and autonomous parastatals regulate HCE programs in Nigeria: The NUC on behalf of the Federal Ministry of Education and the professional regulatory boards under the FMH which include the MDCN, PCN, MRTBN, Optometrists and Dispensing Opticians Registration Board of Nigeria, NMCN, Medical Laboratory Science Council of Nigeria/Nigeria Institute of Science Laboratory Technology, Radiographers Registration Board of Nigeria, College of Biomedical Engineering and Technology, Community Health Practitioners Registration Board of Nigeria and the Veterinary Council of Nigeria. The professional regulatory boards and the NUC provide the oversight function and carry out separate accreditation visits to the universities, but there is an ongoing rift between the two bodies. The NUC in 2016 mandated medical and dental faculty members to have a PhD degree before promotion to senior lecturer and higher academic rank. On the other hand, the MDCN does not require a PhD degree but prefer the clinical fellowship credentials offered through the National Postgraduate Medical College and the West African Postgraduate Medical College. The differing point of view between the NUC and MDCN remain acrimonious and unresolved.

The decline in the standard of HCE in Nigeria is indicative of the shortcomings of the accreditation process of the NUC and the professional regulatory bodies. The accreditation process implemented by the NUC and the professional regulatory bodies only concentrate on inspection of resources (physical, human, equipment, and lab.) and evaluation of the adequacy of the curriculum contents. The process lacked public and stakeholder involvement and self-assessment. Universities in North America and Europe require a comprehensive institutional self-study (assessment), culminating in a detailed report before the campus visit to validate the information presented. The rigorous accreditation process adopted in both countries undoubtedly contributes to the high world ranking of their universities.

Self-study requires an in-depth evaluation of the university/program operations and identifying the program's strengths and weaknesses. The process allows the university/program to develop corrective action plans that promote continuous quality improvement. The self-evaluation process also enables the universities to engage in assessment of student learning to support continuous improvement and demonstrate that they are meeting their mission and acts with integrity and conduct their business ethically and responsibly.

Without further delay, both the NUC and the professional regulatory bodies need to require a self-study process and a detailed report of the evaluation. The student-faculty ratio must be monitored closely, and the programs must be required to demonstrate performance outcomes on student learning. The utilization of benchmarking, as described in Chapter 1 of this book, will enable each HCE program to compare its performance against peer institutions or programs. The universities will be able to identify efficiencies, control costs, and learn from areas of good practice and opportunities for continuous improvement. Overall, such comparison will enable institutions to understand what makes superior performance possible and can appropriately implement reforms that will yield significant improvements in their operations.

Curriculum content deficits

The medical and dental lecturers interviewed in phase two of the investigation stated their curricula have no contents in teaching process, administration/management and health economics. Clinical practice in the country has evolved in scope over the years, and the roles of health care professionals have grown from a clinician to research and teaching (Ojo and Akinwumi, 2015). Unfortunately, most health professionals employed in the top administrative position in government establishments have no basic knowledge of the principles of finance. It is, therefore, not surprising that most large organizations and systems led by health professionals are poorly managed and financially insolvent. A course in organization leadership, health economics or health care financing that covers the fundamental elements of management, accounting, mobilization of funds, distribution of financial risks, allocation and utilization of services, provider payment incentives, costs, pricing, expenditure, essential drugs, supplies, and human resource management, will address the apparent management deficits in the HCE curricula. As the first step toward meaningful reforms, both the NUC and professional regulatory organizations should include the above contents in their accreditation standards.

The remaining section of this chapter will discuss the findings from the unstructured conducted in part three of the investigation – gender inequity, inadequate infrastructure, plagiarism, underfunding, corruption, cronyism and nepotism, sexual harassment, campus cultism, dilapidated facilities, insufficient number of qualified lecturers, poor conditions of service, low remuneration, and the continuous brain drain of faculty to other countries.

Gender inequity

To achieve gender parity in higher education, both the government and the educational institutions play a vital role. Nigeria has a national gender policy that commits to ensuring affirmative action for women, but women's representation remains below the 35% target set by regional and international organizations over the years. The constitutions and manifestos of political parties rarely mention affirmative action for women, and when they do, the commitments are lower than the set benchmark. Laws against early marriage that hinder young girls from pursuing education should be promulgated. The government should scale up financial assistance in the form of scholarships to female students. Aggressive public education at the local level that emphasizes the benefits of education and elimination of cultural and traditional practices that expose young girls to early sex and unwanted pregnancies should be pursued. Such a program will be beneficial in bringing about positive attitudinal change toward gender equality in education at all levels. Increasing the admission of women in postgraduate degree programs should be of paramount importance in the universities.

Most importantly, universities need to develop strategies, action plans, and policies that address gender inequality issues, particularly in the health disciplines that are dominated by men. Each university should set annual targets for equal gender representation at all levels (administrative and academic levels supervisor, senior management, and board leadership). Furthermore, administrators must be held accountable in achieving their set targets. Besides, universities should offer scholarships and develop mentorship programs that pair junior women faculty with senior-level women role models. The plan will increase the visibility and the likelihood that junior faculty will ascend to leadership positions. Universities should promote networking among peer female lecturers and provide value-added training and professional development opportunities across disciplines. These recommendations will ensure that women have diverse experiences and the clinical skills that they need to succeed in the academy.

Infrastructure, university autonomy and campus security

The physical facilities and instructional/research infrastructures at many of the universities are old and, for the most part, nonfunctional. Overcrowded classrooms and residence halls have become a norm in most Nigerian universities, with over 1,000 students enrolled in natural science courses. This unacceptable situation should take priority and addressed through fundraising among alumni, and from local foundations. Funds generated can be used to build new classrooms, laboratory facilities, and residential halls. Without a doubt, more funding is needed to address the multifactorial resource-related challenges. But critics argued that the problems go beyond funding; that the system is corrupt, and the administrative operations are ineffective and incongruent with international best practices. The federal government must finance education at the level that is consistent with UNESCO's budgetary recommendation of 15–20% of the nation's annual budget (Adedigba, 2017). The allocated funds must be utilized for the purpose for which it is designated and not embezzled. Furthermore, the NUC should increase the salary and improve the working conditions of the lecturers in line with the global standard. Implementation of this recommendation will abate the ongoing brain drain in the country. The university administration should engage law enforcement to address the surging cult-related activities on the campuses. Furthermore, the universities should be granted full autonomy and allowed to operate without external political pressure, influence, and interference.

Plagiarism

The use of online and personal plagiarism software can drastically curtail the upsurge in the incidence of plagiarism in the country. The NUC should immediately provide adequate funding to each university to enable them to subscribe to the plagiarism software. The popular institutional-based plagiarism checkers are iThenticate and Turnitin (Sarker, 2018). There are several other online software that can be downloaded on a personal computer for free. The best free plagiarism detectors are Dupli Checker, Copyleaks, PaperRater, Plagiarisma, Plagiarism Checker, Plagium, PlagScan, PlagTracker, Quetext, and Viper (Pappas, 2013).

The iThenticate and Turnitin software allow instructors to perform plagiarism checks, provide feedback on specific phrases or entire assignments, and they can grade submitted documents up to 400 pages. Instructors can check documents submitted by themselves and by students through their accounts. Generated plagiarism reports are available for instructors, and students can view them at the discretion of the instructor. The printouts typically highlight identical or similar text with different colors that correspond to various matching sources, and each source has a similarity matching percentage.

The Premium version of Grammarly is a desktop automated proofreader that corrects grammar, spelling, and punctuation mistakes, and it is also a plagiarism checker. However, it can only upload a document of less than 40 MB in size or check up to 60 pages at a time. The subscription fee is about $139.95 per year for five computers. Grammarly offers a free version that allows for basic grammar and spelling proofreading but does not allow scan for plagiarism.

Corruption

Corruption is the bane of Nigerian health care and education systems. Reforming and expanding the HCE programs in the country is not going to be an easy task because corruption is ubiquitous. The government's absence of political will to fight corruption aided by weak governance, inactive, and fragile internal checks and balance and abdication of external oversight functions are responsible for the poor quality of education in the universities. Institutional corruption breeds the lack of initiative, productivity, and creativity needed to proffer sound policies that will further develop the country.

Fighting corruption should involve the crafting of laws to promote transparency, accountability, and good governance with the support of functional civil societies, an independent judiciary, and an enlightened citizenry. The federal government should increasingly focus attention on strengthening the anti-corruption agencies — the Independent Corrupt Practices Commission, the Economic and Financial Crimes Commission, and the Code of Conduct Bureau and Tribunal.

Conclusion

This chapter provides the recipe for high-quality HCE and discusses the previous attempts at revising the medical and dental curricula at the national level. It also presents the formative and summative evaluations of the HCE system conducted between 2015 and 2019 that includes a written survey and unstructured interviews. The findings from the system assessment form the basis for the recommendations proffered in this chapter. The proposals include the adoption of interprofessional education model and integration of entrepreneurship education in the curriculum, workforce capacity building, upgrade of the NUC and the professional regulatory boards' accreditation process to include a self-study assessment and report detailing remediation plans for the identified areas of weakness. Other recommendations proposed centered on funding, infrastructure, plagiarism, sexual harassment, gender inequity, corruption, university autonomy, and campus security

References

Adedigba, A. (2017) Fact check: Did UNESCO ever recommend 26 percent budgetary allocation to education? *Premium Times.* [online]. Available at: www.premiumtimesng.com/news/headlines/251927-fact-check-unesco-ever-recommend-26-per-cent-budgetary-allocation-education.html (Accessed: 16 February 2020)

Adedigba, A. (2019) Why Nigerian professors aren't getting research grants – TETFund boss. *Premium Times.* [online]. Available at: www.premiumtimesng.com/news/top-news/326893-why-nigerian-professors-arent-getting-research-grants-tetfund-boss.html (Accessed: 16 February 2020)

Alubo, O and Hunduh, V. (2017) Medical dominance and resistance in Nigeria's healthcare system. *International Journal of Health Services*, 47(4): 778–794.

Balogun, JA, Aka, PC, Balogun, AO and Obajuluwa, VA. (2017a) A phenomenological investigation of the first two decades of university-based physiotherapy education in Nigeria. *Cogent Medicine*, 4(1) 10.1080/2331205X.2017.1301183[online]. Available at: https://bit.ly/3nD4WuK (Accessed: 14 February 2020)

Balogun, JA. (2017b) The case for a paradigm shift in the education of health professionals in Nigeria. Second distinguished university guest lecture. Nigeria: UNIMED, Ondo City. May 15, 2017. [online]. Available at: www.researchgate.net/publication/317387397_The_case_for_a_paradigm_shift_in_the_education_of_healthcare_professionals_in_Nigeria (Accessed: 14 February 2020)

Cohen D and Crabtree B. (2006) Qualitative research guidelines project: Unstructured interviews. *Robert Wood Johnson Foundation.* [online]. Available at: www.qualres.org/HomeUnst-3630.html (Accessed: 26 April 2020)

Federal Ministry of Health of Nigeria. (2012) Nigeria undergraduate medical and dental curriculum template. Bethesda, MD: *Health Systems 20/20 Project*, ABT

Associates Inc. [online]. Available at: www.healthsystems2020.org (Accessed: 14 February 2020)

FundsforNGOs. (2019) Grants and resources for sustainability: Latest grants and resources for NGOs and individuals in Nigeria. [online]. Available at: https://www2. fundsforngos.org/tag/nigeria/page/2/ (Accessed: 14 February 2020)

Gill, SV, Vessali, M, Pratt, JA, Watts, S, Pratt, JS, Raghavan, P and DeSilva. JM. (2015) The importance of interdisciplinary research training and community dissemination. *Clinical and Translational Science* 8(5): 611–614. [online]. Available at: www.ncbi.nlm. nih.gov/pmc/articles/PMC4625396/ (Accessed: 14 February 2020)

Ibrahim, M. (2007) Medical education in Nigeria. *Journal Medical Teacher,* 29(9– 10): 901–905. [online]. Available at: www.tandfonline.com/doi/full/10.1080/ 01421590701832130?scroll=top&needAccess=true (Accessed: 14 February 2020)

Institute of Medicine of the National Academies. (2001) Educating health professionals in teams: Current reality, barriers, and related actions. *Institute of Medicine Report,* 1–10.

Institute of Medicine of the National Academies. (2003) *Health Professions Education: A Bridge to Quality.* Washington, DC: National Academies Press.

John, P. (2016). National postgraduate physiotherapy college of Nigeria: Before creating more problems in the health sector. [online]. Available at: www.medicalworld nigeria.com/2016/05/national-postgraduate-physiotherapy-college-of-nigeria-beforecreating-more-problems-in-the-health-sector/#.V0piaDUrJdg (Accessed: 16 February 2020).

Ju, W and Nguyen, M. (2018) The need for entrepreneurship education in medical school and residency training. *Dermatology Times,* 39. [online]. Available at: www. dermatologytimes.com/business/need-entrepreneurship-education-medical-school-and-residency-training (Accessed: 14 February 2020)

Lavin, M, Ruebling, I, Banks, R, Block, L, Counte, M, Furman, GE, Miller, P, Reese, C, Viehmann, V and Holt J. (2001) Interdisciplinary health professional education: A historical review. *Advances in Health Sciences Education,* 6:25–47. [online]. Available at: www.researchgate.net/publication/11857303_Interdisciplinary_Health_ Professional_Education_A_Historical_Review (Accessed:14 February 2020)

Limb, M. (2017) The rise of medical entrepreneurs – How students are turning their ideas into innovative apps and products. *Student British Medical Journal* [online]. Available at: http://student.bmj.com/student/view-article.html?id=sbmj.j1694 (Accessed: 14 February 2020)

Ojo, TO and Akinwumi, AF. (2015) Doctors as managers of healthcare resources in Nigeria: Evolving roles and current challenges. *Niger Med Journal of Medicine,* 56(6):375–80. [online]. Available at: www.ncbi.nlm.nih.gov/pmc/articles/ PMC4743284/ (Accessed: 14 February 2020)

Oleribe, OO, Ezieme, IP, Oladipo, O, Akinola, EP, Udofia, D and Taylor-Robinson, SD. (2016) Industrial action by healthcare workers in Nigeria in 2013–2015: An inquiry into causes, consequences and control—a cross-sectional descriptive study. *Hum Resource Health,* 14(1):46. [online]. Available at: www.ncbi.nlm.nih.gov/pmc/ articles/PMC4962455/ (Accessed: 14 February 2020)

Oleribe, OO, Udofia, D, Oladipo, O, Ishola, TA and Taylor-Robinson SD. (2018) Healthcare workers' industrial action in Nigeria: a cross-sectional survey of Nigerian physicians. *Hum Resour Health,* 16: 54. [online]. Available at: www.ncsi.nlm.nih.gov/ pmc/articles/PMC6192190 (Accessed: 16 October 2020)

OpenLearn. (2015) What are the benefits of interdisciplinary study? [online]. Available at: www.open.edu/openlearn/education/what-are-the-benefits-interdisciplinary-study (Accessed: 14 February 2020)

Pappas, C. (2013) Top 10 free plagiarism detection tools for eLearning professionals (2017 update). [online]. Available at: https://elearningindustry.com/top-10-free-plagiarism-detection-tools-for-teachers (Accessed: 14 February 2020)

Rasheed, AA. (2017) Directory of full professors in the Nigerian university system. *National Universities Commission*, 26: 1–525.

Sarker, A. (2018) Best plagiarism checker? Free or pay? [online]. Available at: www.researchgate.net/post/Best_Plagiarism_Checker_Free_or_pay (Accessed: 14 February 2020)

TY Danjuma Foundation. (n.d.) About the Foundation. [online]. Available at: www.tydanjumafoundation.org/about-the-foundation **(Accessed**: 14 February 2020)

WHO. (1988) Learning together to work together for health. Report of a WHO study group on multi-professional education of health personnel: The team approach. *World Health Organization Technical Report Series*. Geneva: World Health Organization, 769:1–72

Zwarenstein, M, Goldman, J and Reeves, S. (2009) Interprofessional collaboration: Effects of practice-based interventions on professional practice and healthcare outcomes. *Cochrane Database of Systematic Reviews*, 3.

10 Elite Nigerian health care academics in diaspora

Introduction

The mass departure of Nigerian academicians and skilled professionals to the northern countries, a phenomenon called the "brain drain," is one of the most significant obstacles to the development of the country. In the last decade, Nigerians have left their homeland in droves, and today the country has the highest migrant population among the developing nations. Despite the migration, as of April 23, 2020, the people of Nigeria are 205,122,116, and the country remains the most populous African nation (Worldometer, 2020; Multimedia Foundation Inc., 2020).

Before independence in 1960, many Nigerian students go to Europe and North America for their university education and typically return to their homeland after graduation. However, postindependence, there has been an increasing number of Nigerians in the diaspora. The migration trend in Nigeria is associated with socioeconomic instability and calamities at home. For example, the increase in migration in the 1960s was due to civil and political unrest, and many refugees and skilled workers fled the country. And in the 1980s, emigration was due to economic hardship caused by the collapse of petroleum in the global market and the structural adjustment program foisted on the country by General Ibrahim Babangida at the behest of the world bank. In the mid-1990s, many Nigerians fled the country for their safety during General Sani Abacha's reign of terror.

The migration of Nigerians to the United States dates back to the transatlantic slave trade. As of 2016, about 380,785 Nigerians lived in the United States, mostly in the state of Texas, Maryland, California, New York, Florida, Georgia, Illinois, and New Jersey (Minnesota Multimedia Inc., 2020). In 2001, there were 88,000 Nigerians in the United Kingdom, but by 2011, the number has increased to 200,000, representing 0.3% of the 63 million Britons. Because of the large community of Nigerians in London's Peckham, the city is often called "little Lagos." As a group, Nigerians are a significant contributor to the British economy (Blair, n.d.). The mass immigration of Nigerians to Canada started during the Biafra war from 1967–1970, as many Ibos fled to Canada. Between 1973 and 1991, 3,919 Nigerians arrived in Canada, and by 2016, the number soared to 51,800, with over half living in Ontario. On the other hand, the number of Nigerians in Italy and Germany, have declined significantly in the last decade (Multimedia Foundation Inc. 2020). Nigerians are increasingly relocating in large numbers to Australia. As of 2011, there were 4,519 Nigerians in Australia, a two-fold increase from 2006. Nigeria ranks in the top ten nations with the highest number of students in Australian universities (Multimedia Foundation Inc., 2020).

The pertinent question is, what is responsible for the mass exodus of Nigerian health care professionals to other countries of the world? A survey of Nigerian physicians was conducted in 2016 to assess the prevalence with which they pursue work opportunities abroad and the probable reasons. The findings revealed that high taxes and deductions from salary (98%), low work satisfaction (92%), and meager wages (91%) are the primary reasons that made them depart the country (NOIPolls, 2016). About 83% of the study respondents completed their medical education in Nigeria and were registered with the Medical and Dental Council of Nigeria before they left the country. The top suggestions they proffered to address the challenges physicians face include improved remuneration (18%), upgrade of all hospital facilities and equipment (16%), increase health care funding (13%), and enhanced work conditions.

Nigerians in diaspora play a significant role in the development of their homeland through remittance of funds to their relatives and engagement in different entrepreneur development projects (Ayanruoh, 2018). Their payment to the homeland increased from $18 billion in 2009 to $22 billion in 2017, and $6.19 billion of the investment is from the United States alone (World Bank, 2017). The amount is about 50% of Nigeria's earnings from oil export, which stood at $42.4 billion in 2015. The Nigerians in diaspora invest in their country for emotional returns and social rewards (Ayanruoh, 2018), and they have made significant contributions to HCE and clinical practice. Many have become global health experts in their areas of specialization, but their contributions are obscure to the rest of the world. This chapter aims to identify the elite Nigerian health care academics in the diaspora and showcase the scientific impact of their research.

Methodology

The investigation in this chapter was implemented in four phases. In phase one, a detailed search of the literature was conducted on PubMed, CINAHL, and PsychInfo databases using the keywords, Nigeria, academics/lecturers, health fields, and H-index/research productivity, which produced no single relevant "hit." In phase two, a snowball sampling strategy and an exhaustive search of several Nigerian affairs–leaning websites (Garloch, 2008; Ajayi, 2010; Straightnews. ng, 2018; Ranker, 2020; Nwachukwu, 2016; Isaac, 2019; African voice, 2019; The Guardian, 2019; Association of Nigerian Physicians in the Americas, 2020; Oyedoyin, 2019; Akinpelu, 2019; Nigeria Physiotherapy Network, 2020) was conducted to obtain the names of elite Nigerian health care academics in the diaspora. Only scholars who have attained the rank of professor or consultant in a health discipline were considered. The searches produced 126 names from different parts of the world: 72 were from the United Kingdom, one from Australia, Finland, South Africa, two from the UAE, 49 from the United States, and two from Canada.

During phase three of the investigation, which occurred between March 5 and May 29, 2020, the H-index score of the 126 Nigerian health care professionals was obtained from the Scopus database (2019). Scopus was selected among the other bibliometric databases because it does not require scholars to create a profile account. During the H-index search, 11 of the 126 names were not found due to name mismatch or spelling errors. Thus, the sample size whittled down to 115. Following the data collection, the H-index score of the remaining 115 academics was categorized into four groups. First-tier academics have H-index greater than 30 (n = 17), second-tier academics have H-index between 29 and 20 (n = 17), other academics with H-index less than 20 (n = 81).

Phase four involved an unstructured interview conducted with six of the academics to explore if they plan to return to the homeland permanently and their suggestions on what should be done to improve HCE in Nigeria. Attempts were made to let the interview flow like a natural conversation, and the follow up questions modified to suit the respondent's specific experiences (Cohen and Crabtree, 2006). Before the interview, they were assured that their names and identities would not be released in any publications that may emerge from the discussion. The opinions expressed were compiled and analyzed for major themes.

Result

First-tier academics

Summarized in Table 10.1 is the name, country of residence, gender, discipline, H-index score, number of years since first publication, M-quotient, and scientific impact ranking for the first-tier academics. Only 15% of the sample (115) had H-index score higher than 30 and the top six academics - Olopade (84), Rotimi (68) Achilefu (56), Odunsi (55), Johnson (44) Dagogo-Jack (44) – are all from the United States, followed by Uchegbu (42) from the United Kingdom, and Nwariaku/Lucas (38) from the United States.

The overwhelming majority (82%) of the first-tier academics were from the United States, 12% were from the United Kingdom, and 6% from the UAE. Their biographic information and scholarship/service accomplishments were gleaned from different open access sources and presented below; academics with the highest H-index are presented first.

1. Professor Olufunmilayo (Funmi) Ibironke Olopade (Scopus H-index = 84) – United States

Funmi was born in Nigeria in 1957 to an Anglican musician father and graduated from the University of Ibadan (UI) medical school in 1980. She immigrated

Table 10.1 The profile of the first-tier diaspora academics (N = 17)

S/N	Name	Country	Gender	Discipline	H-index	Year since first publication	M-quotient	Scientific impact ranking
1	Olufunmilayo Olapade	USA	F	Medicine	84	1989 (31)	2.709	1
2	Charles Rotimi	USA	M	Public Health	68	1993 (27)	2.519	2
3	Samuel Achilefu	USA	M	Medicine	56	1990 (30)	1.867	3
4	Kunle Odunsi	USA	M	Medicine	55	1994 (26)	2.115	4
5	Samuel Dagogo-Jack	USA	M	Medicine	44	1985 (35)	1.257	6
6	Bankole Johnson	USA	M	Medicine	44	1988 (32)	1.375	5
7	Ijeoma Uchegbu	UK	F	Pharmacy	42	1992 (28)	1.500	7
8	Adetokunbo Lucas	USA	M	Medicine	38	1964 (56)	0.679	9
9	Fiemu Nwariaku	USA	M	Medicine	38	1995 (25)	1.520	8
10	Oluyinka Olutoye	USA	M	Medicine	32	1995 (25)	1.280	10
11	Adewale Adebajo	UK	M	Medicine	31	1988 (32)	0.969	11
12	Adekunle Adekile	UAE	M	Medicine	31	1982 (38)	0.816	12
13	John Igietseme	USA	M	Microbiology	30	1987 (33)	0.909	16
14	Mukaila Raji	USA	M	Medicine	30	1992 (28)	1.071	15
15	Elizabeth Ofili	USA	F	Pharmacy	30	1994 (26)	1.154	13
16	John Ehiri	USA	M	Public health	30	1994 (26)	1.154	13
17	Chukuka Enwemeka	USA	M	Physiotherapy	30	1986 (34)	0.882	17

to the United States in 1983 and worked as an intern/resident/chief resident in the Department of Internal Medicine at Cook County Hospital in Chicago (1984–1987). She joined the University of Chicago in 1991 as an assistant professor in the Department of Hematology and Oncology, and in 1992, she was appointed the director of the Center for Clinical Cancer Genetics. Funmi is internationally renowned in cancer risk assessment and individualized therapy for the most aggressive forms of breast cancer.

She has received six honorary degrees from prestigious universities in the United States, including North Central, Dominican, Bowdoin, and Princeton. Additionally, she has received several academic and professionals honors and awards: Doris Duke Distinguished Clinical Scientist and Exceptional Mentor Award (2000), Phenomenal Woman Award for work within the African-American Community (2003), Access Community Network's Heroes in Healthcare Award (2005), Cancer Society Clinical Research Professorship, Officer of the Order of the Niger Award, Villanova University Mendel Medal (2017), and the Order of Lincoln Award in 2019 – the highest honor bestowed by the government of the State of Illinois. Currently, she serves on the boards of the *American Journal of Internal Medicine*, the National Cancer Advisory, Susan G. Komen for the Cure of Cancer, and the Lyric Opera. Funmi in 2005 received the MacArthur Fellowship ("Genius Grant") award for "translating findings on the molecular genetics of breast cancer in African and African-American women into innovative clinical practices in the United States and abroad." In 1983, she married Christopher Sola Olopade, also a physician at the University of Chicago. The union is blessed with two sons and two daughters (University of Chicago Medicine, 2020; Multimedia Foundation, 2020).

2. Professor Charles Nohuoma Rotimi (Scopus H-index = 68) – United States

Charles was born at Benin City in 1957 as the second oldest of six children. He obtained a biochemistry degree in 1979 from the University of Benin. He graduated in 1983 with a master's degree in health care administration from the University of Mississippi and a PhD in epidemiology from the University of Alabama, and a postdoc at Loma Linda University. He is the director of the trans-National Institute of Health (NIH) Center for Research in Genomics and Global Health. He was instrumental in the launch of the human heredity and health in Africa (H3Africa) with the NIH and Wellcome Trust. Charles' research focusses on genetics and health project disparities, ensuring that African genomes are represented in genome databases. He was employed at Loyola University Chicago, as an epidemiologist, where he investigated the link between cardiovascular disease and obesity amongst Africans in the diaspora. He received the Curt Stern Award from the American Society of Human Genetics in 2019 for his contributions to genetics in African and African-descent populations. And was elected in 2018 to the National Academy of Medicine (NIH, 2019).

3. Professor Samuel Achilefu (Scopus H-index = 56) – United States

Samuel was born in northern Nigeria in 1963, although his parents are from the eastern part of Nigeria. His father worked in the north until the civil war broke out in 1967, and his family migrated to their ancestral home, where they stayed until the civil war ended in 1970. Samuel, after his early education, won a French government scholarship to attend graduate school in France. He received a doctorate in molecular and materials chemistry at the University of Nancy in France and postdoctoral training at Oxford University in the United Kingdom. He joined the Mallinckrodt Institute of Radiology at Washington University in 2001 and established the world-renowned Optical Radiology program at the School of Medicine (Everything Radiography International, 2018). At Washington University, Samuel wears multiple academic and administrative hats: professor of medicine, biochemistry, molecular biophysics, professor of radiology and vice-chair for Innovation and Entrepreneurship, and director of the Molecular Imaging Center and codirector of the Center for Multiple Myeloma Nanotherapy (Washington University School of Medicine, 2020, Multimedia Inc, 2020).

Samuel is a world-acclaimed expert in the development and use of light-sensitive drugs for cancer detection, imaging, and therapy. He has 59 US patents and over 300 publications in peer-reviewed journals. Samuel has received over 30 local, national, international honors and awards: Prestigious Britton Chance Biomedical Optics award (2019), distinguished investigator award from the Academy for Radiology and Biomedical Imaging Research (2018), Carl and Gerty Cori faculty achievement award (2018), Excellence in Healthcare award (2017).

4. Professor Kunle Odunsi (Scopus H-index = 55) – United States

Kunle received his medical degree from the University of Ife (now Obafemi Awolowo University – OAU) and completed the postgraduate education in Obstetrics and Gynecology (O&G) at the Rosie Maternity Addenbrookes Hospitals, University of Cambridge, United Kingdom, and was admitted to the Royal College of Obstetricians and Gynecologists in 1991. He completed a research fellowship in molecular oncology and a PhD at the University of Oxford, United Kingdom. Subsequently, he completed his O&G residency training at the School of Medicine, Yale University New Haven, and clinical fellowship in Gynecologic Oncology at Roswell Park. Kunle dons multiple hats as professor of O&G at the State University of New York, School of Medicine and Biomedical Sciences in Buffalo, deputy director Roswell Park Cancer Institute (RPCI), chair, Department of Gynecologic Oncology RPCI, executive director of the Center for Immunotherapy, and endowed professor of gynecologic oncology.

Kunle pioneered the development of antigen-specific vaccine therapy for prolonging remission rates in patients with ovarian cancer. Kunle is a fellow of several academic and professional bodies worldwide, including the United States National Academy of Medicine in 2018. This distinguished lifetime designation is considered one of the highest honors in health and medicine. Kunle has authored or coauthored more than 340 publications in peer-reviewed journals or book chapters. His work has appeared in several prestigious journals that include the *Proceedings of the National Academy of Sciences (USA)*, *Nature*, *New England Journal of Medicine*, *Genetics*, and *Immunity*. Kunle presently serves on several national academic advisory committees (Unmc.edu. 2019; University at Buffalo, 2020; Roswell Park Comprehensive Cancer Center, 2020).

5. *Professor Bankole Johnson (Scopus H-index = 44) – United States*

Bankole was born on November 15, 1959, and graduated from King's College, Lagos, in 1975. He graduated in 1982 from the University of Glasgow medical school and later trained as a psychiatrist at the Royal London and Maudsley and Bethlem Royal Hospitals. He earned a Master of Philosophy (neuropsychiatry) degree from the University of London Institute of Psychiatry in 1991. He obtained a Doctorate in Medicine (1993) and a Doctor of Science degree in medicine (2004) – the highest science degree granted by a British university – from the University of Glasgow. Bankole joined the University of Texas (UT) Health Science Center, Houston, in 1993 and, in 1998, was appointed chief of the Division of Alcohol and Drug Addiction.

Bankole is a board-certified psychiatrist in the United Kingdom and the United States and chairman of the Department of Psychiatry at the University of Maryland, where he leads a brain science research consortium in the neurosciences. His area of research expertise is the psychopharmacology of medications for treating addictions. In 2001, Bankole received the Dan Anderson Research Award for his significant contribution to scientific knowledge in addiction recovery. A year later, in 2002, he received the distinguished senior scholar of distinction award from the National Medical Association and was inducted, in 2003, into the Texas Hall of Fame for his contributions to science, mathematics, and technology. Bankole is a fellow of the Royal College of Psychiatrists (2007), the American Psychiatric Association (2008), and the American College of Neuropsychopharmacology (2010) (Multimedia Foundation Inc., 2019; Ranker, 2020).

6. *Professor Samuel Dagogo-Jack (Scopus H-index = 44) – United States*

Samuel E. Dagogo-Jack completed his medical education from the UI medical school in Nigeria and completed his residency in internal medicine, endocrinology, and a Master of Science degree at the University of Newcastle (1988), and the Doctor of Medicine at the UI (1994). He is a member of the Royal College of Physicians in 1982, also completed a fellowship training at the School of Medicine, Washington University, St. Louis (1992).

He is an endowed professor in translational research, and chief of the division of endocrinology at the University of Tennessee Health Science Center, Memphis. His research focuses on the interaction of genetic and environmental factors in the prediction and prevention of prediabetes and type 2 diabetes; regulation and metabolic significance of leptin in humans; and mechanisms of diabetes complications, including hypoglycemia-associated autonomic failure (Multimedia Foundation, Inc, 2020; Cardiometabolic Health Congress, 2020).

7. *Professor Ijeoma Uchegbu (Scopus H-index = 42) – United Kingdom*

Ijeoma grew up in southeast Nigeria and obtained her entry-level pharmacy degree at the University of Benin in 1981. She earned a master's degree at the University of Lagos and a PhD at the University of London in 1997. She joined the University of Strathclyde in 2002 as the chair in drug delivery and left in 2006 to join the University College London as professor and chair of the Department of Pharmaceutical Nanoscience. In 2015, she was appointed vice-provost for Africa and the Middle East. She is the chief scientific officer for *Nanometrics*, a pharmaceutical tech company. Ijeoma is globally acclaimed for her work in science, public engagement, equality, and diversity in Science, Technology, Engineering, and Mathematics. In 2017, she won the Royal Society of Chemistry Emerging Technologies prize for the molecular envelope technology. She is the editor-in-chief of *Pharmaceutical Nanotechnology* and on the advisory team of the Engineering and Physical Sciences Research Council. And served on the committee that planned the celebrations of the 2019 National Health Service (NHS) turning event 70.

Ijeoma has published three books and won several awards and honors including the United Kingdom Department of Business, Innovation and Skills, Women of Outstanding Achievement in Science Engineering and Technology (2007), Royal Pharmaceutical Society Pharmaceutical Scientist of the Year (2012), Academy of Pharmaceutical Sciences Eminent Fellow (2013), Controlled Release Society College of Fellows (2013), and Academy of Pharmaceutical Sciences Innovative Science award (2016).

8. *Professor Adetokunbo Oluwole Lucas (Scopus H-index = 38) – United States*

His profile is featured in Chapter 6 of this book.

9. *Professor Fiemu Nwariaku (Scopus H-index = 38) – United States*

Fiemu obtained his primary and secondary education in Nigeria and attended the UI medical school from 1981 to 1987. He completed his internship and residency training in surgery at Baptist Medical Center, Nigeria (1987–1991), and residency/fellowship in general surgery at the UT Southwestern medical school (1995–1998). He joined the UT faculty in 1998. He is currently a professor of surgery at UT Southwestern and holds the Dr. Malcolm O. Perry professorship in surgery. He is also the associate dean of the Office for Global Health, which was established in 2010 to direct and develop training and research initiatives with partners worldwide.

Fiemu research focuses on developing new drugs to treat medullary thyroid cancer. His team previously discover a particular protein that causes medullary thyroid cancer cells to grow. Fiemu has published over 100 peer-reviewed journal articles, 15 book chapters, and three books and has lectured on endocrine surgery and global health topics worldwide. He has received several awards including the Educational Scholarship award (1995), Society of Critical Care Medicine Academic Excellence award (1996), UT Southwestern Medical Center Resident Teaching award (1998), UT Malcolm O. Perry Professorship in Surgery (2007), Australia and New Zealand Chapter of the American College of Surgeons Traveling Fellowship award (2008) (UT Southwestern Medical Center, 2020)..

10. Professors Oluyinka and Olutoyin Olutoye (Scopus H-index = 32) – United States

Oluyinka, and his wife, Olutoyin, graduated from the OAU medical school, in 1988 and 1990, respectively. Oluyinka obtained a PhD in anatomy from Virginia Commonwealth University in Richmond, Virginia (1996), and completed his residency in general surgery at the Medical College of Virginia Hospitals, and fellowship training in pediatric surgery at the University of Pennsylvania School of Medicine. In August 2019, Oluyinka was appointed the surgeon-in-chief of the Nationwide Children's Hospital, Columbus, Ohio, and professor and the chair of pediatric surgery at Ohio State University College of Medicine. (Nationwide Children's, 2019; Akwei, 2018).

Oluyinka received international acclamation in 2016 when he led a team of 22 health care professionals at Texas Children's Hospital, Baylor College of Medicine in Houston, Texas, to perform a delicate surgery on a 23-week old fetus diagnosed with a sacrococcygeal teratoma – a condition that develops before birth and grows from the tailbone. If not treated, the tumor will continue to take the fetus's blood supply and eventually causes heart failure. Oluyinka's team removed the fetus from the mother's uterus and operated upon and returned to the womb to heal and continue to grow until birth at 36 weeks. Olutoyin was the lead anesthesiologist during the surgery (Rilwan, 2016). The surgical feat is a testimony and affirmation of what can be achieved in the Nigerian health care system when professionals have access to appropriate equipment and resources. Oluyinka attributed his success to hard work and God's blessing. He opined that "Nigerians are talented people. If they decide to apply themselves, they can achieve much. When they have access to resources and infrastructure, they can attain even greater heights" (Rilwan, 2016).

11. Professor Adewale O. Adebajo (Scopus H-index = 31) – United Kingdom

Adewale is the clinical director for Research and Development (R&D) at Barnsley Hospital, NHS Foundation Trust in the United Kingdom. He is also associate director of teaching and honorary professor in musculoskeletal health service research at the University of Sheffield and clinical professor of medicine at St. Matthews medical school, Grand Cayman, British West Indies. Adewale has authored over 175 articles in peer-reviewed journals and book chapter publications. His research focuses on psoriatic and rheumatoid arthritis, soft tissue disorders, ethnic minority health, and tropical arthropathies. He is an associate editor for the *Journal of Clinical Rheumatology*, co-editor of the *ABC of Rheumatology Textbook*, and serves on the editorial boards of several other medical journals.

Adewale currently serves on the board of the Devices for Dignity Health Technology Cooperative, and an external assessor for postgraduate degrees at the University of Bradford, regional advisor for the Royal College of Physicians and Surgeons of Glasgow, patient and public involvement advisor, Arthritis Research United Kingdom, a clinical research fellow at Cambridge, diversity advisor to the Department of Health, and associate and strategic lead for the patient and public involvement at the Yorkshire and Humber CLAHRC (University of Sheffield, 2020).

12. Professor Adekunle Adekile (Scopus H-index = 31) – UAE

Adekunle had his secondary school education at Government College, Ibadan (1962–1966), and was admitted at the UI medical school in 1967 and graduated in 1973. He completed the pediatric residency training at the OAU Teaching Hospital Complex. He left the shores of Nigeria in 1980 to pursue a postdoctoral fellowship in pediatric hematology at Howard University Comprehensive Sickle Cell Center. On return to Nigeria in 1981, he joined the Faculty of Health Sciences at the OAU and established a sickle cell clinic at the teaching hospital. He received the Fogarty International Fellowship award in 1990 and worked at Medical College of Georgia, United States. He moved to the University of Kuwait in 1993 and, in 2010, established the Kuwait National Sickle Cell Disease Registry- the first and only such registry in UAE.

Adekunle earned a PhD in cell biology from the University of Maastricht, Netherlands, in 1996. He has authored over 120 publications in peer-reviewed journals around the world. Currently, he serves on the board of the Center for Arab Genomic Studies and Global Sickle Cell Disease Network. Adekunle's landmark academic contributions include the work on the spleen of patients with sickle cell disease and the phenotype in patients with the Arab/India haplotype and elevated HbF. He is the founding president of the Nigerian Society for Sickle Cell Support. During his tenure, the network brought together physicians, nurses, NGOs, and policymakers with interest in the management of sickle cell disease (Sickle Cell Support Society of Nigeria, 2020).

13. *Professor Elizabeth Odilile Ofili (Scopus H-index = 30) – United States*

Elizabeth was born in 1956 and had her medical education at Ahmadu Bello University before migrating to the United States in 1982. She earned a Master of Public Health degree in 1983 from Johns Hopkins University. Elizabeth completed her residency program in internal medicine at Oral Roberts University in Tulsa and was appointed a cardiology fellow at Washington University Medical Center in St. Louis, Missouri. She relocated to Morehouse School of Medicine in 1994 as associate professor of medicine and chief of the cardiology section and was promoted full professor in 1999 (Wikimedia Foundation Inc., 2020).

Elizabeth is an internationally acclaimed cardiologist and the first woman elected in 2000 as the president of the Association of Black Cardiologists. Her research focuses on women's health and the disparities in cardiovascular disease in the African-American population. She has also partnered with NASA in investigating the effects of microgravity on the vasculature. Elizabeth is the recipient of over 20 national and international awards, including the dean fellow, Council of the Association of American Medical Colleges, and Daniel Savage Memorial Science award. She has published over 130 scientific articles in peer-reviewed reputed journals and holds a patent for "a system and method for chronic illness care" (Morehouse School of Medicine, 2020).

14. *John Ehiri (Scopus H-index = 30) – United States*

John was born and received his undergraduate education in Nigeria. He obtained his graduate (MPH and PhD) degrees from Glasgow University in Scotland, an MSc degree in Economics (Health Policy and Planning) from the University of Swansea, Wales, United Kingdom. John is presently a professor, chair, and interim associate dean at the University of Arizona, where he has developed the graduate certificate program in maternal and child health epidemiology and certificate in global health. Before moving to the University of Alabama at Birmingham in 2002, he was the director of the postgraduate program in community health at the Liverpool School of Tropical Medicine. At the University of Alabama, he served as chair of the Framework for Global Health Program.

John is a behavioral scientist with over 25 years of research experience, which focuses on global maternal and child health, and infectious diseases with particular emphasis on HIV/AIDS. He has developed and disseminated numerous policy frameworks for integrated approaches to health system development in low and middle-income countries. His work is cited widely by WHO, UNICEF, the World Bank, USAID, and other leading global health agencies. John has authored a book, numerous book chapters, and over 70 articles in peer-reviewed journals. He is a member of the Global Health Council, and the Global Academy for Tropical Health (University of Arizona, 2020).

15. Mukaila Raji (Scopus H-index = 30) – United States

Mukaila completed a BS degree with first class honors (1984) and a medical degree at OAU (1987). He also earned a MS degree in pharmacology from the University of Alberta, Canada (1994). He had his internal medicine residency at Washington Hospital Center in Washington, DC (1997), and a geriatric fellowship at Duke University in Durham (1999).

He is chief of geriatric medicine at the University of Texas Medical Branch in Galveston. Mukaila has published over 100 manuscripts in peer-reviewed journals and several book chapters in cognitive aging and disability, health policy, and geriatric pharmacology. He has received several academic awards, including the Sir William Osler Excellence in Clinical Teaching Awards (2006 and 2018), America's top doctor in geriatric medicine awards (2017 and 2018), and the top Texas physician awards (2013 and 2018).

16. Professor Joseph Osikhueme Igietseme (Scopus H-index = 30) –United States

Joseph received a PhD in immunology and microbiology from Georgetown University, Washington, DC (1987). He subsequently trained in infection and immunity at the University of Miami School of Medicine, Miami, and the University of Arkansas for Medical Sciences, Little Rock. He joined the University of Arkansas as an assistant professor in 1993 and transferred to the School of Medicine, Atlanta, Georgia, in 1996. He was promoted in 2002 as a professor of microbiology, biochemistry and chief of the molecular pathogenesis laboratory at the Centers for Disease Control and Prevention (CDC), Atlanta.

His research focuses on basic and applied immunology, microbiology, pathogenesis, immunity, and vaccinology. He has published over 200 peer-reviewed articles, and received several awards, including the 2010 CDC Shepard Award for the most outstanding published research, and the 2010 Nakano Citation Award for outstanding research, indicating the national and international recognition of his research work (CDC, n.d.).

17. Professor Chukuka S. Enwemeka (Scopus H-index = 30) – United States

Chukuka was born at Agbor in Nigeria, on March 7, 1953, as the first child of Chief Smart A. Enwemeka and Mrs. Beatrice Enwemeka; he has 17 siblings. Chukuka attended St. Patrick Primary School, and St. Columbus Secondary School, Agbor. He completed his bachelor's degree in physiotherapy at the UI in 1978 and his master's degree in 1983 from the University of Southern California. He earned a PhD in physical therapy from New York University in 1985. He was appointed professor and chairman of the Department of Physical Therapy and Rehabilitation Sciences at the University of Kansas Medical Center (1993–2003), professor and dean of the School of Health Professions at the New York Institute of Technology (2003–2009) and as a distinguished professor and dean of the College of Health Sciences at the University of Wisconsin-Milwaukee (2009–2014). He was appointed the provost and senior vice-president at San Diego State University, California (2014–2018). As the chief academic officer, he achieved recognition for the student success initiatives that he developed, which elevated student graduation and retention rates to record levels and enforced rigorous academic standards.

Chukuka is one of the world's preeminent scientists who first used near-infrared lasers, and monochromatic light to promote collagen polymerization and alignment in animal models of soft tissue injury and for the treatment of chronic ulcers that are unresponsive to antibiotic therapy. His contributions to the science of photo-biomodulation produced significant publications, a patent, journal editorial boards, and academic leadership positions. Chukuka was honored in 2018 with the Lifetime Achievement Award by the North American Association of Photobiomodulation Therapy. He is a fellow of the American Society for Laser Medicine and Surgery and American College of Sports Medicine (James Hope College, 2019).

Second-tier academics

Only 15% of the academics had H-index score between 20 and 29 and they constitute the second-tier academics (Table 10.2).

Sixty-five percent of the second-tier academics were from the United States, and 29% were from the United Kingdom, and 6% from the UAE.

Academics with H-index below 20

The H-index scores for the remaining academics are summarized in Table 10.3. The majority (35%) of them (n = 81) had H-index between four and one, 17% had H-index between 16 and 19; 16% had H-indexes between 12–15, and 10% had H-indexes between 9–11, and 22% had H-indexes between 5–8.

Qualitative findings

Only 5% of the sample interviewed indicated any desire to relocate back to Nigeria in the future. The views expressed by those who reported no willingness to relocate back home were divergent and insightful. Two major themes emerged – security situation in the country and poor work conditions. The quotes below represent typical points-of-view expressed by the academics interviewed.

> "*Look at the number of people killed needlessly in Northern Nigeria by the Boko Haram bandits. … we seem not to value human life, and I do not feel safe working in that type of environment.*"

> "*The high incidence of kidnapping by relatives and the Fulani herdsmen is of grave concern, and the law enforcement seems to be powerless as no one is found responsible.*"

Table 10.2 The profile of the second-tier diaspora academics (N=17)

S/N	Name	Country	Gender	Discipline	H- index	Years since first publication	M-quotient	Scientific impact ranking
1	Nelson Oyesika	USA	M	Medicine	29	1986 (34)	0.853	18
2	Sarki Abdulkadir	USA	M	Medicine	28	1990 (30)	0.933	19
3	Henry Akinbi	USA	M	Medicine	26	1994 (26)	1.000	21
4	John Vincent	UK	M	Pharmacy	26	1996 (24)	1.083	20
5	Babafemi Taiwo	USA	M	Medicine	25	2000 (20)	1.250	22
6	Flora Ukoli	USA	F	Medicine	25	1979 (41)	0.610	23
7	T.O. Obisesan	USA	M	Medicine	24	1996 (24)	1.000	24
8	Adebayo Oyekan	USA	M	Medicine	24	1986 (34)	0.706	25
9	Olumayokun Olajide	UK	M	Pharmacy	23	1997 (23)	1.000	26
10	Oluwafemi Oyebode	UK	M	Medicine	23	1985 (35)	0.657	27
11	Benett Omalu	USA	M	Medicine	22	2001 (19)	1.158	28
12	Ben Nwomeh	USA	M	Medicine	22	1998 (22)	1.000	29
13	Adesuyi L. Ajayi	USA	M	Medicine	22	1985 (35)	0.629	30
14	Soji Olusi	UAE	M	Medicine	22	1975 (45)	0.489	31
15	Timi Edeki	UK	M	Pharmacology	21	1986 (34)	0.618	33
16	Olagunju Ogunbiyi	UK	M	Medicine	21	1993 (27)	0.778	32
17	Anthony Archibong	USA	M	Pharmacology	20	1982 (38)	0.526	34

Table 10.3 The profile of the remaining academics with H-index score below 20 (N = 81)

S/N	H-index category	Name of the academics	N (%)
1	19 – 16	Ohia Sunday, Anthony Okorodudu, James Essien, Ifeanyi Arinze, Ayotunde Adeagbo, Olakunle Akinboboye, Austin Ugwumadu, Joseph Balogun, Dilichukwu Anumba, Roger Makanjuola, Elizabeth Anionwu, Frank Chinegwundoh, Kelsey Harrison, Chike Nzeruke	14 (17%)
2	15- 12	Omene Jackson, Bolanle Adamolekun, John Muir, Emmanuel Okafor, Ifeanyichukwu Okike, Leroy Edozien, Abiodun Akinwuntan, Francis Fatoye, Christopher Okunseri, Titilayo Abiona, Kelechi Nnoaham, Olawale Sulaiman, Charles Ameh	13 (16%)
3	11 – 9	William Ebomoyi, Gabriel Iveijaro, Ferdinand Ofodile, Funmilayo Odejinmi, Adeyemi Coker, Nnamdi Maduekwe, Emmanuel Fadiran, Kayode Adetugbo	8 (10%)
4	8 – 5	Adetokunbo Oyelese, Adebayo Laniyonu, Uche Menakaya, Seyi Ladele Amosun, Eno Ekpo, Adedeji Adefuye, Akinniran Oladehin, Femi Olatunbosun, Bolanle Asiyanbola, Andrew Alalade, Anthony Owa, Cliff Eke, Emeka Nchekwube, Chinwe Ogedegbe, Udo Asonye, Hilary Onyiwke, Victor Chilaka, Abraham Ariyo	18 (22%)
5	4 – 1	Olu Obaro, Esther Kuyinu, Alphosus Obayuwana, Stanley Okoro, Godwin Eni, Victor Obajuluwa, Felix Adah, Emmanuel John, Olurotimi Badero, Ayo Ayoola, Ngozi Ezike, Joanna Umo-Etuk, Aliko Baba Ahmed, Yele Aluko, Rotimi Jaiyesimi, Oluseye Oyawoye, Olubukola Abiona, Dapo Popoola, Uduak Archibong, Olayinka Akinfenwa, Tai Ayodele Ajayi, Julian Mamiso, John Agwunobi, Charmaine Emelife, Nkem Chukwumerije, Oviemo Ovadje, Julius Kpaduwa, Aloysius Anaebonam	28 (35%)

"It is impossible to continue my research in Nigeria because I will not have access to the equipment that I need to do my work."

"At this stage of my career, I do not see myself going back to Nigeria to work. I am open to contributing to national development, not in a salaried position but as a consultant."

"No, I cannot return to Nigeria. I have seen some of my colleagues back to Nigeria and had to return to the USA because peers sabotaged them, and the system messed them up. I cannot afford to ruin my career."

In response to the question on what should be done to improve HCE in Nigeria, the opinions were also divergent and four major themes emerged. The need to revise the curriculum, capacity building, raising the academic bar and accreditation standard. The following are sample responses by the scholars.

> "*To reform the educational system, the University Teaching Hospitals and academic programs in the health fields should be encouraged to seek international accreditation to raise the standard.*"

> "*The curricula should be revised and aligned with the international standard.*"

> "*Emphasis should be placed on capacity building of the knowledge base and clinical skills of the lecturers.*"

> "*I will select one university from each of the six geopolitical zones and develop the universities to international standard levels to serve as a model for the remaining universities.*"

> "*Encourage more international collaboration and faculty exchange with universities from the North.*"

> "*With scarce financial resources and no coordinated family planning program to curtail the booming population growth, the country's future is ominous.*"

Discussion

This chapter identified the elite Nigerians in diaspora from different health fields, which have influenced HCE and clinical practice globally. Many of the academics whose biography were not featured deserve mentioning here because they made Nigeria proud in several ways. The academics from the United Kingdom were among the outstanding health care workers recognized during the 70th anniversary of the NHS in 2019. Many of the individuals honored are trailblazers and leading experts in their professions who have made noteworthy contributions within the NHS.

Among the second-tier academics, three of them deserve special recognition here. Professor of colorectal surgery and consultant surgeon, Olagunju Ogunbiyi, received thunderous applause from his colleagues at Royal Free Hospital, United Kingdom, as featured in a U-tube video that went viral on May 16, 2020, after he was discharged from the hospital. The best physician in the NHS battled very hard to bring him back to life after coronavirus infection. His contribution to NHS was described as "irreplaceable" (Paul, 2020). Another spectacular Nigerian is Professor Bennet Ifeakandu Omalu, a forensic-neuropathologist with seven advanced degrees and board certifications and the first to discover chronic traumatic encephalopathy among American football players (Multimedia Foundation Inc. 2020; ConnetNigeria.com, 2020).

Professors *Olurotimi Badero* has extraordinary educational achievements as the only physician in the world with board certification in cardiology and nephrology. He is among the top interventional cardiologists and nephrologists in the United States with expertise in six specialties – internal and cardiovascular medicine, invasive and interventional cardiology, nephrology and hypertension, interventional nephrology, endovascular medicine, nuclear cardiology, and peripheral vascular interventions. He is one of few blacks in the discipline who received the excellence in cardiology award presented by the Association of Black Cardiologists and named the Jackson, Mississippi's best surgeons in 2008 (Taylor, 2019).

One of the few Nigerians to ever serve in the corridor of power in Washington, DC is Dr. John O. Agwunobi, a pediatrician and member of the United Stataes Public Health Service Commissioned Corps, and a four-star admiral in the United Stataes Navy. He is a graduate of the University of Jos medical school and served as the assistant secretary for health from 2005 to 2007 during President George Bush administration, and on WHO's executive board. He is currently chief executive officer of Herbalife, a multi-level marketing global corporation that develops and sells dietary supplements. (Multimedia Foundation Inc. 2020; White House, n.d.).

Nigeria has several nimble scientists at the forefront of finding a cure or vaccine for COVID-19 – a lethal disease that poses an existential threat to the human race. Professor Babafemi Taiwo, Chief of the Division of Infectious Diseases at Northwestern University, caused a global sensation on April 29, 2020, as he leads a team of scientists at Chicago in a multinational study of the efficacy of an antiviral drug made by Gilead Sciences. In a CNN interview, Babafemi indicated that Remdesivir had "a clear-cut significant positive effect," shortening the time to hospital discharge by four days. About 8% of the patients with COVID-19 on Remdesivir died compared to 11.6% among the control group, but the difference was not statistically significant (CNN, 2020). Another Nigerian scientist Olubukola Abiona and her colleagues at the UT, Austin, made a breakthrough on February 19, 2020, toward producing a vaccine for the COVID-19. They developed the first 3D atomic-scale map of the part of the coronavirus that attaches to and infects human cells (UT News, 2020).

Other Nigerian scientists and inventors at the cutting edge of biomedical research also deserves special mention. A Nigerian plastic surgeon, Ferdinand Ofodile, developed a nasal implant for rhinoplasty for ethnic minority populations. The device produces more natural results that fit Black and Hispanic anatomical features and is named "Ofodile implant" after him. Ferdinand and Olawale Sulaiman have led charity medical missions to several underserved communities around the world, including Nigeria, Mozambique, the Dominican Republic, and Haiti. Olawale typically spends considerable time in Nigeria, up to 12 days each month, providing health care, sometimes for free to the indigent population that cannot afford complex spine surgeries (Akinpelu, 2019; Anonymous, 2015; Salaudeen, 2019; Multimedia Foundation Inc. 2019). In 1989, Colonel Oviemo Ovadje with only $120 invented and patented a low-cost, affordable, and practical Emergency AutoTransfusion System device that saves life in developing countries. As a result of his invention, Oviemo has received several national and international awards, including the

World Intellectual Property Organization and Organization of African Unity Gold Medal in 1995. He is the first African to win the WHO Sasakawa Gold Medal award in 2000. Another Nigerian pharmacist's, Aloysius Anaebonam, Founder and Chief Scientist of BREEJ Technologies, Inc.United States, with 12 patents also developed a cosmetic product used for the treatment of problem skin (Akinpelu, 2019).The list of inventions and academic feat by Nigerians are too numerous to recount in this chapter.

The scholars interviewed referenced the violence and mayhem perpetrated by the jihadist group Boko Haram in the Lake Chad basin in Nigeria as a major barrier to relocating back to Nigeria.Their fear is real since the Boko Haram terrorist group has killed over 30,000 innocent people and displaced more than two million in the last decade.They also referenced the ongoing spates of kidnapping in the country, poor work conditions, and lack of infrastructure that will enable them to continue their research as deterrents to relocating back to the homeland.The recommendations made by the academics on how to enhance HCE are consistent with the views presented in Chapter 9 of this book.

Implications

Despite the academic achievements of the academics in the diaspora, the homeland remain underdeveloped. With the enormous human resources at home and in the diaspora, why is Nigeria not able to transform itself into a nation like Singapore? In 1965, Singapore was expelled from Malaysia and thrust into unwanted independence; it was an impoverished nation with only $500 per capita income.Today, their education and health care systems and economy are the envy of the world. Singapore was able to transform itself with an intentional national plan built upon three simple vision strategies – MPH: Meritocracy, Pragmatism, and Honesty. The Singaporean government intentionally make leadership appointments based on merit and the nation embraced the best of socialist and capitalist ideologies that work for their country and fought corruption head-on (Mahbubani, 2017).The lack of "MPH" is the bane of the Nigerian nation, which has abundant human talents. Sadly, Nigerians rarely bloom on her shores due to a political system that embrace mediocrity, ineptitude, nepotism, and corruption.

The problem causing Nigerian academics to underperform on the homeland, is a reflection of the government severe under-investment in R&D, and the stagnation of the private sector in science and technology development. North America has the highest investment in science and technology, while Africa has the least. In 2010, allocation to R&D in science, technology, and innovation (as a percentage of GDP) was 2.7% for North America, 2.2% for Oceania, 1.8% for Europe, 1.6% for Asia, 0.7% for Latin America and the Caribbean, and 0.4% for Africa (Obasanjo, 2015). In 2019, European Union sets overall R&D investment to 3%, the United States spends 2.7% and over 2% by China.The African region set a benchmark of 1% of its GDP to be invested in R&D, but only

South Africa, Kenya, and Senegal (around 0.8% in the three countries) are close to the target (African Union, 2019).

Complicating the problem is the declining research skills of the burgeoning academics in Nigeria. Many of them employed in the universities and research centers are poorly trained compared to the academics in the 20th century. African academics unlike their counterparts in the North, appears increasingly unwilling to venture into new grounds. For example, in 2014, with over 215,500 new inventions in science and technology, only a dismal 0.01% were from Africa. An interplay of several factors, including poor working conditions and limited infrastructures, may explain the "intellectual timidity" and the limited adventure by homeland academics.

For the country not to be left behind in the 21st century, academics must be engaged in research that will address local developmental challenges. And the government must increase investment in science, technology, and innovation significantly. The government must set a research agenda that is relevant to the needs of the country and monitor its implementation. At least a 15% higher level of investment, progressively increased by 5% every year for the next 20 years, has been proposed (Obasanjo, 2015). Implementation of this proposal will translate to improvement in the quality of life for the Nigerian people. Furthermore, the government must improve the working condition of academics and make it attractive to reverse the brain drain phenomenon. The opportunity for continuous professional development should be a top priority.

Limitations

The apparent limitations of the investigation in this chapter must be recognized, and the theses taken with an abundance of caution. In the absence of a national register of Nigerian academics in the diaspora, there is an excellent probability that several scholars may have been omitted. The use of the snowball sampling method in recruiting academics limits the external validity of the findings presented. It is impossible to determine the sampling error or deduce inferences about populations based on the obtained sample with the snowball sampling. The participants' social networks are usually not randomly drawn. A few cases after referrals, some potential participants refused to participate in the research study. Also, given that people typically refer those they know and have similar experiences, the snowball sampling strategy is fraught with potential sampling bias and margin of error (Statistics How To 2020; Bhat, 2020). Some of the academics that met the study criterion have limited information about them in the open access literature. Hence, vital aspects of their academic accomplishments and biography may not be reflected adequately.

The second limitation is the imperfection associated with the use of H-index to judge research productivity, and scientific impact of the academics is an ongoing debate in the literature (Saleem, 2011; Williams, 2014; Kreiner, 2016). Among the many criticisms of H-index is the view that it does not give an accurate measure for early-career academics, and the fact that it is derived using articles indexed in specific databases-article published in local journals ignored. The M-quotient value was calculated by dividing their H-index index score by the number of years since the first publication and used to determine the scientific impact ranking of academics with the same H-index. The M-index represents the average amount the scientist's H-index has increased per year over the publishing career and can differentiate between two scientists with similar H-indexes but different years of work experience. An H-index of 12 for a scientist with ten years of experience (M-quotient of 1.2) is more substantial than an H-index of 12 for a scientist with 24 years of work experience (M-quotient of 0.5). However, the use of M-quotient can penalize scientists who demonstrate research productivity early in their career (e.g., during undergraduate education) followed by years during which they joined the academy as a full-time faculty (Choudhri et al., 2015).

Another substantial limitation is that H-index cannot be compared across different disciplines, and the scores can be higher in one field (genetics) than in another area (anthropology). Also, H-index is open to manipulation through self-citation, peer citation practices, and ignoring the impact of individual contributions in multiple-authored publications. It does not identify the hierarchy of author contributions. Dominant fields with more researchers produce more articles. Thus, creating more opportunities for citation and higher H-indices. Some academic disciplines emphasize the use of more references than other areas, and H-index changes over time (University of Canterbury, 2020). Therefore, the findings reported in this chapter are the academics' snapshot research productivity as of March 5 and May 29, 2020, when the H-index information was extracted from the Scopus database.

However, despite the above-stated flaws, the H-index and its variants, such as the g-index, m-quotient, hc-index, e-index, and i-10 (i-n) index, are generally recognized in the academy as a viable single robust metric of scholarship productivity (Masic, Begic, 2016; Harzing, 2017; Ciaccia et al., 2019). Askbecker (2019) affirmed that H-index is "an estimate of the importance, significance, and broad impact of a scientist's cumulative research contributions." Harzing (2017) contends that H-index "combines an assessment of both quantity (number of publications) and an approximation of quality (impact, or citations of a publication)."

Conclusion

This chapter contends that Nigeria, as a nation, is endowed with human resources and an avalanche of eminent health care academics contributing to social development in other parts of the world. The elite scholars featured in this chapter worked very hard to elevate the quality of HCE in the countries that they practice. Besides their scholarship activities, many of them still find time to visit their homeland to conduct workshops in the universities and provide free health care services to the vulnerable populations in Nigeria and other developing countries. Undoubtedly, Nigeria has several talents in the diaspora, and the government can harness their skills to revitalize the crumbling HCE and health care systems. The prevailing insecurity manifested by the wave of kidnapping and poor work conditions are challenges that must be overcome for the elite Nigerian health care academics in the diaspora to relocate to the country. The information contained in this chapter can be utilized for investment schemes development and enhance collaboration with highly skilled academics in the diaspora.

References

Adefusika, JA. (2010) Understanding the brain-drain in the African diaspora: Focusing on Nigeria. The senior honors projects *University of Rhode Island*. Paper 164. [online]. Available at: https://digitalcommons.uri.edu/cgi/viewcontent.cgi?referer=&httpsredir=1&article=1166&context=srhonorsprog (Accessed: 26 April 2020)

Adeniyi, KO, Sambo, DU, Anjorin, FI and Aisien, AO, Rosenfeld, LM. (1998). An overview of medical education in Nigeria. *Journal of the Pennsylvania Academy of Science*, 71(3): 135–142. [online]. Available at: www.jstor.org/stable/44149234?readnow=1&seq=1#page_scan_tab_contents (Accessed: 26 April 2020)

African Union. (2019) Third ordinary session for the specialized technical committee on education, science and technology (STC-EST), December 10–12, 2019, Addis Ababa, Ethiopia. [online]. Available at: https://au.int/sites/default/files/newsevents/workingdocuments/37841-wd-five-year_science_technology_and_innovation_plan_en.pdf (Accessed: 26 April 2020)

Africanvoice. (2019) Final list of Nigerian healthcare professionals nominated for NHS @70 excellence awards. [online]. Available at: http://africanvoiceonline.co.uk/final-list-of-nigerian-healthcare-professionals-nominated-for-nhs-70-excellence-awards/ (Accessed: 26 April 2020)

Ajayi, LA. (2010) Nigerian biomedical leaders in America- based on verifiable contribution to knowledge and impact celebrating Nigeria's global accomplishments in its Jubilee year! [online]. *Chicago Inquirer*. Available at: https://groups.google.com/forum/m/#!topic/yorubaaffairs/53wpAKnYVWw (Accessed: 26 April 2020)

Akinpelu, O. (2019) 7 Nigerian scientists you have probably never heard of a year ago. *Legit*. [online]. Available at: www.legit.ng/1206274-7-nigerian-scientists-heard-of.html (Accessed: 26 April 2020)

Akwei, I. (2018) Meet Dr. Oluyinka Olutoye, a black trailblazer in medicine. [online]. Available at: https://face2faceafrica.com/article/meet-dr-oluyinka-olutoye-a-black-trailblazer-in-medicine (Accessed: 26 April 2020)

Anonymous. (2015) Successful Nigerian academics in the world's top universities. – Education. [online]. Available at: www.nairaland.com/2273563/successful-nigerian-academics-worlds-top (Accessed: 26 April 2020)

Askbecker, K. (2019) H-index. [online]. Available at: https://beckerguides.wustl.edu/authors/hindex (Accessed: 26 April 2020)

Association of Nigerian Physicians in the Americas. (2020) [online]. Available at: https://anpa.org/about/board-of-directors/ (Accessed: 26 April 2020)

Ayanruoh. (2018) Why does Nigeria diaspora invest in their country of origin? Engaged management scholarship conference: Philadelphia, PA. *Fox School of Business Research*, Paper No. 18–027. [online]. Available at: https://papers.ssrn.com/sol3/papers.cfm?abstract_id=3240861 (Accessed: 26 April 2020)

Azuh, B. (2019) Rising emigration of pharmacist. *The Guardian Newspaper.* [online]. Available at: https://guardian.ng/features/health/rising-emigration-of-pharmacists/ (Accessed: 26 April 2020)

Balogun, JA. (2011) Our American journey: Challenges, threats, and opportunities. *Journal of the Nigerian Society of Physiotherapy*, 18/19: 59–67. [online]. Available at: www.researchgate.net/publication/280024014_Joseph_A_Balogun_Our_American_Journey_Challenges_threats_and_Opportunities_Journal_of_the_Nigerian_Society_of_Physiotherapy_Vol_1819_59-67_2011 (Accessed: 26 April 2020)

Banke-Thomas, A. (2018) The emigration of doctors from Nigeria is not today's problem, it is tomorrows. [online]. Available at: https://blogs.lse.ac.uk/africaatlse/2018/10/15/the-emigration-of-doctors-from-nigeria-is-not-todays-problem-it-is-tomorrows/ (Accessed: 26 April 2020)

Bhat, A. (2020) Snowball sampling: Definition, method, advantages and disadvantages. [online]. Available at: www.questionpro.com/blog/snowball-sampling/ (Accessed: 26 April 2020)

Blair, T. (n.d.) Why are there so many Nigerians in UK? [online]. Available at: www.quora.com/Why-are-there-so-many-Nigerians-in-UK (Accessed: 26 April 2020)

Cardiometabolic Health Congress. (2020) Biography: Samuel Dagogo-Jack, MD. [online]. Available at: www.cardiometabolichealth.org/sam-dagogo-jack.html (Accessed: 26 April 2020)

Centers for Disease Control and Prevention. (n.d.) Joseph U Igietseme. [online]. Available at: https://loop.frontiersin.org/people/428030/overview (Accessed: 26 April 2020)

Choudhri, A.F, Siddiqui, A, Khan, N.R and Cohen, H.L. (2015). Understanding bibliometric parameters and analysis. *Radiographics*, 35(3): 736–746. [online]. Available at: https://pubs.rsna.org/doi/10.1148/rg.2015140036?url_ver=Z39.88–2003&rfr_id=ori%3Arid%3Acrossref.org&rfr_dat=cr_pub%3Dpubmed (Accessed: 10 March 2020)

Ciaccia, EJ, Bhagat, G, Lebwohla, B, Lewisa, SK, Ciaccic, C and Green, PH. (2019). Comparison of several author indices for gauging academic productivity. *Informatics in Medicine Unlocked*, (15): 100166. [online]. Available at: www.sciencedirect.com/science/article/pii/S2352914818302363?via%3Dihub (Accessed: 26 April 2020)

CNN. (2020) Nigerian doctor in US: Babafemi Taiwo leads major study on Antiviral Covid 19 drug remdesivir. [online]. Available at: https://video.search.yahoo.com/yhs/search?fr=yhs-symantec-ext_onb&hsimp=yhs-ext_onb&hspart=symantec&p=babafemi+taiwo#id=3&vid=dfec98a37666d2e4b5460fc896141eb3&action=view (Accessed: 26 April 2020)

Cohen D and Crabtree B. (2006) Qualitative research guidelines project: Unstructured interviews. *Robert Wood Johnson Foundation.* [online]. Available at: www.qualres.org/HomeUnst-3630.html (Accessed: 26 April 2020)

ConnetNigeria.com (2020) Bennet Omalu. [online]. Available at: https://connectnigeria.com/articles/2016/07/top-ten-nigerian-scientists-today/ (Accessed: 26 April 2020)

Duncan, J. (2019) 400 Nigerian physicians and dentists arrive in Kelowna today. *KelownaNow.* [online]. Available at: www.kelownanow.com/watercooler/news/news/Kelowna/400_Nigerian_physicians_and_dentists_arrive_in_Kelowna_today/#fs_85295 (Accessed: 26 April 2020)

Duvivier, RJ, Burch, VC and Boulet, JR. (2017) A comparison of physician emigration from Africa to the United States of America between 2005 and 2015. *Human*

Resources for Health, 15(41). [online]. Available at: https://human-resources-health. biomedcentral.com/articles/10.1186/s12960-017-0217-0 (Accessed: 26 April 2020)

Everything Radiography International. (2018) Samuel Achilefu: The Nigerian born radiographer who invented the cancer goggle. [online]. Available at: https:// everythingradiography.com/index.php/2018/05/27/samuel-achilefu-the-nigerian-born-radiographer-who-invented-the-cancer-goggle/ (Accessed: 26 April 2020)

Garloch, K. (2008) Nigerian doctors in the U.S. never forget home. *The Charlotte Observer*. [online]. Available at: www.charlotteobserver.com/living/health-family/ article8988767.html (Accessed: 26 April 2020)

Harzing, AW. (2017) Research in international management. Metrics: h and g-index. [online]. Available at: https://harzing.com/resources/publish-or-perish/tutorial/ metrics/h-and-g-index (Accessed: 26 April 2020)

James Hope College. (2019) Professor Chukuka S. Enwemeka. [online]. Available at: www.jameshopecollege.edu.ng/professor-chukuka-s-enwemeka-phd-facsm/ (Accessed: 26 April 2020)

Kreiner, G. (2016) The slavery of the *h-index*—measuring the unmeasurable. *Frontiers in Human Neuroscience*, 10: 556. [online]. Available at: www.ncbi.nlm.nih.gov/pmc/ articles/PMC5089989/ (Accessed: 26 April 2020)

Mahbubani, K. (2017) Why Singapore is the world's most successful society? *HuffPost News*. [online]. Available at: https://bit.ly/3iYYD1f (Accessed: 26 April 2020)

Masic, I and Begic, E. (2016) Scientometric dilemma: Is H-index adequate for scientific validity of academic's work? *Acta Informatica Medica*, 24(4): 228–232. [online]. Available at: www.ncbi.nlm.nih.gov/pmc/articles/PMC5037980/ ml (Accessed: 26 April 2020)

Multimedia Foundation, Inc. (2019a) Bankole Johnson. [online]. Available at: https:// en.wikipedia.org/wiki/Bankole_Johnson (Accessed: 26 April 2020)

Multimedia Foundation, Inc. (2019b) Olawale Sulaiman. [online]. Available at: https:// en.wikipedia.org/wiki/Olawale_Sulaima (Accessed: 26 April 2020)

Multimedia Foundation, Inc. (2020a) Bennet Omalu. [online]. Available at: https:// en.m.wikipedia.org/wiki/Bennet_Omalu (Accessed: 26 April 2020)

Multimedia Foundation Inc. (2020b) John O. Agwunobi. [online]. Available at: https:// en.wikipedia.org/wiki/John_O._Agwunobi (Accessed: 26 April 2020)

Multimedia Foundation Inc. (2020c) Nigerian Americans. [online]. Available at: https:// en.m.wikipedia.org/wiki/Nigerian_Americans#US_states_with_the_largest_ Nigerian_populations (Accessed: 26 April 2020)

Multimedia Foundation Inc. (2020d) Nigerian Canadians. [online]. Available at: https:// en.m.wikipedia.org/wiki/Nigerian_Canadians (Accessed: 26 April 2020)

Multimedia Foundation, Inc. (2020e) Olufunmilayo Olopade. [online]. Available at: https://en.wikipedia.org/wiki/Olufunmilayo_Olopade (Accessed: 26 April 2020)

Multimedia Foundation Inc. (2020f) Samuel Achilefu. [online]. Available at: https:// en.wikipedia.org/wiki/Samuel_Achilefu (Accessed: 26 April 2020)

Multimedia Foundation Inc. (2020g) Samuel Dagogo-Jack. [online]. Available at: https:// en.wikipedia.org/wiki/Samuel_Dagogo-Jack (Accessed: 26 April 2020)

Morehouse School of Medicine. (2020) Elizabeth Ofili. [online]. Available at: www.msm. edu/about_us/FacultyDirectory/Medicine/ElizabethOfili/index.php (Accessed: 26 April 2020)

Nationwide Children's. (2019) Oluyinka O. Olutoye, MD, PhD, Appointed surgeon-in-chief at nationwide children's hospital. Renowned fetal surgeon to lead nationwide children's surgery programs. [online]. Available at: www.nationwidechildrens.org/ newsroom/news-releases/2019/08/olutoye-announcement (Accessed: 26 April 2020)

Negin, J, Rozea, A, Cloyd, B, Martiniuk, ALC. (2013) Foreign-born health workers in Australia: an analysis of census data. *Human Resources for Health*, 2013 (11): 69. [online]. Available at: www.ncbi.nlm.nih.gov/pmc/articles/PMC3882294/ (Accessed: 26 April 2020)

Nigeria Physiotherapy Network. (2020) [online]. Available at: www.nigeriaphysio.net/ en/Home (Accessed: 26 April 2020)

NIH. (2019) Charles Rotimi. [online]. Available at: https://irp.nih.gov/pi/charles-rotimi (Accessed: 26 April 2020)

NOIPolls. (2016) Emigration of Nigerian medical doctors' survey report. [online]. Available at: www.researchgate.net/publication/319546512_Emigration_of_ Nigerian_Medical_Doctors_Survey_Report (Accessed: 26 April 2020)

North American Association of PhotoBiomodulation Therapy. (2018) NAALT honors Professor Chukuka Enwemeka, PhD. [online]. Available at: www.naalt.org/news/ naalt-honors-professor-chukuka-enwemeka-phd/ (Accessed: 26 April 2020)

Obasanjo, O. (2015) The African scientist in a fast-changing world. *Premium Times*, February 27. [online]. Available at: https://opinion.premiumtimesng.com/2015/ 02/27/the-african-scientist-in-a-fast-changing-world-by-olusegun-obasanjo/ (Accessed: 26 April 2020)

Obinna, C. (2020) Brain drain: Less than 4,000 physiotherapists in Nigeria. *Vanguard*. [online]. Available at: www.vanguardngr.com/2020/03/brain-drain-less-than-4000-physiotherapists-in-nigeria/ (Accessed: 26 April 2020)

Oyedoyin, T. (2019) Night Nigerian healthcare professionals in United Kingdom honored their own. *The Guardian*. [online]. Available at: https://guardian.ng/ features/night-nigerian-healthcare-professionals-in-united-kingdom-honoured-their-own/ (Accessed: 26 April 2020)

Paul, U. (2020) A priceless Nigerian professor of colorectal surgery, survives Covid-19 in England. TNG May 16, 2020. [online]. Available at: www.youtube.com/ watch?v=etdZBSJfFVs (Accessed: 26 April 2020)

Ranker. (2020) Famous professors from Nigeria. [online]. Available at: www.ranker. com/list/famous-professors-from-nigeria/reference (Accessed: 26 April 2020)

Rilwan, R. (2016) My story – US-based Nigerian surgeon who operated on unborn baby. [online]. Available at: https://face2faceafrica.com/article/us-based-nigerian-surgeon-operates-on-23-weeks-old-foetus (Accessed: 26 April 2020)

Roswell Park Comprehensive Cancer Center. (2020) Kunle Odunsi. [online]. Available at: www.roswellpark.org/kunle-odunsi (Accessed: 26 April 2020)

Salaudeen, A. (2019) Nigerian neurosurgeon takes pay cut to perform free operations. [online]. Available at: www.cnn.com/2019/10/03/africa/dr-sulaiman-free-surgeries-intl/index.html (Accessed: 26 April 2020)

Saleem, T. (2011) The Hirsch index – a play on numbers or a true appraisal of academic output? *Int Arch Med.*, 4: 25. [online]. Available at: www.ncbi.nlm.nih.gov/pmc/art-icles/PMC3224391/ (Accessed: 26 April 2020)

Scopus website. (2019) [online]. Available at: https://www2.scopus.com/freelookup/ form/author.uri. (Accessed: 26 April 2020)

Sickle Cell Support Society of Nigeria. (2020) Adekunle Adekile. [online]. Available at: https://scsn.com.ng/our-leaders/adekunle-adekile/ (Accessed: 26 April 2020)

Statistics How To. (2020) Snowball sampling: Definition, advantages and disadvantages. [online]. Available at: www.statisticshowto.com/snowball-sampling/ (Accessed: 26 April 2020)

Straightnews.ng. (2018) First Nigerian professors in various disciplines. [online]. Available at: https://straightnews.ng/first-nigerian-professors-in-various-fields (Accessed: 10 March 2020)

Tankwanchi, ABS, Özden, Ç, Vermund SH. (2013) Physician emigration from sub-Saharan Africa to the United States: Analysis of the 2011 AMA physician Masterfile. *Public Library of Science (PLOS) Medicine*, 10(9): e1001513. [online]. Available at: www.ncbi.nlm.nih.gov/pmc/articles/PMC3775724/ (Accessed: 26 April 2020)

University at Buffalo. (2020) Jacobs School of Medicine and Biomedical Sciences. Adekunle Odunsi. [online]. Available at: http://medicine.buffalo.edu/content/medicine/faculty/profile.html?ubit=aoodunsi (Accessed: 26 April 2020)

University of Arizona. (2020) John E. Ehiri. [online]. Available at: https://profiles.arizona.edu/person/jehiri (Accessed: 26 April 2020)

University of Canterbury. (2020) Measure impact: Author impact metrics. [online]. Available at: https://canterbury.libguides.com/impactmeasure/impactauthor (Accessed: 26 April 2020)

University of Chicago Medicine. (2020) Olufunmilayo I. Olopade. [online]. Available at: www.uchicagomedicine.org/find-a-physician/physician/olufunmilayo-i-olopade (Accessed: 26 April 2020)

University of Sheffield. (2020) Prof. Adewale O. Adebajo, PhD. [online]. Available at: www.catch.org.uk/team-member/dr-adewale-o-adebajo/ (Accessed: 26 April 2020)

Unmc.edu. (2019) CV for Kunle Odunsi. [online]. Available at: www.unmc.edu/_documents/Odunsi_Kunle_CV.pdf (Accessed: 26 April 2020)

UT News. (2020) Breakthrough in coronavirus research results in new map to support vaccine design – UT News. [online]. Available at: https://news.utexas.edu/2020/02/19/breakthrough-in-coronavirus-research-results-in-new-map-to-support-vaccine-design/ (Accessed: 26 April 2020)

UT Southwestern Medical Center. (2020) Fiemu Nwariaku, M.D. [online]. Available at: https://utswmed.org/doctors/fiemu-nwariaku/ (Accessed: 26 April 2020)

Washington University School of Medicine. (2020) Samuel Achilefu. [online]. Available at: www.mir.wustl.edu/research/research-laboratories/optical-radiology-laboratory-orl/people/achilefu (Accessed: 26 April 2020)

Wikimedia Foundation, Inc. (2020) Ijeoma Uchegbu. [online]. Available at: https://en.wikipedia.org/wiki/Ijeoma_Uchegbu (Accessed: 26 April 2020)

Wikimedia Foundation, Inc. (2020) Elizabeth Ofili. [online]. Available at: https://en.wikipedia.org/wiki/Elizabeth_Ofili (Accessed: 26 April 2020)

White House (n.d.) Admiral John O. Agwunobi. [online]. Available at: https://georgewbush-whitehouse.archives.gov/government/jagwunobi-bio.html (Accessed: 26 April 2020)

Williams, S. (2014) Four reasons to stop caring so much about the h-index. *London School of Economics and Political Science.* [online]. Available at: https://blogs.lse.ac.uk/impactofsocialsciences/2014/03/31/four-reasons-to-stop-caring-so-much-about-the-h-index/ (Accessed: 26 April 2020)

World Bank. (2017) Migration and remittances data. [online]. Available at: www.worldbank.org/en/topic/migrationremittancesdiasporaissues/brief/migration-remittances-data (Accessed: 26 April 2020)

WHO – World Health Organization. (2014) Migration of health workers: the WHO code of practice and the global economic crisis. [online]. Available at: www.who.int/ hrh/migration/14075_MigrationofHealth_Workers.pdf (Accessed: 26 April 2020)

Worldometer. (2020) Nigeria population (Live). [online]. Available at: www. worldometers.info/world-population/nigeria-population/ (Accessed: 26 April 2020)

Index

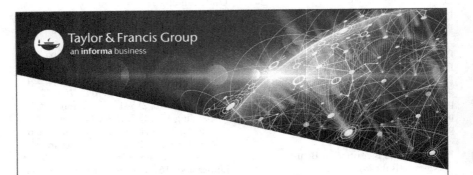

Printed in the United States
By Bookmasters